I0819665

Praise for *When Memory Fades*

"In *When Memory Fades* Dr. Chin skillfully bridges the gap between clinical knowledge and the lived experience of dementia—whether one is navigating the condition personally or supporting another individual. Drawing on his own experience as a family care partner, he brings empathy to his expertise, conveying complex medical information in a way that is both accessible and compassionate. This book is an outstanding resource for anyone seeking to better understand dementia and to live as well as possible with its challenges."

—Teepa Snow, MS, OTR/L, FAOTA, founder of Positive Approach to Care®

"*When Memory Fades* is a humane and rigorously informed guide to cognitive aging and Alzheimer's disease that balances clinical clarity with deep compassion. Drawing on his experience as a physician, researcher, and son, Nathaniel Chin illuminates each stage of the disease with honesty and empathy, while engaging readers on a human level. It is a book that informs without overwhelming, invites reflection, and offers steady guidance for families at every point along the journey."

—Bruce Miller, MD, A.W. and Mary Margaret Clausen Distinguished Professor in Neurology and director, Edward and Pearl Fein Memory and Aging Center, University of California, San Francisco

"*When Memory Fades* is a wonderful book for individuals and caregivers to educate, support, demystify, and navigate the journey through Alzheimer's disease. Dr. Chin beautifully weaves together science, medicine, and his own experiences as an Alzheimer's specialist and caregiver for his father to create this practical guide. The many lessons are clearly taught with a heartwarming and hopeful perspective. I will be recommending this book for my patients and their families."

—Allan Levey, MD, PhD, Robert W. Woodruff Professor of Neurology at Emory University and director, Goizueta Alzheimer's Disease Research Center

"Alzheimer's is a disease we all fear yet for which we are never prepared. Dr. Nathaniel Chin offers an intimate and empathic—yet practical and essential—guide to the decisions each of our families will face in our personal journeys." —George Vradenburg, UsAgainstAlzheimer's

"*When Memory Fades* stands out for its rare blend of scientific rigor and lived experience. Drawing on his work as an Alzheimer's doctor and his deeply personal role as a son who cared for a father with Alzheimer's, Dr. Nathaniel Chin offers succinct and compassionate guidance with a clear understanding of the critical decisions families face and are often unprepared for. The result is an excellent road map for anyone living through a dementia diagnosis that helps patients and families move forward with honesty, clarity, and purpose."

—Deborah Kan, founder and executive editor, Being Patient

"Dr. Chin has produced a thoughtful, compassionate, and highly instructive how-to guide for families with concerns about a loved one's cognition. Weaving in personal stories that let the reader feel like they are in a private conversation with this experienced specialist, Dr. Chin bears his soul while providing practical, informative, and state-of-the-art information that is sure to be of immense value for the growing number of people dealing with the challenges of age-related diseases that cause dementia."

—Joshua Grill, PhD, professor and director, Institute for Memory Impairments and Neurological Disorders, University of California, Irvine

"*When Memory Fades* is the kind of book clinicians wish they could place directly into every family's hands. With a rare blend of extraordinary clinical expertise and deep compassion—born not only from his leadership in the field but also his personal experience as a caregiver—Dr. Chin walks alongside patients and their families through the Alzheimer's journey, bringing clarity and steadiness to the maze of decisions families face. Dr. Chin shines a light on the humanity at the center of Alzheimer's care, offering guidance that is both clinically precise and profoundly reassuring. *When Memory Fades* is an indispensable companion that empowers families and professionals to navigate memory loss with wisdom, hope, and heart."

—Michelle Braun, PhD, ABPP-CN, author of *High-Octane Brain: 5 Science-Based Steps to Sharpen Your Memory and Reduce Your Risk of Alzheimer's* and founder of High-Octane Brain Fitness®

"*When Memory Fades* is the rare book about Alzheimer's disease that offers both practical advice for families struggling with the impact of this illness and up-to-date clinical and research information on advances in the field. Dr. Nathaniel Chin approaches Alzheimer's disease from his many experiences as a son, geriatric physician, dementia specialist, science communicator, and clinical researcher. The result is a wonderful, comprehensive guide that is eminently readable, poignant, and informative."

—Reisa Sperling, MD, professor of neurology, Harvard Medical School, and director, Center for Alzheimer Research and Treatment at Brigham and Women's Hospital and Massachusetts General Hospital

"*When Memory Fades* is an essential guide for the Alzheimer's journey—blending medical expertise, practical caregiving wisdom, and the emotional truth of loving someone through cognitive change. Dr. Nathaniel Chin helps readers recognize early warning signs, prepare for an effective evaluation, and understand why symptoms extend beyond memory. The strength of this book is its usefulness: concrete strategies for communication, routines, safety planning, and caregiver resilience, alongside validation for the uncertainty families often carry in silence. Chin also explains the promise and limits of today's treatments and the vital role of clinical research—without hype, and with respect for individual goals. Most of all, this book reinforces a message we share at the Alzheimer's Association: No one should face Alzheimer's alone. *When Memory Fades* helps families move from fear to informed action, and from isolation to support."

—Maria Carrillo, Chief Science Officer and Medical Affairs Lead, Alzheimer's Association

WHEN MEMORY FADES

WHAT TO EXPECT AT EVERY STAGE, FROM EARLY SIGNS TO FULL SUPPORT FOR ALZHEIMER'S AND DEMENTIA

NATHANIEL CHIN, MD
WITH GEORGE SPENCER

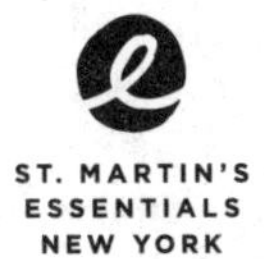

ST. MARTIN'S ESSENTIALS
NEW YORK

First published in the United States by St. Martin's Essentials,
an imprint of St. Martin's Publishing Group

EU Representative: Macmillan Publishers Ireland Ltd, 1st Floor, The Liffey Trust Centre,
117–126 Sheriff Street Upper, Dublin 1, D01 YC43

www.stmartins.com

Designed by Steven Seighman

The Library of Congress Cataloging-in-Publication Data is available upon request.

ISBN 978-1-250-40085-7 (hardcover)
ISBN 978-1-250-40086-4 (ebook)

First Edition: 2026

10 9 8 7 6 5 4 3 2 1

For my dad, whose passion for medicine and healing became my own. You taught me the value of family, food, travel, and living with purpose. My work is—and always will be—in your honor.

For my wife and my boys, who are the foundation of my happiness and meaning in life. You remind me every day to live in the moment and appreciate what's right in front of me.

Contents

Introduction

"What would you do if this were your father?"

This is a question I'm often asked in the memory clinic. I diagnose Alzheimer's disease regularly, and people look to me for answers. I help families navigate one of the most challenging, disorienting chapters of their lives. I offer recommendations about diagnostic tests, referrals to specialists, medications, lifestyle changes, clinical trials, and even care facility options.

But this question stands apart. It's never asked casually. It's not theoretical. It's raw, urgent, personal. Just like the disease itself.

Many of my patients know my story. My father, Moe Chin, MD, practiced family medicine for forty years. He was diagnosed with Alzheimer's on a hot, humid August morning in 2012, retired the next day, and died in 2018. I was in my second year of internal medicine residency and had planned to specialize in infectious diseases. But everything changed when my mother told me he was ill. I chose to become a geriatrician—not necessarily to help my father, but to help patients like him, and families like ours. My calling became supporting people facing this disease and standing alongside caregivers like my mother. More than that, I wanted to contribute to finding a cure for Alzheimer's, or at least treatments that could slow or delay its progression.

I don't hide my father's story from my patients. I carry no shame, though sadly I know many caregivers who do. Embarrassment, guilt, fear—they weigh heavily on families confronting Alzheimer's. I use my story to educate and, I hope, to inspire action. I tell my patients what I did when the disease struck my own father. I share my family's struggles, our missteps, and our moments of grace. I speak with the confidence of someone who has walked this road and with the humility of someone who knows he didn't do it perfectly.

* * *

In this era of novel therapies and groundbreaking clinical trials, the question "What would you do if it were your father?" carries even more weight. My patients want more than textbook answers. They crave something real, something grounded in experience. The question they ask isn't hypothetical for me. It never was.

Two years before my father's diagnosis, when I was an intern, I experienced a chance event late one night that I would later understand as a kind of revelation—unexpected and profound. At the time, I was blind to what it meant. But in hindsight, it was the first instance that truly showed me a glimpse of the emotional weight of dementia—and offered a peek at the kind of care that would define my career. It was an encounter that lingered long after the night was over.

Let me explain. It was well past midnight. The hospital smelled like sweat and antiseptic, and I was deep into a thirty-hour shift. As the overnight cross-cover intern, I was responsible for every patient ward, fielding pages from nurses and managing issues while the primary teams slept. At the University of California–San Diego, this was a rite of passage, and it came early in my intern year. I was excited by the medicine—the tests, the treatments, the pathologies—but I was scared, too.

I was twenty-six years old and had just finished four years of medical school. People's lives were on the line. My pager rang nonstop. The situations I found myself in challenged everything I had learned from classes and textbooks. One minute I faced a low hemoglobin issue, the next chest pain, then came a patient with a fast heart rate, and another with shortness of breath. My mind leapt from one crisis to the next.

In the middle of the chaos, I got a page from a nurse. When I called, her voice was tight. "Can you come to my floor? *Now.* There's a patient who's confused and agitated. He pulled out his IV."

I was annoyed. I had other patients, and the notes were piling up. Going to this patient's bedside would take time. But I could hear something in her voice—real fear. I told her I'd be there shortly and pulled up his chart.

This seventy-six-year-old man had been admitted for pneumonia. On the problem list: dementia.

My gut reaction was irritation. *Why am I being asked to evaluate confusion in someone with dementia?* I thought. *They're all confused. That's what dementia is.* I had no real experience with the condition. My grandparents died of heart disease and cancer. I'd never had a geriatrics rotation in medical school. I knew what the textbook said about dementia, but I'd never stood at the bedside of someone living with it.

I thought this was a waste of time. I wanted to deal with *real* medicine issues. Still, I went to the unit, where the nurse and other staff met me. They looked shaken. "He's been yelling. We're worried he'll fall or hurt someone," the nurse said.

I gave her an intern spiel: "This is delirium on top of dementia. It could be the pneumonia, sleep deprivation, or meds. There's not much I can do."

Their faces dropped. "You can order Haldol or Ativan," said the nurse, suggesting drugs that would calm the man.

I shook my head. I knew better. Sedation isn't the answer unless the patient is a real danger to himself. "No," I said. "But I'll go in and see him."

The nurse rolled her eyes at me, yet another cocky intern on her watch. I walked in. The man was sitting up—lanky, disheveled, with sun-darkened skin and a scruffy shadow from not shaving. A slight sour odor clung to him, and he started yelling as soon as I came in.

"Mary?" he shouted. "Where's Mary?"

"I'm Dr. Chin. What seems to be the problem?"

A ridiculous question, in hindsight. It was 2 AM. I was exhausted and leaning on habit. His answers were fragmented, but beneath them I realized he wasn't angry. He was scared.

I pulled up a chair. I asked him where he lived, who he lived with, and what he did for fun. Slowly, his aggression faded. He answered in pieces, offering snippets about his family, his old job, surfing on Sundays.

Then he called me by his son's name. I recognized it from the chart.

I didn't correct him. "What do you love about your family?" I asked. He talked, and I listened.

Halfway through, he reached for my hand. Inside I flinched, but I didn't show it. I'd cared for dozens of patients that night, but I'd barely touched any of them beyond the exam. This was different. This was personal.

He held my hand, still talking to me as if I were his son. My pager buzzed in my pocket. More work. More patients. But I stayed. His yelling had stopped. His fear had ebbed like waves after a storm.

When he paused, I told him I had to go. He squeezed my hand. "Thanks for coming to visit, son."

I swallowed hard. "You bet," I said, and walked out.

When I left his room, I realized that the nurse who'd paged me was in the doorway. She had seen and heard everything. She gave me a hug. I was startled. I didn't understand why this moment affected her so much.

To me, this had been the dullest visit of the night. It wasn't medically interesting. I simply sat with this man. But he went to sleep, and I didn't get another call from that floor.

I didn't think about that encounter for years. Back then, I didn't see dementia care as real medicine. It wasn't what I valued. I had other plans.

Only later—after walking with my own father through his Alzheimer's—did I realize how meaningful that moment had been. I'm embarrassed I couldn't see it then, but I'm grateful I do now.

This memory lives differently in me today. I come to this book not only as a memory-care specialist and researcher but also as a son—someone who has lived and is still living with the personal cost of Alzheimer's.

I now understand that moment in a new light—through loss, through family, through years of listening. I thought I was just getting through the night. I didn't know that encounter would foreshadow my life.

Looking back, I realize the man in that hospital bed could have been my father, years after his diagnosis. Sitting there holding that man's hand—something I thought little of at the time—became the very instinct that now defines how I provide medical care, especially for Alzheimer's. Where there is no cure, we can always offer compassion. We can always connect and be present. Million-dollar MRI scanners do wonders, but the human touch is priceless. What I once dismissed as insignificant became the heart of my life's work.

I hope that by sharing my advice and stories in this book, I will not only make a diagnosis of Alzheimer's more bearable for the next person who receives it but also illuminate the deep honor I've felt in showing up both for my family and for my patients. Whether you're wearing a white coat or sitting at a loved one's bedside, you have immense power to shape the life of someone with memory change.

* * *

Today, as a geriatrician specializing in memory care, I work closely with patients and their families as they navigate the challenges of cognitive decline. I serve as the medical director of the Wisconsin Alzheimer's Disease Research Center (ADRC), where I help oversee the scientific program, provide medical guidance, and direct participant care. I am also the medical director and co-principal investigator of the Wisconsin Registry for Alzheimer's Prevention (WRAP), a landmark study focused on identifying early risk factors for Alzheimer's disease. In addition, I host *Dementia Matters*, a long-running podcast where I interview leading Alzheimer's researchers from around the world.

My most cherished purpose, however, is being a partner to my wife, Erin, and a father to two beautiful boys, Augustine and Bennett.

I like to think I'm fulfilling the commitments I made to myself when I first started: to care for those with cognitive disorders, to teach, and to conduct meaningful research.

* * *

This book has three main threads.

First, it offers advice, focused on the critical period immediately before, during, and after an Alzheimer's diagnosis. This book can also be helpful to those worried about their own cognition or simply interested in how memory changes over time.

Second, it weaves together my personal family stories and our experiences surrounding my father's illness. I have lived Alzheimer's disease—as a family member—from diagnosis to death and through the years of caregiving in between. I have what you might call "street credibility." I have walked the talk and stood in the footsteps of the patients and families who see me. That life experience pulses through the care I give.

Third, this book illustrates hope. I want to share the incredible advances happening in Alzheimer's research. In my lifetime, I firmly believe that Alzheimer's will be treated the way cardiovascular disease is—as a condition that can be managed over many years and may even be reversed.

If you are reading this because you're worried about a loved one or yourself, or navigating a new diagnosis, I hope what you're about to read is helpful and reassuring. And for all readers, I encourage you to consider volunteering for Alzheimer's research, whether or not you have symptoms. Without people who volunteer their time, sweat, and, yes, blood, our progress will be limited. With them I believe real breakthroughs are within reach.

* * *

This book's nine chapters are designed to walk you through the formative stage surrounding an Alzheimer's diagnosis. Chapter 1, "What Is Happening to My Mind?," puts you in the shoes of someone worried that their cognition is declining. Next comes "I Didn't See It Coming," which explores the often difficult but essential family meetings held to discuss a loved one's changing brain. In the third chapter, "What Are You Testing Me For?," I guide you through what happens as your loved one goes through the evaluation process with a geriatrician or neurologist, where a diagnosis is eventually made.

But what happens after a diagnosis? Chapter 4 is summed up by two words: "Have faith." In this chapter I discuss ways you can muster the courage to move forward. (Hint: You don't have to go it alone, and support is available. I cover these two subjects in depth in chapter 7.) This theme continues in chapter 5, which is about living "the Good Life" following a diagnosis. I've seen this happen many times. People can and do thrive, even while living with this disease. Next comes a chapter on "the Bright Future" of Alzheimer's research and the promise of new disease-modifying drugs like lecanemab and donanemab.

Chapter 8 highlights the vital role patients, caregivers, and community members play in advancing research, and it details the different types of studies they can join. The book concludes with a chapter on what is likely to happen as death nears. If death and dying seem unusual in a book about living well with Alzheimer's, I've found that honest conversations about the end of life are among the most needed, quietly longed for, and meaningful you can have. Death is a deeply human part of this journey, and it deserves to be discussed openly and compassionately.

A note: No medical or pharmaceutical companies were involved in the creation or writing of this book. I use generic names for all medications. Although I'm proud to work at the University of Wisconsin, the university did not participate in or influence the writing of this book either. That said, I believe some of the world's best Alzheimer's research and care happens at our program, and I'm happy to sing our praises.

I made a few linguistic choices to keep the text clear, respectful, and accessible. I've made an effort to alternate between "he," "she," and "they" when referring to patients and doctors throughout the book. This is meant to reflect balance and inclusivity, and to avoid favoring one gender over another.

While I clinically adhere to the biological definition of Alzheimer's disease—the confirmed presence of amyloid and tau proteins in the brain—I occasionally use the term more broadly to refer to cognitive impairment in general. The same is true with the words "memory" and "cognition," which I sometimes use interchangeably. I made these decisions to keep the language approachable and avoid excessive technicality. Please forgive the imprecision.

Finally, this book is not intended to replace medical care or offer prescriptive solutions. While my advice is grounded in sound clinical practice, it should not be followed without consulting your own healthcare team. Every individual's situation is unique, and your medical providers are best equipped to guide you.

* * *

Often during visits with patients, I end up holding their hands. It's not something I plan. It just happens. This simple gesture emerges naturally in those quiet moments when words fail.

These times always take me back to one specific day with my dad. It was a beautiful summer afternoon in Madison, Wisconsin. The kind of day where the breeze carries birdsong, the sun sits gently in the sky, and the world feels—if only briefly—at peace.

My wife Erin and I had moved home from San Diego two years earlier, thinking we would stay long enough to help my mom settle into the steady rhythm of caring for my father. I didn't know then that I would stay longer, that we would build a life here.

On that day, my mom and Erin went to run errands, a rare reprieve for my mom, who carried the immense weight of caregiving. Dad stayed with me at our rental house. By then, he was in the moderate stage of dementia. He didn't talk much, but he could still walk steadily when he held onto someone's arm.

We sat together in the living room, the quiet folding around us. It wasn't planned, but I decided to tell him what was in my heart. I told him how much I loved him, how grateful I was for the life he and my mom had given me, how proud I was to be his son. I reminded him of our travels together, our shared adventures. I promised him I would walk this road with him, and I would help Mom. I knew he worried about her.

He said nothing, but his tears spoke everything. I wept, too, but I kept going, holding his hand, determined to leave no words unspoken. When my mom and Erin returned, they quietly stepped back and let us have our moment.

Later, I hugged my father, and we went out for a walk and some lunch, as if nothing extraordinary had happened. I never spoke about that afternoon I spent with my father with my family. Those moments were his and mine—a sacred, unspoken bond between father and son.

Even now, as painful as it is to recall, I'm grateful I said those things when I could. Even in sadness, there is joy. There is honor in showing up, in offering care, in simply being present. I learned that from both my parents—my father, the devoted physician, and my mother, his tireless caregiver.

This book is a continuation of that moment. Through my stories and my recommendations, I want to offer that same sense of gratitude, that same resolve to act, to those who are beginning this journey.

In many ways, my father is still holding my hand, guiding me as I walk alongside others.

Nathaniel Ark Chin
Madison, Wisconsin
July 2025

1

"What Is Happening to My Mind?"

THE UNCERTAINTIES OF AGING

How Brain Cells Work • Normal Brain Changes in Aging • Symptoms of "Abnormal" Thinking • Barriers to Medical Evaluation • The Stigma of Alzheimer's • What Your Primary Care Provider Can Do

Life is the dynamic process of aging. Between birth and middle age, most of us move rapidly through the years with an expectation of wellness. As we grow older, the vagaries of illness, both chronic and acute, can catch up with us. My job as a board-certified geriatrician is to evaluate these changes and make recommendations to improve health and address disease. When it comes to normal brain aging and possible Alzheimer's disease, I strive to differentiate between the two.

You are reading this book because you are worried—about yourself, your spouse, a parent, a loved one, or a friend. Maybe that person has been diagnosed with a cognitive disorder. Maybe your loved one has yet to see a doctor. What you need to understand is the difference between the signs of normal and abnormal aging. The brain and human behavior are complex and interrelated. Test results can be inconclusive and symptoms misleading. Mental status tests, called cognitive screeners, can misdirect. Diagnosing Alzheimer's is time-consuming, complex, and always difficult. Every physician wants to be careful—and caring—when determining the cause. A proper evaluation takes time because too much is at stake to get it wrong.

By the time a diagnosis is made, patients and families have spent hours, days, and months sitting through appointments, doing online research, and fearing the worst, all of which takes a toll. Think of this book as a map, a guide to a place you hope is not your final destination. With the help of this book and your medical team, the journey will become easier, I promise, and you will discover some essential truths along the way.

This chapter includes several key tasks. It will explain how normal cognitive aging differs from premature, accelerated cognitive decline caused by Alzheimer's. (*Cognitive* means mental processes related to how the brain acquires, stores, manipulates, and retrieves information.) This chapter will also describe how brain cells function—and how they fail in disease. I'll cover normal changes, such as short-term memory lapses, and why these occur as we grow older. The early signs of Alzheimer's get a close look, along with the challenge of determining when aging crosses the line from expected to concerning.

I will also address the barriers patients face when seeking a dementia evaluation. The shame and stigma surrounding a dementia diagnosis are agonizing and can be detrimental to finding solutions. We have all experienced the awkwardness and discomfort of looking away, ignoring, or quietly distancing ourselves from people behaving in a peculiar fashion. Since the Covid-19 pandemic, even a simple cough can make us hyper-alert to a person nearby. Now imagine living in a world where sudden, unexplained, uncharacteristic behavior is your daily reality. We rarely recognize how tightly scripted our lives are until they're not. Worry, fear, and uncertainty prevent people from seeking an assessment, leading to delays in both diagnosis and treatment. This chapter also offers practical guidance on how to make the most of a primary care visit for memory screening, including when and how to request a referral to a geriatrician, neurologist, or other memory specialist.

"Do one thing every day that scares you," said First Lady Eleanor Roosevelt. You have courage. Let it shine a light on your worries. The more you learn, the brighter the future may look, and the more you will be able to help yourself and others.

THE AMAZING BRAIN

Before diving into what is normal and abnormal in the cognition of older adults, it's helpful to start with the basics of how the brain works. As you read, it will become clearer what happens when this incredible thinking engine begins to stall, sputter, or misfire. Cars need regular maintenance and occasional repairs, and it's the same for humans. Sometimes we need a checkup when something is just not right.

This takes me back to the anatomy class I attended during my first year at the University of Wisconsin School of Medicine and Public Health in Madison. Some precepts in anatomy are easier to grasp than others. You can see that the knee is a joint where bones partner with tendons and ligaments in order to bend. The inner ear has a tiny, drumlike membrane that catches sound waves. The heart is a cluster of tireless pumps made of muscle. The kidney is a sponge.

The universe is full of wonders and mysteries, and the human brain is one of them. Medical students don't explore this organ during the first part of the semester. Dissection comes months into the course, only after mastering the delicate skills and physiological understanding needed to approach it properly. When the time does come, you immediately sense the brain's distinctness—foreign, yet profoundly sacred. It is protected by the cranium, an almost all-encompassing helmet of dense bone designed to prevent intrusion and preserve the essence of who we are.

When at last you peer into its cavernous depths, the brain gives up no secrets. To the untrained eye, it is a purplish-gray mass, inert and quiet. Like a dense pudding, it pushes back when touched. To the skilled surgeon, however, the brain is a work of art and absolutely beautiful. Covered with nets of blood vessels that nourish it, the living brain looks robust. It's pink. It glistens. Unlike a knee, there is no indication of how it works. No sign appears that says, "This is the place where recipes are stored" or "This region remembers how to ride a bicycle."

You sense that the brain is magical. Here is how neurosurgeon Frank Vertosick Jr. describes it in his book *When the Air Hits Your Brain*: "The soul's tapestry lies woven in the brain's nerve threads. Delicate, inviolate, the brain floats serenely in a bone vault like the crown jewel of biology."

When you see a living brain as I have, you ask yourself, "How is it that my thoughts, my identity, are in this thing?" We know a great deal about how other organs work, but much about the brain remains undiscovered. Only half of neuropathology autopsies reveal the cause of late-life cognitive decline, a surprising fact based on studies of brains of people who donated their bodies to science. For us humans, understanding our brains remains a frontier to be explored.

Weighing about three pounds, a typical human brain contains nearly one hundred billion neurons—the individual nerve cells that send and receive electrical and chemical signals. That's roughly the same as the number of stars in the Milky Way, according to NASA. Those neurons form vast networks with *trillions* of connections. In fact, young children create more than a million of these new connections not every day or hour . . . but every *second.*

The brain quadruples in size during the toddler years. By first grade, it reaches 90 percent of its adult size. For years, experts believed that the brain cells you were born with were all you would ever have. Now we know that's wrong. New neurons are formed throughout life, in a process known as *neurogenesis.*

The problem is that as we age, the rate of loss begins to exceed the rate of gain. On average, adults lose about fifty thousand neurons each day. That's normal. What's abnormal is when we lose significantly more than we should, or when the neurons we have fail to behave as they should when healthy.

Let's also paint a picture of what each brain cell—a neuron—looks like and how it teams up with others. Each neuron has a nucleus—the director—telling it what the cell should do. Extending from the main cell body are frizzy, finger-like projections called *dendrites* and a single, slender stem called an *axon.*

Neurons don't touch each other directly. Instead, they connect across tiny gaps called *synapses.* Information travels in one direction—from an axon to a dendrite—never the other way. The synapse is not a physical bridge but a microscopic space where an electrical signal arriving at the end of one neuron triggers the release of chemical neurotransmitters, which cross the gap and spark a new electrical signal in the next neuron. Without this lightning-speed communication, there would be no thoughts, shopping lists, arithmetic, or marvels like Beethoven's Ninth Symphony and the Golden Gate Bridge.

If a neuron loses its axon, the party's over because that's the only way it can send its "knowledge" to another neuron. True communication, though, happens at the synapse level. To me, this is where all the magic lives. Our emotions, thoughts, memories, and even how we view the world all zip across these tiny junctions, allowing meaning to be conveyed. Some researchers believe that early stages of cognitive change—those subtle disruptions in thinking—may begin with synaptic dysfunction. Neurons don't have to die for thinking issues to arise.

Luckily, billions of years of evolution have created a protective system for neurons. To defend axons from damage, the brain provides each with bodyguards called *glial cells*. There are two key types of these glial helper cells. The first is an *astrocyte*. It improves the flow of blood and nutrients to the neuron, helps it excrete waste matter, and fights intruders. The second is the *oligodendrocyte*. It wraps a sheath called *myelin* made of a white fatty substance around the axon. (The expression "gray matter" to describe the brain came about because other parts of neurons are gray. The brain gets its outer pink appearance thanks to its tough covering called the *dura*, but cells beneath it look different.) Think of myelin as being like the rubbery material that encases an electric wire in a power cord. Not only does myelin insulate the axon, it also speeds transmission of its "data." Unfortunately, these coatings fray over time, a trend that's believed to be accelerated by excessive alcohol use, among other factors. That unraveling leads to poorer processing speed.

Each part of the brain has a different function, but they all work together like an orchestra. Music utilizes an arrangement of notes, tempo, and rhythm. Similarly, our bodies depend on eleven major organ systems to function fully. The brain is part of the nervous system and is composed of four lobes. Each lobe focuses on distinct duties, ones different from the others. Executive functions—thinking, planning, and problem-solving, abilities that distinguish us from other animals—happen in the largest lobe, the frontal lobe located behind the forehead. This lobe develops last, during the teenage years, giving us clues, or to some extent scientific excuses, as to why behavior at this age can be reckless. In our later years, we ideally take the sum of our experiences and broaden our view. Wisdom truly does come with age.

Contrary to popular belief, the brain remains dynamic throughout life, capable of adapting and reorganizing its connections. Even functions such as judgment, perspective, and emotional regulation can continue to mature and strengthen with experience. Understanding where these abilities originate helps explain how this remarkable organ coordinates everything we think, feel, and do. The parietal lobe, located at the top of your brain, interprets feelings and senses. Nestled between the frontal and parietal lobes, near the crown of the head, are the motor and sensory cortices. The motor cortex governs movement while the sensory cortex interprets touch and physical sensations. The temporal lobe, found behind the ears, processes sights, smells, and sounds and plays a key role in memory. The occipital lobe, at the back of the head, governs visual processing and spatial thinking. Deep within the brain are smaller structures, including the pituitary gland, pineal gland, thalamus, and hippocampus—this last structure plays a crucial role in memory storage, a topic discussed later in this chapter.

Frequently engaging in activities like writing, singing, or even brushing your teeth trains your brain in a process called—quite fittingly—entrainment. Memories aren't stored in just one neuron or even one hundred neurons. They live in shape-shifting networks composed of thousands, possibly millions, of neurons. These networks can shrink or grow, naturally causing memories to become richer or fade in detail over time.

When you learn new information, your brain wires fresh connections. Using a memory regularly—say, how to brush your teeth—sparks the neurons in that network to fire, reinforcing and cementing that network. (I can still remember struggling to learn how to tie my shoes when I was in kindergarten. What an ordeal! Now, of course, it's a rote task that I literally don't think about.) Studies have shown that well-practiced activities like brushing your teeth do not require active, "new" thinking. They're automatic. The neural pathway is already well established. And that's not necessarily a bad thing. If your brain becomes damaged and part of the network goes offline, it may not impact your overall ability to brush your teeth. Even if the damage does cause disruption, other networks can be created through cognitive rehabilitation to help you regain the skill. The brain is plastic. It evolves, adapts, and rewires itself, an incredible capacity referred to as *neuroplasticity.*

In Alzheimer's disease, plaques made of a protein called *amyloid* begin to appear between synapses just as dental plaque (a completely different but equally destructive substance) builds up between teeth. Amyloid acts like chewing gum jammed into a lock. It prevents the key—the neuron's "data" traveling along the axon—from turning the lock at the dendrite. Worse, these plaques contribute to the premature, accelerated death of neurons, creating deficits in the neuron's cargo of data, or neurotransmitters. Multiply this by millions of neurons, and symptoms begin to appear. Eventually, even the most deeply ingrained tasks, like tying shoelaces or brushing teeth, can be forgotten.

A year before my dad's diagnosis, I remember my dad telling me he was thinking about skipping a medical conference he had already registered for. It was surprising—he loved going to conferences and had taken the day off from work to attend. When I asked him why, he said the conference center was in a "tricky location" and he wasn't confident he could get there. That struck me as odd. He had been to that same venue several times before. He even had printed out the MapQuest route, and this was a man with an incredible sense of direction.

I reminded him of that, gently encouraging him. He explained that the off-ramp was confusing, and he didn't want to deal with the stress of missing it or being late. Eventually, he decided to go, and he made it there on his own. I was on standby, waiting by my phone just in case. Looking back, I realize this could have been the first quiet sign of his change. Maybe he sensed it, too.

Alzheimer's attacks a key part of the brain responsible for short-term memories. Near the center of the brain sits the hippocampus, a two-inch-long seahorse-shaped structure. (Technically, it's the hippocampi because it has two halves, one for each of the brain's hemispheres.) The hippocampus is the brain's librarian. It decides where and how memories are encoded, stored, and retrieved. Besides cataloging the facts of a memory, such as where you were or the time of day, the hippocampus stitches together all the different experiential sensory details, such as what a rose smells like or how a piece of sandpaper feels.

Unfortunately, if the librarian is ill, no new memories are properly stored. The shelves of the mind—the neurons and their networks—remain empty. This is why someone with Alzheimer's may not remember what they did a minute ago. Even significant events, like a recent trip to Disney World or a grandchild's high school graduation, may prove elusive. The memory was never *made*, that is, it never got stored. In a sense, it went in one ear and out the other. Even in a healthy brain, the hippocampus shrinks with age, affecting memory creation and storage, but not nearly to the degree seen in Alzheimer's disease.

WHAT EXACTLY IS DEMENTIA?

The more you learn about the brain—how its neurons and hippocampus work, and what can go wrong—the more confidence you'll bring to conversations with doctors, nurses, and relatives. You'll better understand what medical professionals are saying because you'll be able to speak their language. This will help elevate your discussion to a more productive, less frustrating, and ultimately more satisfying level.

With this in mind, it's key to understand terms like *dementia*, *Alzheimer's*, and *mild cognitive impairment* the way a doctor does.

First, dementia is not a disease. It is a syndrome—a label, a way of describing what someone is experiencing and what others are observing. It's an umbrella term. Similar to the word *transportation*, which covers types of movement ranging from cars to planes to pogo sticks, dementia is a broad category. Here is a formal definition of dementia: a clinical syndrome of acquired and persistent declines in both cognitive and functional abilities. The word *functional* refers to specific daily activities such as cooking or sewing. For a dementia diagnosis, two criteria must be met. First, the declines in cognitive and functional ability must be reported by the patient, family, or clinicians. Daily functional changes are often observed by family or friends because the patient may not always have insight into the problem. Second, the cognitive decline must be confirmed through formal cognitive testing. From a doctor's point of view, both are essential. Tests must confirm observations.

Most importantly: Dementia is not normal. It is not a normal part of aging. I want to emphasize this point because it's so often misunderstood—dementia is not simply getting old. It's not a psychiatric illness, a kind of delirium, or an inevitability. Most of all, it is not the same as Alzheimer's disease.

Alzheimer's is one of a handful of specific diseases that fall under the dementia umbrella. The six most common include Alzheimer's disease, cerebrovascular disease, Lewy body disease, frontotemporal disease, limbic-predominant age-related TDP-43 encephalopathy (LATE), and Parkinson's disease. Mixed dementia is also part of this classification, meaning multiple brain diseases are involved in causing the cognitive and functional symptoms. Doctors are increasingly recognizing that as people get older, dementia is often the result of multiple overlapping pathologies rather than a single process operating on its own. For example, a person may have both Alzheimer's *and* vascular cognitive impairment, or Alzheimer's *and* Lewy body disease at the same time. Despite their differences, all brain diseases under the dementia umbrella share three key features: (1) they are persistent; (2) their symptoms are consistent; (3) and they cause progressive declines in ability over time. While the symptoms vary depending on the disease, these three facts unite them.

Most lessons about dementia arrive not in the clinic but in the quiet, personal spaces where life and death meet. I had studied mixed pathology dementia in textbooks and lectures, but I didn't truly understand it until I lived it with my own family. When a brain is to be studied postmortem, it must be cooled immediately after death to preserve it. When my mom called me before dawn to tell me that my dad had died, I wasn't in a state of mind to think so practically. It was my wife who reminded her of the need to chill Dad's head. She was the one who calmly called the university's brain retrieval team, the funeral home, and the hospice before we got in the car to see him.

Attendants from the funeral home in my parents' small town picked up my dad and took him to the hospital for the brain-removal process. They asked if we wanted the linens from my father's bed that they had used to help lift him onto the gurney. It was one of those strange moments, given the gravity of the situation, where you wonder if this could really be happening, and it is difficult to focus on answering such a question. In hindsight, however, it was a blessing that the attendants suggested it. Printed on the bedsheet was a tapestry of farm animals that my mom later made into quilts for her grandchildren.

Though my dad was in hospice care and had not had anything to eat or drink in a week, the news of his death felt like a blow to my heart. On the day he died, I said goodbye to his body, but I also needed to say goodbye to the part of Dr. Moe Chin that made him *my father*. The hospital, at my request, conducted an autopsy. We knew the cause of death was dementia, but an examination of the brain remains the only way doctors can without a doubt identify what type or types of dementia a person had.

As a professional courtesy, the pathologist allowed me to attend. I wasn't sure if I could watch without being overcome. I greatly admired my father's intellect, his compassion, and his love for his family—those qualities that came from his mind, the sum total of his brain's workings that made him who he was.

As the pathologist and I expected, his brain was smaller than normal, shrunken by the atrophy of dementia. It contained voids that were created when the brain receded. It no longer hinted at the miracles deep within its tissues where his love of family, food, and hobbies had mingled.

During this gross (large-scale) examination, the pathologist collected tissue samples. Microscopic examination later revealed that my dad had mixed Alzheimer's and Lewy body disease. This finding had enormous importance for our family. It explained his more unusual symptoms—acting out his dreams, difficulty judging distances, and rigidity in his arms—as well as the dementia's early onset and fast progression. Studies now show that people with multiple brain diseases often experience faster decline compared to those with one. This deeper understanding of what my father went through anchored us and brought us solace as we grieved.

The final crucial term to understand is *mild cognitive impairment* (MCI).

Like dementia, MCI is a condition, not a disease. Put simply, it refers to a person experiencing notable cognitive disruption while still functioning independently, albeit with mild outward changes. For a patient to be diagnosed with MCI, two main criteria must be met. First, there must be a symptom (or symptoms) present that the patient, close family, friends, or the healthcare provider notices. Second, objective cognitive testing must reveal a lower result than would be typical for a person of the same age or compared to how the person previously scored on the identical test. Such lower scores occur when a person struggles to answer questions and puzzles correctly or is unable to respond at all. Once again, what's observed must match what's measured. MCI is not part of normal aging. At the same time, it's not a form of dementia, but it does represent a decline from a person's prior baseline—not the average performance of all people of the individual's age but of that individual's own prior ability.

Here's the key point to remember about MCI—there is no impairment in a person's day-to-day functioning, only a lessening of abilities. The person can still do everything they've always done. They might take longer, make occasional mistakes, or rely on compensatory strategies like writing to-do lists on Post-it notes, but they remain independent and do not need assistance.

In my clinic, almost half the patients who come in are diagnosed with MCI. They present with (i.e., exhibit) mild or subtle symptoms. They score at subpar levels on cognitive tests, but they live their daily lives and accomplish all their tasks as they have always done. They might make mistakes or find subtle ways to adapt—keeping more notes, setting reminders, or simplifying tasks—but they are not dependent or disabled. Crucially, the overwhelming majority of these people, if not all of them, retain insight into their condition. Some may initially be in denial, but when we review their cognitive test performance using visual graphs to display the changes in how they perform, most will tell me, "Yes, that's true, Dr. Chin. You're right."

Researchers estimate that about two in ten people aged sixty-five and older with MCI will progress to dementia within one year. At the same time, however, some people with MCI get better or maintain the same mental ability. This can happen when the symptoms are caused by modifiable conditions—such as sleep apnea or a thyroid disorder—because treating those underlying issues can restore, or at least improve, cognitive function. In fact, as many as 20 percent of people over sixty-five may have MCI. There's no specific treatment for it except to address any reversible causes and to redouble one's efforts to get enough sleep, eat well, exercise, and follow other advice doctors have for staying physically and mentally fit. (See the sidebar "Modifiable Risk Factors" on page 34 for more on this.)

The brain at age seventy-five is not the same as it was at twenty-five. Just as we begin losing around 1 percent of our muscle mass per year starting in our thirties and forties, our brains gradually get smaller, too. Brain cells die. Connections between living cells (i.e., synapses) vanish in the normal course of aging. Tiny blood vessels in the brain get even smaller, and they die as well, which means brain cells receive less oxygen and fewer nutrients. (Yes, new brain cells get created all the time. The problem when we're older is that more cells die than are replaced.)

Most people reach their peak cognitive performance in their mid-twenties. That's when subtle mental declines begin, though they usually go unnoticed. We gradually become slower at taking in, processing, and responding to information, and tasks that once felt effortless—like multitasking or holding a phone number in mind while dialing—begin to require more focus. It can also become harder to sustain attention, filter out distractions, or adapt quickly to new rules or environments, reflecting a gradual decline in cognitive flexibility. Around age sixty to sixty-five there's an inflection point where a very gradual downward slope in cognitive sharpness begins to take shape. This is when people start noticing problems with their thinking. It becomes harder to find the right word during a conversation. We become more sensitive to distractions. We need a quieter space to learn or finish tasks. Learning new information takes longer. We need more repetition to retain that new information. Our mental processing speed and reaction times slow down, but we can still make complex decisions.

I remember when I first began to recognize my dad's symptoms as the consequence of disease and not just his age. He would pause midsentence, searching for a word that once came effortlessly. He would ask me the same question later in a conversation, as if he hadn't heard my story the first time. Without his diagnosis, I would have brushed it off. I would have told myself it was just part of getting older. That's the power of a diagnosis—it changes what you notice and how you interpret it.

Gradually, these moments became more frequent and routine in our conversations. I found myself finishing his thoughts to spare him the frustration of a word that wouldn't come. I patiently retold stories from my day at work, sometimes more than twice in a single exchange, knowing now that this wasn't inattentiveness. It was the disease, unfolding quietly between us.

The difficulty in differentiating abnormal from normal aging is why I'm an outspoken advocate for repeated cognitive testing over time. It allows doctors to track how a person is doing relative to themselves—not compared to other people. Everyone has different cognitive baselines and varying abilities. What's normal at seventy is not the same as what's expected at age thirty. One often-used memory test gives a person fifteen words and asks them to recite as many as possible thirty minutes later. For a seventy-year-old, remembering eight out of fifteen is normal. For a thirty-year-old, that same score would suggest borderline or mild impairment. Older patients—especially scientists, lawyers, doctors, and others with advanced degrees—are sometimes stunned when their cognitive test score is lower than what they expected, even when the results are still within normal limits for their age demographic. Unless that lower score is part of a downward trend over time, it's not regarded as impaired. After all, if you took the SAT test today, would you do as well as when you were studying geometry?

MAKING SENSE OF SYMPTOMS

Early symptoms of decline can be tricky to decipher. Forgetting words might be completely normal—or it might not be. It depends on the person. Historically, diagnosing Alzheimer's starts by ruling out other possible causes. In fact, until recently, it was referred to as a diagnosis of exclusion (see chapter 8 on how biomarker tests are changing this paradigm).

There can be many other causes for mental fogginess. They include stress, poor sleep, obstructive sleep apnea, medication side effects, drug interactions, alcohol or drug use, poor eating habits, psychological issues such as depression and anxiety, head injuries, blood clots, brain tumors, infections, and medical conditions like thyroid, kidney, or liver problems. As a doctor, I go through a mental checklist of all these possibilities when I see a patient. It's like being a detective. That's why physicians often ask questions that seem odd or order tests that, at first glance, may appear unrelated to what the patient thinks is relevant. Every piece of information can be a clue.

What are some of the most frequently observed early symptoms of cognitive decline? It often depends on which part of the brain is most affected. Symptoms generally fall into five main categories:

1. **Memory:** Forgetting recent events or conversations, repeating stories and questions, frequently losing items.
2. **Language:** Difficulty finding the right words, understanding words or a conversation, challenges with reading and writing.
3. **Visual-spatial:** Getting lost in familiar places, trouble recognizing people, not comprehending spatial relationships.
4. **Attention:** Problems focusing, staying on task, or following conversations.
5. **Executive function:** Trouble with reasoning, problem-solving, organizing projects or tasks, or multitasking.

When a person has Alzheimer's, it tends to affect memory first, causing them to forget such things as the details of recent conversations or someone's name. But Alzheimer's can also cause early changes in problem-solving and planning (executive functions) or in language abilities. Subtle difficulties, compared to more obvious changes, can be addressed early. The mantra "Earlier is better" is true in the world of Alzheimer's whether it's a diagnosis or a lifestyle intervention.

I want to dispel a myth. The most common and earliest sign of Alzheimer's is not a functional mistake such as getting lost while driving or leaving the stovetop on after cooking a meal. These situations, while common and concerning, indicate more advanced progression. That said, if the symptoms being noticed are dangerous, take action. Have that family meeting. See a doctor. This bears repeating: If a loved one is engaged in a dangerous activity or is experiencing a day-to-day functional disability and you think the cause is a brain health issue (or any other cause, for that matter), make sure they get medical attention right away.

Alzheimer's tends to affect memory first because the temporal lobes—where the learning and memory storage processes start—are often the first brain regions impacted by the buildup of tau protein. Tau, the second defining protein in Alzheimer's disease, accumulates within a brain cell, leading to neuronal death and synaptic dysfunction. This initiates the beginning of noticeable symptoms. But Alzheimer's doesn't always manifest first as memory loss. In some cases, early symptoms include difficulty with language and expressing oneself, a condition known as *logopenic primary progressive aphasia.* In another less common situation called *posterior cortical atrophy,* Alzheimer's manifests its presence through changes in visual-spatial perception when people struggle to see things in front of them or misjudge spatial relationships.

Even when Alzheimer's is considered "typical," or memory predominant, the next symptoms to develop are not predictable. Once established in the brain, it can rampage from one lobe to the next, causing difficulties in executive function that affect judgment and reasoning or in one's ability to pay attention, such as being able to follow conversations and process information. The course of the disease is one of decline, but how each person experiences that decline is unique to them.

By the same token, if the neurodegenerative disease is frontotemporal dementia, it might affect language first, notably the ability to find the right word or understand the meaning of words. This disease process afflicts a different part of the brain, leading to a different presentation of symptoms. Alternatively, this same condition might instead cause disturbing changes in behavior, like hypersexuality or extreme self-centeredness.

A separate brain pathology called Lewy body disease tends to affect younger adults and often reveals itself in visual-spatial testing. For example, when asked to copy a complex figure with overlapping lines and shapes, a person with Lewy body disease may produce a disorganized image or omit entire sections rather than crafting a reasonably neat rendering. Outside of cognitive testing, Lewy body disease has several classic features. These include Parkinson's-like movements, acting out dreams (which may involve having full conversations or making dramatic arm or leg movements during sleep), and well-defined visual hallucinations—often of children or animals—that are usually not frightening to the person. Another hallmark of the disease is fluctuating mental abilities, attention span, and awareness of time. Cognitive ability can vary significantly, even within the same day.

The first symptoms and changes in cognitive testing can be incredibly helpful in discerning the underlying cause, because not every case is Alzheimer's and therefore not all initial symptoms involve memory loss.

When evaluating memory issues, here are some useful questions to consider:

Is the person forgetting recent events?
Can he no longer recall conversations?
Is she repeating stories, forgetting that she told them a few minutes ago, or is she unable to tell a well-worn family story?
Is the same question asked over and over, such as "What is our neighbor's name?" or "When are we going to visit so-and-so?"

Louie, the son of one of my patients, first became worried that his mother had Alzheimer's when she lost the ability to tell funny, dramatic stories about her youth.* He told me she had been a master storyteller. She was like an actor performing a soliloquy. Every word of every line was deep in her brain and delivered with exuberant flourishes and pauses. Then one day he noticed that while telling a story to friends she lost track of what she was saying, as if the script of the play had been destroyed. Soon she began to lose confidence in her storytelling gift and shared an-

* The names and identifying details of all persons mentioned in this book have been changed to conceal their identities.

ecdotes less often. None of her listeners—except her children and closest relatives—would have ever noticed her trepidation.

Sometimes the earliest symptom is one of the classics, but it still might take an astute observer to recognize it. My mom was the first, years before anyone else, to notice changes in my dad. They enjoyed watching old crime shows before bedtime, with my father usually falling asleep toward the end but loving the entertainment nonetheless. My mom started to notice he couldn't follow plots and didn't ask questions, which is a telltale sign. He didn't respond when she'd say things like, "Wow, can you believe Sherlock Holmes did that?" She started to pay more attention to him during the shows to see what he understood. Her gut told her something her brain wasn't ready to process.

Problems with language can be another area of concern. Struggling to find the right word happens to the most cognitively healthy of us and is often referred to as the tip-of-the-tongue phenomenon. It happens to everyone as a part of normal aging, but when it occurs more often and regularly it could be a sign of underlying disease. Ask yourself: Is the person having a hard time understanding ordinary words (not obscure terms or current slang)? Is she having a hard time reading or writing, whether on a keyboard or with a pen or pencil?

I had a patient in my memory clinic who was sharp as a tack, with no signs of short-term memory loss. He was an English teacher who excelled in reading and writing. His concern stemmed from increasing difficulty to express himself. He knew exactly what he wanted to say but couldn't "get the words out" during conversation. What troubled him most was that he was confusing the meaning of words, substituting words for what he wanted to say (often incorrectly), stuttering, and unable to finish his sentences. He decided to see me when he started to struggle with reading and writing, too.

To evaluate language issues, some researchers use what they call "the cookie theft test." A patient is shown a picture of a boy about to put his hand into a cookie jar and is given one minute to describe what they see. The goal is to find out if those who have early changes describe the scene differently than those with unimpaired brains. More typical tests include naming a long list of common everyday objects, repeating words and sentences, and coming up with one's own list of animals, fruits, and words that start with a certain letter. Cognitive testing often involves more than one task because no test can assess one brain function (i.e., memory, language, attention, etc.) in isolation.

Beyond words, people can also have difficulty working with numbers. I have had retired accountants, bankers, and stockbrokers as patients who suddenly start having trouble doing their taxes, keeping their checking account balanced, or paying credit card bills. Margaret, the child of an accountant who was my patient, said to me, "Oh, Dad is seventy-five. It's time to have a CPA assume these responsibilities." I thought, *Possibly, but her father had strong math and numbers skills his entire life. What's happening now may represent a pathological decline from what was normal for him.* Again, the key is what was normal for that person, not what's typical for everyone else.

Visual and spatial misperceptions are worrisome, too. Is she getting lost? Is he unable to recognize people he once knew? Is she having difficulty keeping things arranged? Is a formerly immaculate kitchen or desk now a mess? Losing or misplacing common household items again and again can also be an early symptom. Most of us on occasion can't find our cell phone or purse, but when that happens three times a week or the items, such as a wallet, are found in bizarre places, like the freezer, that's concerning.

Because my dad also had Lewy body disease, additional brain changes occurred outside his memory center. Lewy body disease damaged the visual-spatial part of his brain (i.e., occipital lobe) at the same time Alzheimer's was harming his hippocampus. My father always had a great sense of direction. He could easily navigate the streets of a European city during a family vacation after one look at a map. Despite not playing a lot of sports, his hand-eye coordination was fantastic. So, it was odd when he couldn't find things that were in front of his face in the cabinet or when he got into a bike accident because he misjudged his distance from a car. At the time, our family didn't think much of it, but then again, we, like most people, would have been on the lookout for memory loss, not changes in spatial abilities.

Symptoms can also show up as declining attention and executive functioning. Ask yourself:

Is she having trouble staying focused long enough to solve a problem?
Is he having a hard time following a conversation, assuming there is no hearing issue?
Does it take longer for him to process information and complete complex tasks?
Is she having a hard time using reason to reach a conclusion or troubleshoot issues that arise during the day?
Is juggling two or three steps of a recipe at once in the kitchen becoming impossible?

Here's a story to illustrate executive-function problems. My patient Leo cooked so well he could have been an executive chef at a five-star restaurant. He learned the culinary arts from his grandmother, who had immigrated from Italy as a child. He made his own pasta, sauces, desserts, meatballs, and even wine. His daughter told me that she and her siblings couldn't wait to get home for the holidays because they knew their dad would create feasts that would remind them of when they were little kids.

Then one Christmas the spaghetti sauce was too salty. Everyone ate it, but without much joy. The pasta dough was too tough. The ravioli wouldn't seal. The meatballs fell apart while cooking. Even worse, when his daughter Elinor tried to help Leo in the kitchen, he got furious, said something hurtful, and stormed away. Leo had never behaved this way before. There could have been causes for these foul-ups, like stress, depression, or other possibilities, but his children, knowing him as they did, were troubled and even frightened by the behaviors they were witnessing.

Cerebrovascular disease not only co-occurs with Alzheimer's disease but can also mimic the same symptoms. In addition to forgetfulness, people may experience slowed thinking ability, inattention, trouble with concentration, and poor reasoning. The specific symptoms depend on where the disease is located within the brain. One particularly common and frustrating behavioral change in cerebrovascular disease is apathy—a lack of motivation, drive, or concern. It is distinct from depression. People with apathy may still enjoy activities when engaged but often lack the interest or initiative to start or repeat them. Families, not realizing their loved one isn't trying to be obstinate, often struggle with this without realizing this is the disease manifesting itself.

Different Types of Memory Loss—Depression and Sleep Apnea

Dr. Victoria Williams, an assistant professor at the University of Wisconsin School of Medicine, is a clinical neuropsychologist and researcher. I recently asked her about different types of memory loss that can mimic the symptoms of Alzheimer's. Speaking with her made me remember when my mother first told me she thought my father had Alzheimer's. Upon hearing her concerns, I immediately thought that surely something else must be behind his memory woes. Here is Dr. Williams's response to my inquiry:

Dr. Williams, part of making an Alzheimer's diagnosis is ruling out other possible causes of memory loss, such as sleep apnea, depression, and vascular problems, perhaps caused by a stroke. How does the memory loss these conditions cause differ from the memory loss of Alzheimer's disease?

Sleep apnea happens when pauses in breathing during sleep prevent the body from supplying enough oxygen to the brain, a condition known as hypoxia. *In addition, people frequently wake up (called microawakenings), preventing them from getting a good night's sleep. Fragmented sleep impacts optimal functioning of the prefrontal cortex, which plays an important role in cognitive control and attention. Individuals with sleep apnea often complain of difficulty with attention and memory.*

Alzheimer's, on the other hand, is characterized by difficulty with encoding—the initial formation of a memory—stemming from damage *to the hippocampus. In people with sleep apnea, memory changes can be linked to* prefrontal dysfunction, *which causes inefficient learning and retrieval. So, whereas Alzheimer's damages brain cells, sleep apnea merely causes otherwise normal brain cells to function poorly.*

Mood disorders, like depression and anxiety, impact how the brain works in an entirely different way. Research has shown that depression is linked to an imbalance of neurotransmitters as well as atypical patterns of connectivity between brain regions. Both impact how the brain processes information. Slowed processing speed and executive dysfunction contribute to less efficient learning and retrieval, but when someone with depression learns information, he or she generally remembers it.

Depression is another reversible cause of memory and thinking changes. As one's mood improves, there's a corresponding improvement in cognition. This is why assessing mood disorders is a critical component for a dementia workup. It should be ruled out as a cause for memory concerns before a neurodegenerative process such as Alzheimer's disease is considered.

Vascular dementia has been defined as dementia caused by a brain injury from an event like a stroke. Research, however, has shown that subtler brain function changes stem from an accumulation of milder vascular injuries to smaller brain capillaries. The narrowing in these small blood vessels leads to widespread changes in the white matter. The white matter of the brain is the highway system that connects various brain regions.

When this network breaks down, communication between brain regions slows. The consequence is reduced processing speed and deficits in higher-level cognitive abilities (i.e., problem-solving, multitasking, reasoning, etc.). The deterioration of the brain's information highway impairs the frontal lobe's ability to integrate information and control other brain areas, leading to executive dysfunction.

Overall, although various conditions create symptoms of memory loss, there are key differences in the ways in which these conditions cause memory to break down. Memory loss in Alzheimer's disease is unique—direct damage to the hippocampus causes an inability to form new memories.

A caveat: Two less common hippocampus dysfunctions mimic Alzheimer's symptoms. One is an inflammation of the hippocampus called hippocampal sclerosis. *The other is LATE (limbic-predominant age-related TDP-43 encephalopathy), a buildup of the TDP-43 protein in the hippocampus.*

If noticed early in the course of disease, a person's symptoms may reflect mild cognitive impairment (MCI), a stage that comes prior to dementia. There is also a new category of symptoms called mild behavioral impairment (MBI), where the first noticeable changes are not in thinking ability but in mood and behavior. Not all doctors agree that these presentations are unique and different from mood disorders like depression or anxiety, but there is research evidence that some people experience behavioral changes before they experience memory loss. If you or a loved one are suddenly apathetic or clearly anxious for no reason, such puzzling and unexpected mood shifts might be an early warning sign of brain disease.

One symptom can be caused by multiple deficits occurring in the brain. While each region of the brain has unique functions, none works in isolation. And not every decline is due to memory loss. For example, being unable to find your car keys can indicate any, some, or all of the following: memory loss, lack of attention when putting down the keys, an issue with spatial orientation when searching for them, or a loss of problem-solving ability if the strategy being used to find the car keys is inappropriate.

Geriatricians like me hear family anecdotes every day. As an outside observer, I sometimes find it hard to determine "the truth." Loved ones may worry too much. Sometimes a seasoned actor has a bad night, or a great chef prepares a disastrous meal. Everyone is entitled to have a bad day, and there can be many causes besides Alzheimer's. That's why I urge you, if you have a loved one you suspect may be showing early signs of Alzheimer's, keep a diary. Use it to record specific events or situations that concern you. Show it to your loved one's doctor. Believe me, she will appreciate it. It will help her make a more accurate diagnosis. (For more on recordkeeping, chapter 2 discusses it in detail.)

One helpful way to determine if a medical evaluation is needed (i.e., addressing the question of normal versus abnormal aging) is to look for three key characteristics. Determine if the symptoms are consistent, persistent, and getting worse. First, forgetting what you need from the grocery store is a fairly common complaint. It's more concerning when you consistently return home without the items you intended to purchase and routinely need to make trips back to the store. Second, are these lapses persistent? Do they occur regularly, even when you aren't stressed or busy, and possibly despite your efforts to correct them? That's a red flag, but by no means conclusive. Third, are these issues starting to affect your life in meaningful ways? Have you begun to shun social events or change your plans to avoid confronting worsening problems? Has your job performance noticeably declined? Have your day-to-day habits and routines changed in ways that are worrisome (e.g., my dad not following a TV plotline, causing my mom to watch him instead of the show)? If you answer these questions in the affirmative, it's time to be concerned. When someone comes to me exhibiting all these signs, it will prompt me to perform a full evaluation.

Finally, a word about the medical community. Society often puts physicians on a pedestal, but we and other healthcare professionals are far from perfect. The results from standard mental tests used by general practitioners can be misleading or flat-out wrong. Busy doctors might miss important findings or fail to fully consider all pieces of data from multiple sources. They form their own assessment, but those conclusions are subjective. That's why getting a second opinion can be important. Let me assure you that it never offends me—and it should not offend any doctor—when a patient would like another viewpoint. Whether you have back trouble, cancer, metabolic disease, or dementia, if you visit four specialists in a field—even within the same medical practice—you could easily get four different opinions and four different treatment plans. The best action you can take is to educate yourself about the medical issues. The more you understand, the better equipped you are to make sound judgments.

Modifiable Risk Factors and How Knowing Them Will Help You

It is a myth that getting Alzheimer's or dementia is inevitable. In fact, nearly half of all cases of dementia can be prevented or at least delayed. There are fourteen risk factors you can change in your life to reduce the odds of getting the condition, according to a 2024 report in the British medical journal *The Lancet*. "It's never too early—or too late—to take action," says the study's lead researcher, Gill Livingston, a professor of psychiatry of older people at University College London.

Steps you can take to protect yourself include:

1. Prevent or control diabetes. Keeping blood sugar in a healthy range helps protect your brain and body.
2. Manage cholesterol. Keep LDL, triglycerides, and total cholesterol low to reduce risk. Keep HDL levels high to protect your brain, too.
3. Minimize high blood pressure. Aim for healthy blood pressure levels. Lower is better, but not so low that you feel dizzy or weak.
4. Maintain a healthy weight. Reduce obesity and avoid excess body fat, especially around the abdomen.
5. Prevent and treat depression. Addressing mental health is essential for brain health and quality of life.
6. Prevent and manage hearing loss. Get regular hearing checks and use hearing aids if needed.
7. Address vision problems. Correct vision changes to stay safely engaged in daily life.
8. Avoid tobacco products. Do not smoke or use other forms of tobacco.
9. Limit alcohol use. Keep alcohol intake to a minimum to protect cognitive function. If it's not important to you, then don't drink at all.

10. Reduce exposure to air pollution. Limit exposure when you can, especially in areas with poor air quality. Wear a mask if needed.
11. Prevent head injuries. Wear a helmet when biking or riding a motorcycle, and always use a seatbelt.
12. Stay physically active. Regular movement helps keep both your body and brain healthy. Strive to partake in consistent physical activity—such as walking—on most days of the week.
13. Be a lifelong learner. Engage in mentally stimulating activities throughout life. It's never too late to learn something new.
14. Stay socially active. Maintain meaningful social connections and avoid isolation.

Chapter 5 offers practical, understandable ways to incorporate these lifestyle interventions into your daily life.

ENDING THE STIGMA OF ALZHEIMER'S

Stigma. The word comes from ancient Greek. It meant a mark or indentation made by a pointed instrument. It could also refer to a disfiguring scar or wound, but this meaning has evolved over two thousand years. Today the word *stigma* refers to a psychological mark of disgrace or shame, a burden that weighs down the soul.

Attitudes toward Alzheimer's today are comparable to how society felt about cancer in the decades before World War II. Doctors had few, if any, effective treatments for cancer. It terrified people. No one in government, medicine, or the media wanted to talk about it. The English word *cancer* comes from a Latin word that meant "crab." It's easy to picture the similarity between a spreading, tenacious, malignant growth and an ugly sea creature whose fearsome claws refuse to let go.

In the early 1950s, Fanny Rosenow, a cancer cure advocate, called *The New York Times* about placing an ad for a support group for women who had breast cancer. For some reason, the newspaper's receptionist transferred her phone call to the society editor. After a long pause, the editor told Rosenow, "I'm sorry, but the *Times* cannot publish the word *breast* or *cancer* in its pages." Since then, health groups have spent millions on changing public attitudes toward the disease, and the federal government has spent billions on cancer research. Cancer treatments are light-years beyond where they once were.

Today, however, 56 percent of American adults feel there's a similar stigma surrounding Alzheimer's, according to a 2021 AARP survey of 3,022 Americans aged forty and older. By contrast, only 23 percent of those polled thought a stigma surrounded heart disease, which is a far more common ailment. Sadly, 48 percent (nearly half!) of people surveyed thought they might get Alzheimer's, when in reality only about 12 to 15 percent will.

Attitudes toward Alzheimer's are changing, though slowly. Countless news stories trumpet the latest research findings. Organizations like AARP, the Alzheimer's Foundation of America, and the Alzheimer's Association are moving heaven and earth to educate people and push the boundaries of research. Movies and TV shows routinely feature characters who have the disease. Julianne Moore won an Oscar for her performance in the 2014 film *Still Alice* in which she plays a Harvard professor diagnosed with early-onset Alzheimer's. (I strongly recommend the movie, as well as the novel of the same name by neuroscientist Lisa Genova; each depicts a family's Alzheimer's journey in a heartfelt and realistic way.)

The stigma around Alzheimer's is lifting, but its doleful influence remains strong with many patients, loved ones, and even doctors. Almost all who have mild cognitive impairment or who have progressed into the mild stage of dementia are noticing changes in their mental status. They are typically self-aware, even if they don't talk about it. They may initially attribute their experience to normal aging. Some may suspect the truth but would just rather not confirm it. Many may suffer from disbelief or denial. Worse yet, they may think their children will use the diagnosis to rob them of their freedom, make decisions for them, misuse their financial assets, or put them in a nursing home. I see patients who don't want to know their diagnosis because they think their lives will lose all meaning. The sad fact is they're living with the symptoms regardless, but as a result of their denial, they are not getting the help they require.

Statistically, between 30 and 48 percent of dementia residents are in nursing homes today. Given those numbers, I understand my patients' fear that they might be forced to leave their homes. Though I have an abiding commitment to the wishes of my patients, at times there is no alternative to recommending a long-term care facility.

After my father was diagnosed with young-onset dementia (diagnosis before the age of sixty-five), I went with my parents to visit both adult day centers and long-term facilities. No one knows in the early stage of the disease what type of care will be required later. Seeing the environment was jarring for me and my father and mother.

Women are more impacted by Alzheimer's than men. They are more likely to become caregivers to those with the disease and are at higher risk of developing it themselves. Fortunately, women schedule more routine doctor appointments and are therefore more likely to bring up concerns that help identify the earliest symptoms. Meanwhile, men, in general, are less likely than women to seek medical care. So if you're a man reading this, good health is the foundation of everything in your life—see a doctor for regular checkups, if not for yourself then for your family's peace of mind.

Dementia does not affect all racial groups equally, and experiences and attitudes of communities of color vary when it comes to seeking medical care. Studies show that the overall prevalence of dementia is higher in African American, Hispanic/Latino, and Native American populations compared to white and Asian populations. African Americans are twice as likely as whites to be diagnosed. Latinos are one-and-a-half times as likely. It's important to note that this increased risk is not necessarily driven by Alzheimer's disease alone—other conditions like cerebrovascular disease and Lewy body disease may contribute significantly.

No one knows exactly why these disparities exist. It could be factors (now called social determinants of health) such as life experience, income, environmental exposure, access to healthcare, and the opportunity to engage in healthy lifestyle habits. There are also deeper cultural barriers. African Americans, for example, have historically distrusted the medical system more than other racial groups due in part to well-documented abuses like the Tuskegee experiments, where Black men were deliberately denied medical treatment. In that forty-year study, hundreds of men with syphilis were misled into believing they were receiving care, while researchers intentionally withheld penicillin—even after it became the standard treatment—to observe how the disease progressed. This violation of trust caused needless suffering and left a deep and lasting scar on the relationship between Black communities and the medical establishment. A great deal of work needs to be done to restore trust in these communities, and not just because it is the right thing to do—it is also because the health implications will affect generations to come.

Some cultures even lack a word for dementia. The term *dementia* comes from the Latin word *demens*, meaning "out of one's mind." In Wisconsin, where I live, there is a large Hmong population, people from rural Laos who immigrated here after the U.S. withdrawal from Vietnam in the mid-1970s. They have no term for dementia in their language, nor do some American Indian tribes. Adding to the challenge, Alzheimer's and related causes of dementia are thought to be more prevalent among Indigenous Americans than other groups. Recent population-based research suggests that as many as one-third of Native Americans are likely to develop Alzheimer's disease. This estimate is consistent with smaller community-based findings, including research involving the Oneida Nation in Wisconsin. Like African Americans, many Native Americans also report feeling that doctors treat them with less respect than they do other groups, which can further discourage people from seeking medical care.

For loved ones, stigma is often entangled with denial. No one wants to have dementia, and most understand that it is a long and arduous journey. Some may quietly fear that they won't be able to handle the demands of being a future caregiver. Others may worry that their family will suffer social embarrassment, lose friendships, become isolated, or even be forced to move away from the place they call home.

Stigma may also arise because the family is dysfunctional, and they sense that a diagnosis might cause ruptures. Tenuous relationships often worsen because of a dementia diagnosis. The condition tests people's fortitude. Despite this potential fraying of family connections, in my experience I often see the strength, courage, and creativity of families. (For more on ways to support caregivers and family, see chapter 7.)

Lack of access to healthcare, especially in underserved populations, only deepens stigma. If you don't have a trusted family doctor, who do you turn to when memory changes begin? It is not uncommon to feel ostracized by family or community, and not having a regular doctor can intensify feelings of isolation, helplessness, and shame.

What about doctors and other health professionals? Do their attitudes about Alzheimer's influence whether a patient gets timely treatment? After all, there is often a huge delay—sometimes years—between the first time a patient or loved one reports symptoms and the moment a diagnosis is finally made. That's why learning to advocate for yourself—or someone you love—is essential. It can make all the difference in getting the right care at the right time.

Take Action

That's the advice of Sarah Lenz Lock, who at the time served as senior vice president for policy at AARP, and executive director of the Global Council on Brain Health. During our conversation, I asked her what advice she has for anyone who is concerned about their mental status.

Cognitive decline is not inevitable. You can be proactive about your brain's health and make a difference for yourself as you age.

The sooner you find out what's going on, the better off you're going to be. If there's a possibility that medications can assist you, you want to know early, because they're not effective later. It's a myth that nothing can be done if you get a diagnosis of dementia.

An early diagnosis isn't about just medications. You can delay the onset of Alzheimer's through lifestyle modifications. Seeing a doctor isn't about just diagnosing you to see if you have Alzheimer's disease. It's diagnosing you to find out if you have other conditions that can be corrected.

If you wait too long, not only will you not be eligible for some of the new medications but you're going to be unable to put plans in place to help yourself manage this disease if you have it. The longer you wait, the less opportunity you will have to enjoy your life.

The reluctance of individuals to go to the doctor and seek a diagnosis is something we must get a handle on. Everyone agrees—both clinicians and the general population—early diagnosis is key.

When you have an opportunity to make decisions about your healthcare, your personal finances, and how you want to live the rest of your life, you can be part of the conversation and retain control over what matters most.

AARP has an online program called Staying Sharp that teaches healthy habits and is available free to nonmembers. Besides offering advice on healthy living for your brain, it also shares news on brain health, advice for caregivers, and listings of local events.

MAXIMIZING THE DOCTOR VISIT

Clinicians can unintentionally become a barrier to an early diagnosis. As a memory specialist, I know why the patient is coming to see me, and the universe of things I have to think about and look for is more contained than for some physicians. In my practice, we spend the entire visit focusing exclusively on cognitive concerns and related factors. Unlike a busy primary care physician, I'm not trying to solve ten different ailments in an eighteen-minute window. I also have full access to the patient's complete medical records on my computer.

Before meeting a patient, I will spend an hour "precharting," a process where I review their history so I can be well prepared. One of the most valuable tools I use is a simple search for the word "memory" in the patient's electronic medical file. This function streamlines and coordinates all appointments, labs, brain scans, and hospitalization records that mention my targeted word. Invariably, I find a complaint containing the word in their record. Someone—a speech therapist, physical therapist, doctor, spouse, or child, or sometimes the patient themselves—reported a memory problem, often years earlier.

Yet too often, no healthcare providers acted on those early concerns. Some may have been nervous about making the diagnosis. Others may not have known what to do next. Many physicians work in silos, not by choice but because the healthcare system rarely allows for the time or structure needed to address the whole person. Older adults in particular often present with complex layers of medical, cognitive, and psychosocial issues. As treatment options have become more specialized, so too has the care—fragmenting responsibilities and making it harder for any one provider to step back and see the full picture.

An AARP study found that while 91 percent of adults surveyed would want to be told if they had dementia, only 78 percent of clinicians said they always told patients the truth. In one survey, 97 percent of primary care providers admitted waiting for their patients to make them aware of memory symptoms or request an assessment.

But that wait can be dangerous. In a separate community-based study, only 40 percent of people said they would talk to their doctor immediately if they were experiencing memory loss. Even more concerning, among respondents who had symptoms suggesting dementia, 41 percent didn't talk to their provider at all. Doctors shouldn't wait for their patients to report a memory complaint because the majority won't, even when the condition has progressed significantly. We have to do better.

It is no secret that primary care doctors are more stressed for time than ever. Medical practices often track the time providers spend with each patient, and doctors are pressed to see as many patients a day as possible. In these conditions, one can imagine a checkup or yearly physical where the patient and doctor spend most of their time on urgent or chronic health problems. Toward the end of the visit, the patient mentions, "By the way, my memory's not what it used to be." It's not hard to see how a doctor might reply, "Well, you are seventy. It's normal to have some memory decline. I'll make a note of that, and we'll talk about it next time." Unfortunately, the next time might be years later, when symptoms will no longer be subtle.

By the time this patient sees me, I'll often find a note from his primary care doctor saying that the patient reported his memory was worse and that he had had a recent car accident or been the victim of a financial scam. Sadly, this patient could have benefited from treatment sooner—and perhaps avoided a car crash.

Now imagine the same scenario, but instead the doctor replies, "Hmm, memory problems. That's a concern. Let's set up a visit for next week so we can dive into what you're experiencing, examine how serious the changes are, and look for potential reversible causes. Let's also have you take this memory test. We won't have an answer right away, but we'll get to the bottom of this." That kind of response can change the entire course of care.

A Scary Moment in the Car

My father, Dr. Moe Chin, was a family doctor in Watertown, the small Wisconsin town where I grew up. He was diagnosed with early-onset Alzheimer's and passed away in 2018. Throughout his illness, my family experienced moments that were confusing, frightening, wonderful, and unforgettable. One of those moments stayed with my mother, Karen Chin, and marked a turning point for her. This is her story, in her own words:

We all make mistakes when we're driving, but early one spring morning in 2012, my late husband Moe made a mistake that was so scary, I knew something was deeply wrong. This was not a normal error. It was something else. It happened months after I had already started to worry about him, and it became a turning point for me.

Moe was going to a medical conference on an early morning flight. We lived so far from the airport that we had to leave at 3 AM. It was pitch black out in the farm country where we lived. He wanted me to drive.

The timing couldn't have been worse. I had just come home from the hospital after an appendectomy and didn't want to make the trip. I wasn't exactly feeling like a million bucks! But Moe absolutely insisted. He said he didn't want to leave the car in long-term parking. He had always been frugal, but something seemed funny about his attitude and determination to have me drive.

We agreed I would go, but only if he took the wheel. As we got closer to the city, we were cruising along at a good clip. Even though there were streetlights, I sensed he was going to miss the airport exit. "Turn! Go! Turn now!" I yelled.

Moe reacted quickly. He turned, but instead of taking the exit he drove onto nearby railroad tracks. If a train had come at that moment, it would have been all over. Luckily, he didn't drive far onto the tracks and we didn't get stuck. He was flustered, even discombobulated, and honestly, so was I. Moe managed to back off safely, and we got to the airport fine.

I've never forgotten that moment. Six months later, when I took Moe for his neuropsychological evaluation, which was a key part of the process leading to his diagnosis, the neuropsychologist said, "Let's talk about some instances where you believe Moe's judgment was not appropriate."

After I told the train story, the doctor smiled and said, "I don't know, Karen. If you'd said 'Turn!' exactly the same way to me, I might have turned just as sharply at your command, too."

The way the neuropsychologist replied gave me the impression he didn't want Moe to feel bad. He was bolstering Moe's dignity. It was lovely, even if it wasn't entirely true.

Soon thereafter, our geriatrician told Moe, "You have early-onset Alzheimer's." Two seconds after that Moe said, "But I don't have Alzheimer's." I turned to him and said, "I'm sorry, but you do. He just told us that you have Alzheimer's disease." It was very hard for Moe to accept that diagnosis. Little by little, all the professionals at the clinic helped him adjust. They were patient and gentle. I will always be grateful for their kindness.

I'd be remiss if I didn't also acknowledge the many personal notes and phone calls I've received alongside consultation requests from primary care doctors. "I've taken care of Mrs. Smith and her family for decades. They are good people who are understandably concerned by what may be a difficult period ahead. Please keep me informed." These thoughtful gestures remind me that delays in diagnoses aren't because primary care providers don't care about their patients. They do care—deeply. But they are working within a system that too often pushes them toward speed over thoroughness. When we slow down and truly listen, we have the opportunity to make a meaningful difference.

Expert Advice: Goodbye to the Stigma of Alzheimer's?

There is good news about Alzheimer's, according to clinical neurologist Dr. Serge Gauthier, a professor emeritus of neurology and psychiatry at McGill University in Montreal, Canada. Gauthier served as coauthor of the World Alzheimer's Report in 2021 and 2022 for Alzheimer's Disease International. He often speaks to lay audiences about progress in the fight against the disease. I spoke with him for this book. Here is what he had to say:

People are seeking an earlier diagnosis when they have mild symptoms. There's been a shift. Before it was "Let's wait. Let's hide. Let's pretend." People used to come for consultations only when they had moderate-stage dementia and behavior problems. Most clinics now have to adapt to younger people in their sixties rather than their eighties. Sometimes they now only have subjective complaints or mild changes that are real but are not interfering with daily life.

This is a challenge for family practitioners who are not equipped to test people with such mild symptoms. There's probably still a tendency to dismiss mild complaints as just normal age-related things.

But the public is requesting more, so that's probably leading to more consultations in neurology, psychiatry, geriatrics than before.

Sometimes older physicians, doctors who have had someone as a patient for many years, begin to think of that person as a friend. But when that person exhibits cognitive changes, the doctor can be afraid to tell them. The other thing is that if you tell someone they have mild dementia, there will be a list of things you have to do beyond the five-minute checkup. So there are consequences for a diagnosis that some physicians don't have the training or time for.

Talk to your family doctor. If you don't have one, get one. Don't wait until you have symptoms that lead to mistakes in your work or daily life. On the other hand, we all forget with age, so let's not get carried away. There can be a gray zone of many years between benign forgetfulness and a possible diagnosis, or that forgetfulness may never turn into something that needs to be treated.

A blood test to screen for Alzheimer's in the general population is on the horizon, building on current tests already used in people with cognitive impairment. Alzheimer's is also becoming much more treatable. Its progression can be delayed if it's caught early enough. In the next decade it has the potential to become a chronic, not fatal, illness.

There once was a time when no one talked about cancer. Today people are quite open about it. They're proud to say, "I'm a cancer survivor." It gives them a stake in life to say they survived. Maybe Alzheimer's will become like that.

Cognitive screening tests are designed to *screen for*, not diagnose, cognitive impairment. In this context, "to screen" means to quickly assess for the possibility of a condition, not to confirm its presence, much like a metal detector signals the potential for metal without identifying its exact nature. Many were designed to identify *possible* dementia and have limited ability to capture milder conditions like MCI. Three of the most commonly used tools in clinic are the MoCA (Montreal Cognitive Assessment), the Mini Mental State Examination (MMSE), and the St. Louis University Mental Status (SLUMS) Examination. Each has a total of thirty points and typically takes less than twenty minutes to complete. In my opinion, the more difficult the test, the more useful it will be. If we're hoping to catch people early in the course of their disease, the test should not be too easy.

One major problem with cognitive screening tools is they cannot identify true impairment in people just starting to have declines. Most tools currently used by doctors were not designed to detect subtle declines and the earliest signs of impairment. Unfortunately, many providers conflate this screening with diagnostic testing. They are not the same. I frequently diagnose people with dementia who have near-perfect scores on the screening test. Only with a neuropsychological battery are we able to see lower-than-anticipated scores that truly reveal impairment. Highly educated people with lots of cognitive reserve (extra neural networks built from mentally stimulating and challenging activities) can still score well despite having real declines. My own father scored a perfect thirty out of thirty on the MMSE in his PCP office. Just a few months later, he was diagnosed with mild-stage dementia.

I wish primary care providers would stop relying so heavily on these brief screening tools. They often delay referrals to specialists who can conduct a far more complete evaluation. This typically includes hours-long testing by a neuropsychologist who gives an array of tests that gauge performance in all the brain areas—executive function, language, visual-spatial, and more. The result? Obvious impairments will be revealed.

Even neuropsychological testing is imperfect. When the tests were designed, their creators often failed to consider cultural, racial, and social differences. Such blind spots can lead to misleading scores, too. For that reason, there's a big push to revise the assessments to be more culturally sensitive. (I will say much more about these tests and medical evaluations in geriatric clinics in chapter 3.)

So what should you expect a doctor to do when you express concerns about memory changes? First and foremost, if the doctor dismisses the symptoms as "just normal aging" without doing any kind of evaluation, you or your family should push the issue. I have learned that patients and loved ones often need to advocate for themselves.

Tell the doctor you want a more in-depth investigation. Ask for blood work to check for underlying issues like thyroid, liver, and kidney dysfunction, as well as abnormal calcium or sodium levels and vitamin deficiencies. Blood-based biomarker testing for Alzheimer's is now available, but it's best to wait for a full clinical assessment first to ensure the test is ordered and interpreted in the right context. That context matters because the accuracy and interpretation of the results depend not only on where along the continuum of cognitive change someone is but also on other health conditions that can directly alter the biomarker levels, and on the possibility that other brain diseases may be contributing to the symptoms. (See chapter 8 on Alzheimer's clinical research for more on the incredible advancements in the field.) Bring up all current medications and supplements, and ask the doctor to carefully review possible interactions and side effects. Request a cognitive screening test and a brain scan. Make sure to discuss daily functional abilities. It's critical to know if the cognitive changes are impacting your ability to take medications independently, handle finances, go to appointments, drive, cook, clean, and use a computer.

Here's a cautionary note—you should not expect a primary care provider to diagnose Alzheimer's. The painstaking evaluation process can take hours and requires specialized experience. What you can reasonably expect are multiple visits with your primary care doctor, a thoughtful exploration of the symptoms, and answers to a substantial number of questions. Your doctor may not know everything, but if you clearly communicate how worried you are and describe what you're seeing, she is unlikely to brush it aside. Most doctors will take your concerns seriously and will likely make a referral to the specialist.

A memory evaluation is not a secretive or proprietary process guarded by the healthcare establishment. Not only are medical teams trained to administer and interpret these evaluations but they also bring clinical acumen and experience working compassionately with patients. Their role is to help individuals feel more comfortable and steady during what can be an emotional process. Understanding what goes into the medical workup can remove the mystery and anxiety from the clinic visit. Being well informed allows you to prepare and maximize your time with your doctor.

An assertive patient is no different from a confident consumer looking for a house or car. Few people would buy a home without researching it, asking questions, and consulting experts. Home buyers are not intimidated by realtors. They view them as allies and utilize their skills to achieve their goal. Similarly, if you moved to a new town, you'd probably visit elementary schools to see which would be best for your children. You would feel at ease talking with principals, teachers, and other parents. When you get down to it, doctors are people like you, and medical care is no different than other services. Do for yourself what you would for your children. Be prepared, ask questions, and make informed decisions.

2

"I Didn't See It Coming"

How to Plan and Run a Family Meeting • What You Need to Know to Share Your Concerns • Building the Foundation for Successful Caregiving

Looking back, I didn't see it coming—the day my mother delivered the news that she thought my father had Alzheimer's. For months she had been preparing for the moment she would finally share her worries with me and my older sister, Maggie.

Since my father's passing in 2018, I've spent a lot of time reflecting on the journey—from the time of my mother's initial concern in 2010 right through to his death. It has been a painful and sobering look back. There are things I wish I had done differently, words I would have said or left unsaid. I wish I knew then what I know now. I believe I could have made a bigger impact back then. Those feelings are what have motivated me to write this book.

If you're reading this, chances are you're standing at the threshold of uncertainty. Maybe someone you love is forgetting details, repeating themselves, or seeming "off" in a way you can't quite explain. Maybe you've tried to raise your concerns but haven't been heard—or perhaps you haven't found the words to start the conversation. Wherever you are,

I know how heavy that unease can feel. You don't know what next steps to take.

You are not alone.

My family went through what you are going through. Losing my father, Moe, to Alzheimer's disease showed me firsthand what families endure before they ever reach my memory clinic. Like every patient I see, he was more than his disease. My father was an old-school family doctor, the kind who made house calls in a small town in Wisconsin. My mother spent months quietly worrying about him before she shared her concerns with Maggie and me.

I'd like to use this chapter to walk you through the process of what my mother did—planning and holding a family meeting to share concerns. In fact, there are usually two important family meetings. The first is just for the close family members and friends; the second includes the person you are worried about. The first meeting is essential to open the door to honest conversation and helps create allies.

I know all about such family meetings. My mother held one in which she shared her worries about our father. It was one of the most emotional moments of my life. I've replayed that discussion over and over since it happened. I can close my eyes and be right back there, completely unaware of how much my life was about to change. How was I to know what was about to unfold in July 2012?

At the time, I was finishing my second year of residency at the University of California San Diego. I was working close to eighty hours a week. I had been married for two years, but I was completely focused on myself—my work, my career, learning the endless array of details it takes to become a good doctor. Infectious diseases fascinated me, not cognitive disorders. I had spent most of my education since college preparing to specialize in that field.

My sister and I have been following in our father's footsteps since we were children. He never once told us he wanted us to be doctors like him. We never felt any pressure to pursue his career. Yet we both chose the life of medicine, probably because he was the finest physician we knew, and it was clear he loved his work.

Dad was a geriatrician, like I am now, but he did everything else from delivering babies to seeing children to caring for adults. It wasn't a job to him; it was his calling. My sister and I marinated in that environment for eighteen years. It was inevitable we would come to consider it for own lives.

That July, my mother invited Maggie, a general practitioner in Seattle, and me to come home for the holidays. I imagined she simply wanted a joyous family reunion—at least, that's what I thought. As the days grew closer to my flight home to Wisconsin, I looked forward to catching up, swapping stories about my medical training.

I grew up in Watertown, an hour west of Milwaukee, a classic small town of twenty thousand people. My father, Moe, was a first-generation American. His parents and his three older brothers emigrated from China to the West Coast in the late 1940s. He was the only member of his family born after they arrived in the United States. He never learned to be fluent in Cantonese. His family wanted him to live the American dream, which meant shedding the past. Like so many immigrants, my father worked relentlessly. His efforts culminated when he earned his MD at the University of Washington.

For forty years, Moe Chin was a family doctor of the sort you rarely see anymore. He worked seven days a week. It's impossible to count how many evenings the phone would ring as I sat doing homework, eating dinner, or watching TV. Without hesitation, he'd put on his coat and head out the door into whatever conditions—snow, rain, frigid temperatures—awaited him on those Wisconsin nights, carrying his scuffed and tattered black leather doctor's satchel. (These days the satchel has a place of honor on a bookshelf in my office.) Watching him go out, I knew he was on his way to deliver a baby, visit a home where a child had suddenly fallen ill, or attend to an emergency at the hospital.

I grew up wanting to be like my father. He was a rock, a pillar of the community, a fixed star shining brightly in my imagination. He was my hero, my idol.

So I came home. I didn't think anything of it. My sister was there. My mom and dad were there. We had a great time—sharing meals, running errands, and doing things around the house. I had no reason to suspect

I would be blindsided by my mother's news. This felt like a standard visit home, a chance to tell stories and catch up. Everything seemed normal with my father. Granted, he didn't talk a lot, but he never did. He was always a quiet man.

Then one day, when my father went out, my mom asked me and my sister to sit down for a family meeting. At first, I didn't think anything was wrong. But as the conversation unfolded, all those rosy feelings went away. My mom had crafted the moment so gently that I didn't sense what was coming at first. She led us to the sunroom on the side of the house, where light poured in all around us. We could see the beautiful rolling Wisconsin hills and farmland.

My mom arranged the room in a way so that it felt like we were sitting in a circle, like you would in a formal meeting. I didn't pick up on that at all. I don't know if it was intentional, but when I sat down my mom was directly across from me. We were sipping coffee.

I'll never truly know what it felt like for my mother in the moments before she shared her conclusions with us. Years later, she told me about her nervousness and apprehension. She was confident in what she had observed in my father and in her own diagnosis of what was happening to him. But she was restless, worried about the resistance she assumed would come from her children. And of course, she was right. More than anything, she felt sad for us. She knew how this would affect our lives, and the sorrow we would now carry. Even in the depths of her own stress and grief, she was thinking about her kids. That's a reflection of the amazing woman and mother she is.

People living with dementia and their families often feel isolated and alone. They can become trapped by worry about the future, so much so that they forget to live in the present. Those who can stay present are giving themselves a gift. They understand that the future is uncertain—the challenges that may or may not await them have not yet arrived. If you can find the strength to live in the present moment, you will discover a sense of control. After all, none of us can control the future, but what we can do is control how we respond to what is right here, right now, in front of us.

So, as you read this chapter, remember to breathe. Remember to focus.

Remember to be in the moment. You'll feel better, and doing so will help you to act and to make plans.

When talking about serious matters—especially something as delicate as cognitive change—it's important to create an environment that feels safe and welcoming. My mother, Karen, understood this instinctively. She put care into the small details, beginning with what felt like a commonplace moment: "Let's go sit in the sunroom and have coffee." It made perfect sense, since we were there to spend time together.

As we settled into conversation, the calm familiarity of the moment began to shift. Suddenly, my mom started to share her fears—something was wrong with Dad. And then she began to cry. This single act of emotion—crying—is my kryptonite. In the comics, kryptonite is the key substance in the universe that can stun Superman. Her tears had that effect on me. I froze, tense and unable to think. After all, my mother comes from a German American farm family—tough, stoic people. My mom doesn't cry. She doesn't show that kind of emotion in public, which, of course, includes me and my sister. She cried when our dogs died, but other than that, I never saw her weep. To me, seeing her cry was more traumatic than hearing her observations about Dad's mental lapses.

Her words were cut-and-dried. Hearing her was so jarring that all I can clearly recall of my immediate reaction was feeling warm. I said something like, "You don't know what you're talking about. He's fine. He's practicing medicine. I saw him earlier this morning and he's doing great. There's nothing to be concerned about." I don't remember what she said in response.

Despite my defensive retort, she remained calm. Her face held a motherly compassion and softness. Her observations were certain, and she understood, even anticipated, my reaction. She felt sympathy for me, but she displayed resolve and wouldn't be deterred. The warmth in my body only intensified, and was now mixed with tears streaming down my face. A gnawing sensation grew in my stomach, a sick feeling triggered by fear.

That day feels like a blur. I suspect my brain and psyche are protecting me. I was there. I know that. I cried a lot. I know that, too.

Immediately Maggie and I peppered our mother with questions like, "What's your proof? Why do you think this?" It's embarrassing to admit, but even after years of medical training, I didn't know much about

Alzheimer's disease. I was in shock. I thought, *There's no way he's got dementia. He's a fully functional person.*

But my mother had done her research. She certainly was prepared. This meeting was intentional and the reason she wanted us home that week. She waited until my father was out of the house. She came to the meeting with a notebook.

She told us specific instances where my father had experienced deeply troubling mental lapses, none of them work related. As the unofficial office manager of my dad's private medical practice, she had a front-row seat to his professional life. His staff were close and had worked with him for years. They would have felt comfortable speaking to her if they had seen anything concerning. Yet the issues she noticed—the moments that worried her—only happened at home.

Even so, I rebelled at the thought that my father was ill. After all, my dad had never been the most functional or capable person outside work. My mom had always done everything for our family. Maggie and I pushed back. "Dad's stressed," we said. "He's switched from his private practice to the hospital practice. He's busier than ever. He's working a hundred hours a week."

That was our reaction—as two doctors, no less! We denied it. Mom kept pushing back. She wouldn't give an inch. She's not someone to be bullied. She wasn't being mean, just tough and realistic.

She kept going, calmly explaining, patiently laying out what she had seen. I remember hearing her and crying. Even though I was denying it with every word I said, I knew deep inside she was right.

She had her say, but the fact of the matter is, she didn't sell her case well—at least not to me. I didn't leave the room convinced she was right. I simply left the room in complete denial. I didn't want to hear what she had to say. I didn't want to believe that my hero was not only wounded but also mortally injured, and in the same house as me that weekend.

At the same time, I knew my mother was not only very smart but also incredibly observant.

That was my experience of a family meeting. My mother had prepared and managed it well, but still, I walked away doubting. No matter how your loved ones react, this kind of family meeting is a first step that needs to be taken.

Here is my advice for how you can plan such a meeting.

STEPS TO TAKE—OBSERVE, READ, AND WRITE

The number one reason people contact me—by cell phone or email—is to ask: "How do I talk to my loved one? I believe there's a problem. What do I do?"

Unless you are a patient of mine, there's only so much that I, or any other doctor, can do outside the formal doctor-patient relationship. I can be a good listener. I can refer you to resources like the Alzheimer's Association and the Alzheimer's Foundation of America. I can offer expressions of concern, but I cannot make a diagnosis or give medical advice.

What I'd like to do in this chapter is empower you. I want you to take concrete steps toward getting help for your loved one, if that kind of support turns out to be necessary. What follows is a step-by-step guide—a prescription, as it were—to prepare for and hold not one family meeting but two. This two-part conversation creates space to share concerns about a loved one and to begin thinking about an action plan.

The first meeting is just for family members. The second meeting includes the person you're worried about—the one who may have Alzheimer's. This two-step process is crucial because it helps get everyone on the same page—or at least attempts to—before approaching your loved one directly.

The earlier you initiate these meetings, the better. You're reading this book because you have concerns. That alone is a good first step. But don't let years or even months slip by. If you've just started to notice memory changes in someone you love, don't wait until they begin having functional problems in their daily life. You want to start seeking help before that happens. Still, it can be hard for many people to fully believe what they're seeing or feeling. Most people wait until an undeniable event—a car accident or another bright red flashing warning sign—happens before they act.

When Functional Changes Are Already Happening

Sometimes families wait to have a meeting because they aren't sure what they're seeing or they hope symptoms will improve. This is completely understandable. If you have waited, start where you are; it's never too late to come together and make a plan.

When functional changes manifest—when the person begins to struggle with daily tasks—you are in a different situation than when cognitive symptoms like memory lapses first appear. These changes affect how safely and independently a person can live day to day.

Here are some examples of functional changes that may signal it's time to act:

- Financial management: unpaid bills, unusual purchases, confusion about bank accounts, giving away large sums of money
- Medication management: missed doses, taking the wrong medication, confusion about pill schedules, repeated trips to the pharmacy for the same prescription
- Driving: getting lost on familiar routes, difficulty following directions, fender benders, near misses, or increased anxiety while driving

WHAT TO DO NOW

Act with urgency, not panic.
A person exhibiting functional changes may already be in unsafe situations. The family meeting should quickly move toward action—medical evaluation, safety planning, and support services.

Prepare to lead the decision-making.
Early meetings invite partnership. Late meetings may require the family to take a stronger leadership role to ensure safety, even if the person resists.

Expect resistance.

When daily life is impacted, people are more likely to feel threatened or defensive. They may worry about losing their independence. Focus on safety, emphasize your love, and bring specific examples of concerning situations. Remind the family member that you want them to remain as independent as possible, too.

Be direct and compassionate.

"We're seeing things that are now affecting your daily life and safety. We need to make some changes, and we'll do this together."

KEY TAKEAWAY

The longer you wait, the less the meeting will be about "if something is happening" and more about "what must happen now."

SUPPORTIVE NEXT STEPS

- Schedule a medical evaluation with the person's primary care doctor. Tell the doctor that you have concerns about cognitive changes.
- Consider a home safety assessment through a local health provider, social worker, or occupational therapist.
- Start by determining what areas the person needs help with in order to function fully (e.g., cooking meals, doing laundry, driving, etc.), stay engaged in the activities that matter most to them, and experience joy in daily life. Then identify sources of daily support, such as family members, friends, or professional caregivers.
- Contact a local organization like Alzheimer's Association, Alzheimer's Foundation of America, or an Area Agency on Aging for community resources.
- Make a plan for high-risk activities like driving and managing medications.
- Meet with an occupational or speech therapist to improve upon and maintain functional abilities.

If you visit any Alzheimer's-focused website, you'll likely find a page listing "The 10 Signs of Dementia." While I think knowing these signs is useful, I'm against relying on them as the primary guide. Such changes usually appear later—after other subtle, persistent signals have been present for some time. You don't want to wait until your loved one is showing four, five, or seven major signs before seeking help. The earlier an evaluation is done, the sooner steps can be taken to slow the disease's progression, if Alzheimer's turns out to be the diagnosis. Even a few years ago, we didn't have treatments capable of doing that.

Today, FDA-approved drugs such as lecanemab (also known as Leqembi) and donanemab (known as Kisunla) can target and remove amyloid plaques, the first protein of Alzheimer's, but they work only in the disease's earliest stages. That's one reason why national associations and clinicians need to encourage people in the community to keep an eye out for the earliest possible changes. This is a hard task because the earliest signs are often subtle and easy to miss.

As we learned in chapter 1, Alzheimer's disease is not the same as dementia, though in the past these terms were used synonymously. Alzheimer's is defined by the presence of abnormal levels of amyloid and tau proteins stuck in the brain. Amyloid forms first, and then years later tau develops, all while the person has no symptoms. Symptoms arise after brain cells start to die and synapses (connections between brain cells) begin to malfunction due to the buildup of tau protein.

We are living at the dawn of a revolution in Alzheimer's treatment. These novel disease-modifying therapies are now FDA approved. Only a few years ago, they were just a dream. These early drugs, which are likely the spearhead of a legion of new therapies, successfully remove the first Alzheimer's disease protein, and they do their job well. Unfortunately, they do not stop the disease or prevent a person's symptoms from progressing. People on these therapies decline at a slower rate, but studies show that these drugs do modify the disease process itself. This is known as disease-modifying therapy. While we have not yet achieved our ultimate clinical goal of preventing Alzheimer's and halting its progression, disease-modifying therapy is new for the field and offers a platform to build on. (More on different types of disease-modifying therapy in chapter 6.)

I compare the current state of Alzheimer's treatment to where rheumatoid arthritis treatment was just a few years ago. Older people suffered greatly from rheumatoid arthritis for decades. Their fingers grew crooked and stiff. Their hands refused to open. Now, thanks to monoclonal antibody treatments like rituximab, a commonly used immunosuppressive medication, younger patients with rheumatoid arthritis are far less likely to develop such debilitating problems.

It's worth repeating: The best time to begin treatment with lecanemab or donanemab is early in the Alzheimer's disease process. However, it's also important to recognize that these medications may come at a cost, and not just financially. There are real side effects to consider, some of which are not minor or harmless, like stomach upset. (More on this in chapter 6 as well.) The sooner an Alzheimer's diagnosis is made, the better, and that's the goal of this book.

PREPARING FOR THE FAMILY MEETING

Unfortunately, many families never have a "family meeting." Understandably, they feel overwhelmed by their loved one's changes, worried about discussing their observations with others, and unsure of how to broach the subject without upsetting anyone.

But when these meetings don't happen, care and support are delayed, conversations can go poorly, feelings get hurt, and families experience even more stress because they are unprepared and lack a shared plan. Planning ahead and taking a thoughtful approach will lead to better outcomes—for you, your family, and your loved one.

Ideally, these meetings are held in person. When that's not feasible, a hybrid or virtual gathering will have to suffice. The most important aspect is to be present, emotionally and mentally. Being able to see the person is usually better than speaking by phone. I apply the same principles when discussing sensitive issues with my patients.

Even when people hold family meetings, I would guess that most of the time they haven't sought any advice beforehand, making it much more likely for the discussion to blow up and go wrong. When friends or neighbors reach out to me, it's usually because they don't know what to do. That uncertainty freezes people. It leads to delays because they desperately want to protect their family relationships. They worry the meeting could go poorly. There's often a fear that a partner could lash out or grow resentful. A concerned child might hesitate, worried that a parent will shut them out, perhaps believing the child is motivated by financial gain, not love.

There will be two meetings you need to have. The first is with your family, friends, or anyone who will be involved in talking to the person about the symptoms. The meeting with your loved one comes later.

Both meetings will carry a lot of emotion. The goal of the first meeting is to align everyone on the concern. You must explain what's on your mind, what you've observed, and why you've come to your conclusions.

When you prepare for a family meeting, the first and most important step is to begin the habit of writing down what you observe: events, behaviors, and statements. Why? Because you want to understand what's happening to this person you love.

You might record an example like, "On this day, while we were [at home, out shopping, or wherever] my loved one did [such and such] at [such and such] time." You put it on paper so you can see it and go back to it later. Yes, doing this will be emotional. You may be so consumed with fear—fear of what the memory loss means—that you can't believe that the event recorded in your written recollection actually happened. But if you don't commit the event to writing, you will end up second-guessing yourself.

Concerned families have asked me whether they should record their loved one. It's a tricky question. While I loved the movie *The Truman Show*, the main character's shock and deep sense of violation when he realized his entire life had been filmed without his permission is exactly what I would fear for the loved one in this situation. No one wants this to happen to them, even when the intention is good.

The purpose of writing down observations is not to force your version of reality onto someone else—it's to confirm your own concerns and remind yourself why you have them. Logistically, it would also be difficult to record in the moment. You can't anticipate when an early symptom will appear, and you wouldn't want your loved one to realize you're recording them right then and there. Getting caught would likely require an explanation you're not ready to give.

That said, some people respond better to visual or audio documentation than to subjectively written notes. If you think your loved one or family will be more receptive if they see a video or hear the symptoms, you could try—but it wouldn't be my first choice.

Keeping a diary is one of the most helpful practices you can adopt. It allows you to objectively confirm the changes you're noticing. Write everything down. That said, don't treat your notes as if they're ironclad evidence being used in a courtroom to convince your loved one she has a problem. You're not a lawyer trying to prove a case. Instead, think of the diary as a way to better understand what's happening. Over time—you might do this for several months—your record will build a comprehensive picture that you, your family, and your medical care team will greatly value.

Yes, it's very much a secret endeavor. You're keeping a secret from your loved one, something you may be unaccustomed to doing. That can be hard. Fight through the sense of betrayal you may feel. You're doing the right thing for your loved one and yourself.

Keeping quiet over the period of observation is important for two main reasons. First, you may not feel ready to approach your loved one with your concerns. Perhaps you still doubt whether what you're seeing is truly abnormal, whether it's occurring often enough to reflect a real change, or whether it represents a genuine decline from the person's baseline.

Second, if you're trying to understand whether there's a real problem, you don't want your loved one to change their behavior just to appease you. If they know they're being watched, they may act differently or start hiding things from you. This is known as the Hawthorne effect—a phenomenon where people modify their behavior simply because they know they're being observed. If that happens, it may delay a diagnosis.

This can be especially true when someone is beginning to notice their own cognitive struggles but isn't ready to talk about them. Instead of asking questions that will reveal they've forgotten a prior conversation or an upcoming event, they may stay quiet and try to follow along. If finding words in conversation becomes difficult, they might avoid telling stories or participating in spontaneous discussion, choosing instead to listen or give short responses. In social settings, where the risk of being caught off guard is higher, they might begin declining invitations or drifting away from group interactions altogether. Even at home, they may begin secretly writing things down, rereading emails multiple times, or looking up information on their own—trying to compensate without drawing attention.

These shifts can be subtle at first, but they are meaningful. The effort to cover up mistakes or confusion may itself become a source of stress and isolation. And while these compensatory behaviors can delay recognition of a problem, they also offer important clues—if we're paying attention.

(I do have a caveat. Your situation is unique. You may want or need to have a conversation, or several, with your loved one before the family meeting. As you read on, you'll see that this is something my mother did. Bottom line—do what feels right and good for you.)

Not only should you observe and write down what you see, but you should also try to get a sense of what's happening more broadly in the person's life. Presumably, you know this person well because they're your spouse, partner, parent, or friend. Looking back on my situation with my father, even well-intentioned and medically trained people, including his family physician, kept saying to my mother (who was also his patient), "He's just going through a change in his medical practice. His work is demanding. The hospital is asking more of him. He's just super stressed. That's probably all it is."

Yes, those observations were all true about my father, but they weren't the full picture. By keeping a diary, you're trying to understand: *Are there other potential causes at play? Is my husband, wife, or parent on a new medication? Is he sleeping well? Is she drinking too much? Does he seem depressed?* The goal is to widen your lens and consider all possible explanations, not just the most obvious ones.

You're looking for the lowest-hanging fruit among alternative explanations. And in many cases, this search can lead to very good news—the kind of news doctors are eager to deliver and that patients and their families long to hear. Sometimes mental fogginess turns out to be a result of sleep apnea. Imagine not getting a good night's sleep for days, weeks, or months. Your thinking would be in poor shape, too. The same is true for unintended prescription drug interactions, which have side effects that impair brain function.

Most Common Reversible Factors That Can Cause Memory Loss

Depression, anxiety, or significant emotional stress
Side effects of medications
Excessive alcohol use or recreational drugs (like marijuana)
Poor sleep quality
Obstructive sleep apnea
Thyroid disorders (hypothyroidism or hyperthyroidism)
Acute kidney or liver dysfunction
Imbalances in electrolytes (e.g., high calcium or low sodium)
Hearing or vision loss
Chronic infections (e.g., Lyme disease, syphilis, HIV, or Covid-19)
Acute infections (e.g., urinary tract infection, pneumonia, or skin infections like cellulitis)

Subdural hematoma (bleeding between the brain and skull after a head injury)

Concussion

Normal pressure hydrocephalus (a buildup of fluid in the brain)

The second step is to read up on cognitive changes in older adults. Doing so will give you more perspective on the patterns and behaviors you've been recording. As you read and reflect, ask yourself: *What is normal aging? What is abnormal aging? What is this "mild cognitive impairment" that experts talk about? What exactly is Alzheimer's disease, and how does it differ from other types of dementia?* You can be your own best teacher.

However, the value of what you learn depends on the quality of your sources. Be cautious when researching any medical condition online, especially Alzheimer's and related brain diseases. I tell my patients to avoid internet forums and stick to reputable, evidence-based websites.

Trusted Resources for Understanding Cognition and Brain Diseases

National Institute on Aging (NIA)
https://www.nia.nih.gov
A comprehensive federal resource on brain aging, dementia research, and caregiving.

Alzheimers.gov (managed by the NIA)
https://www.alzheimers.gov
Focused on research, clinical trials, and support for patients and families.

Alzheimer's Association
https://www.alz.org
Offers information, a 24/7 helpline, support groups, and local chapter connections.

Alzheimer's Foundation of America (AFA)
https://www.alzfdn.org
Caregiver education, memory screening tools, and practical guidance.

Alzheimer's Disease Research Centers (ADRCs)
Including: Wisconsin ADRC—https://adrc.wisc.edu
Academic centers advancing dementia science and offering study opportunities.

Mayo Clinic—Dementia Center
https://www.mayoclinic.org
Authoritative, up-to-date medical summaries, patient education, and care options.

***Dementia Matters* Podcast**
Hosted by the Wisconsin ADRC—https://www.adrc.wisc.edu/dementia-matters
Accessible interviews with researchers, clinicians, and caregivers.

Lewy Body Dementia Association (LBDA)
https://www.lbda.org
Trusted source specific to Lewy body dementia, including patient stories and medical updates.

Frontotemporal Dementia (FTD) Disorders Registry and the Association for Frontotemporal Degeneration (AFTD)
https://www.theaftd.org
Dedicated to advancing research, awareness, and support for people living with FTD and their families.

National Library of Medicine—MedlinePlus
https://medlineplus.gov
Offers plain-language explanations of conditions, medications, and test results.

Family Caregiver Alliance (FCA)
https://www.caregiver.org
Offers legal, emotional, and practical support for caregivers of cognitively impaired adults.

Use your diary to also keep track of information you come across about Alzheimer's or aging—whether from newspapers, magazines, podcasts, or reliable websites. Besides building up your own base of knowledge, these materials can be valuable when speaking with your doctor or having conversations with other relatives. Whether you jot down notes or print out materials, I implore you to study normal versus abnormal aging. The more you learn, the better equipped you'll be. Become your own expert.

I'm not asking you or your family members to become clinicians. But it's helpful to take in the full picture—the dynamics of your loved one's life beyond the visible symptoms. Even the best doctors spend far less time with your loved one than you do. Time is limited in the clinic, often less than twenty minutes in primary care and about an hour in specialty care. That's not enough to capture the nuances of day-to-day life. In my clinic, families often tell me that their loved one "puts on a show." They summon their energy to present their best self, minimizing the symptoms. I've had families tell me how amazed they are to see how well their loved one performs in the exam room. I'm always appreciative of that effort—and I also understand that what I see may not reflect the fuller reality the family lives with every day.

Once you've read up on aging and cognitive health, you'll be better prepared for conversations with family members, doctors, or other caregivers. You can say, "Okay, well, this is what I found online, or in this book by Dr. Chin, or in the National Institute of Aging's newsletter. That's what these expert sources say. It's not just me saying these things." Credible information gives weight to your concerns and helps you feel more confident speaking up.

GETTING READY TO TALK

Now that you've been observing, documenting, and educating yourself, the next step is to gently widen the circle. You've been carrying the weight of concern quietly, but this burden is not meant to be shouldered alone. You don't need to have all the answers before involving others, but you do need enough clarity to communicate what you're seeing and why it matters. This is the time to think about who else should know, who can support you, and how to begin those first conversations, whether with a doctor, a family member, or a professional outside your immediate circle. You're not sounding an alarm; you're laying groundwork. And you're doing it with care.

When you bring this kind of material to a doctor's visit, it can make a real difference. From a clinician's perspective, the background knowledge is helpful. Despite the jokes about Dr. Google or ChatGPT being better than your doctor, most physicians appreciate proactive patients and families. It shows you're thoughtful and engaged—and that you've done your homework. It also helps your doctor more quickly grasp the situation and offer clearer next steps.

That said, I do offer a word of caution. Online searches can sometimes lead people to the most alarming or misleading information, which may increase anxiety and distract from what's actually useful. I encourage patients and families to start with trusted sources—those that are evidence based, scientifically sound, and person centered. See the resources section on page 64 for a list of these recommended sites.

When I say "going to see a doctor," I recognize that, in most cases, you won't be able to see your loved one's provider and deliver your concerns directly. Doctors generally won't meet with family members unless they are with the patient. That said, you can always talk to your own practitioner. And just as important, you should still call your loved one's doctor. Families do this all the time. In fact, in my experience, concerned calls from relatives are among the most common reasons a cognitive evaluation is triggered.

And remember—there are other medical experts available to you as well. I have found that many people are unaware of these incredibly valuable sources of wisdom and comfort. For example, in Wisconsin, every county has a Dementia Care Specialist, usually a social worker, who is employed by the local government. Your state or city probably has similar specialists who work for the local health department. A quick internet search for your Area Agency on Aging or a simple phone call to the county or city offices can lead you to them.

Plus—and this is a big one—organizations like the Alzheimer's Association or the Alzheimer's Foundation of America are ready and waiting to help. Both offer free hotlines staffed by trained professionals who've heard every kind of question before. When you call, you might say, "I'm observing this and that, and this, too. What do you think?" It's a safe, confidential way to get guidance without involving your loved one or anyone else just yet. You don't need to be ready to take a public step in order to reach out.

Yes, during this period of gathering information, you are in a sense putting on "a show" for other people and your loved one. You're engaging with them as usual while quietly observing and studying them in a new way. I know this can be a very difficult experience, an emotional roller coaster. Let me reassure you—you are doing the right thing. Your patience, dedication, and behind-the-scenes efforts are all powerful expressions of love.

The third step comes after you've done your research and educated yourself. Now it's time to talk to your core group, which might include your children, your siblings, and even a parent. You know best who belongs in that trusted inner circle.

As for how many people constitute (or make) a quorum, there's no fixed rule. Ideally, you want everyone who is essential to your loved one's care and future well-being—those who know them well, see them regularly, or play a role in caregiving or decision-making. Family often comes first, but close friends who feel like family may belong, too. What matters most is having the people who truly need to be part of the conversation gathered together, whether in person or virtually.

Here's the bottom line: You're going to need support. Ideally, you'll have *a team* behind you. Long term, you shouldn't do this alone. (See chapter 7 for more on the importance of caregiver support.) As flight attendants always insist, put on your own oxygen mask first. If you fail to take care of your vital needs first, you won't be able to care for someone with even greater ones—like an ailing parent.

Take a deep breath. Here at the outset, you don't know if the symptoms point to Alzheimer's. Still, the worry is already taking an emotional toll. You're not even living the life of a caregiver yet, but fear is consuming you. The whole time you're keeping your diary, your mind keeps spinning: *Is this Alzheimer's disease? What am I going to do? What does this mean for the family? Can this person still work? Can I leave her at home?* You might be jumping to conclusions, even though you know you shouldn't.

While planning your family meeting, you should still be trying to enjoy your time with this person you care about. You don't want them to feel ashamed or self-conscious about whatever's happening. You're doing your best not to confront them. You're trying not to say, "You just asked me that," or "Why are you misplacing these items?" or "I already told you this."

When you feel that impulse, take a step back. Remove yourself from the situation. Though easier said than done, prepare strategies in advance to help prevent frustration from spilling out. Try taking slow, deep breaths and counting them in your head. Or excuse yourself—say you need to use the bathroom—and find a quiet space to collect yourself.

If you can't walk away in the moment, try gently exploring the issue instead of answering or correcting them. Respond with, "Why are you asking, dear? Are you worried about something?" Or you might say, "Would it be helpful to have a place for your important items, so they're easier to find?"

I can't imagine what that's like on a frequent basis. I experienced these challenges with my father, but I didn't live with him. I wasn't his primary carer, so as frustrated as it may have made me to hear him retell a story, help him locate his wallet, or help him find a word, I only did this for hours at a time. You can see why there's such a true emotional toll on care partners. It doesn't begin with the diagnosis; it happens well *before* the diagnosis.

Empower yourself. First, keep a diary. Second, read up on Alzheimer's and how normal aging affects the brain. Third, seek expert advice. Just keeping a notebook of your observations—blended with authoritative insights you've gathered—can give you some emotional distance from your feelings. You'll feel steadier. You'll feel more confident. The result? You'll be better able to face the next day.

The Family Meeting—Nine Things to Remember

1. Write down specific behaviors or changes you've observed before talking to other family members or your loved one.
2. Learn about the earliest cognitive changes, and don't assume Alzheimer's is the cause.
3. Ask trusted friends or relatives if they've noticed anything concerning.
4. Step back from the symptoms and consider other possible life factors that could explain the cognitive changes.
5. Ask how your loved one is feeling and whether they've noticed any changes. Invite the conversation, but don't force it.
6. Decide who else should speak with your loved one.
7. Choose a safe, comfortable, and private space for the family conversation.
8. Focus on support. Help your loved one understand what may be happening. Share your research on other reversible causes of cognitive decline.
9. Schedule a professional evaluation to clarify the diagnosis, explore potential causes, and receive expert guidance.

THE SPIKES APPROACH

You're about to share difficult and painful information. It's perhaps one of the toughest conversations you'll ever have. Delivering emotionally charged news to family members about a loved one's potential decline is never easy. And it will be equally hard for them to hear and absorb it.

Doctors are trained to deliver bad news, but most approach it with quiet reluctance. Even with years of experience, it's never easy to sit across from someone and watch their world change with a few words. It remains a sobering responsibility—one that calls for clarity and compassion.

Over my years in practice, I've grown more confident in how I approach these conversations, but the weight of the moment never disappears. That's why I turn to structured communication models like SPIKES—a powerful guide that can help *anyone*, not just clinicians, navigate emotionally fraught conversations with greater confidence and grace.

You can do this, too, both in the first family meeting and later with your loved one. So, take a deep breath and carefully consider the SPIKES approach. SPIKES is a structured medical protocol for delivering difficult news with skill and sensitivity. It stands for Setting up, Perception, Invitation, Knowledge, Emotions with Empathy, and Strategy (or Summary). The model was developed by Dr. Walter Baile and colleagues at the MD Anderson Cancer Center in Houston, Texas. While originally intended for clinical settings, its principles are broadly applicable. A simplified version of SPIKES consists of these actions:

Set the scene thoughtfully. As noted earlier, hold the meeting at home and not in a public place. Choose a cozy, familiar room like the kitchen, den, or dining room—somewhere people are used to relaxing and enjoying time together. Turn off the television and try to minimize other distractions. If there are children in the family, consider arranging for them to visit friends or play elsewhere during the conversation. The time of day matters, too. Avoid holding the meeting late in the evening when people are tired or have had a drink.

Reflect on your loved ones' perception of the situation. Before diving into details, take a moment to consider what your family members already know—or think they know—about the situation. Respect their emotional bandwidth and avoid overwhelming them. Share only as much as you believe they can absorb. Keep the tone calm, grounded, and friendly, and steer clear of medical jargon that might confuse or distance them.

Know the medical facts and their implications. You don't want to come off as a know-it-all, but your research will have prepared you to share facts, offer context, and explain basic medical knowledge you've gained. This allows you to gently correct misinformation or address concerns that others may express. If someone says, "I think you might be right. Dad might have a problem, but nothing can be done," you can respond, "But it might not be Alzheimer's. It could be one of several other issues like X, Y, or Z that are reversible if treated. And even if it is Alzheimer's, there are interventions, including new medications, that can help slow its progression."

If you've spent months learning about Alzheimer's as if you were taking a college course, you might be tempted to share it all at once. Resist that urge. You're not here to impress anyone, and you don't want to swamp your family with too much technical detail. Stay grounded and speak with humility, especially when it's time to talk with the person you're most concerned about.

Be prepared for emotional reactions. Anger, sadness, weeping, and silence are all normal responses to bad news. Your posture, tone of voice, and demeanor can make a significant difference in how people react. Try to minimize any evidence of your nervousness. Sit rather than stand while speaking. Place both feet flat on the floor, ankles together, and rest your hands, palms down, on your lap or thighs. This grounded, neutral position can help calm you internally and also make you appear nonthreatening to others. A composed, steady presence will help your loved ones feel safer in processing whatever emotions arise.

Be empathetic. Many of us have relatives who know exactly how to "push our buttons." When that happens, pause. Choose to respond thoughtfully rather than reacting reflexively. You are delivering difficult news. Even if a particular sibling is not your favorite person, they are still human—and likely hurting just as you are. Some of the strongest reactions may come from those who live far away or haven't been closely involved. Try to find a place of compassion in your heart for those who are dismissive, angry, or confrontational. If someone insults you, let it go. It's not *you* they're upset with; it's the information you're sharing. Messengers who deliver bad news often absorb the impact of the message. Be strong, but also be kind.

TALKING WITH YOUR LOVED ONE

This second meeting is just as essential as the first—perhaps even more so. When you sit down with your loved one, the stakes can feel higher and the emotional weight heavier. It's also easier to get off track, so it's important to stay focused and be concise. As with the initial family meeting, your goal is to create a calm, unhurried atmosphere that fosters trust. Take your time. Make sure your loved one feels safe and supported. You're holding this meeting in a private, familiar setting, free from distractions—ideally their home, not a restaurant or other public place.

There's a lot at stake in meeting with your loved one. In some aspects, it resembles what's known as an intervention, the kind of meeting families convene to encourage someone with alcohol dependency to seek treatment. But this conversation is a softer, more compassionate version of that process. What do the two types of meetings have in common? You're initiating this meeting without the person's prior knowledge, and you're bringing up deeply personal concerns. This is not a confrontation. It's a caring, honest conversation about your observations and worries—grounded in love, not judgment.

You don't want to spring a meeting on anyone. It's much better to say something like "Our family is going to meet later today to talk about some changes we've noticed." This avoids the surprise factor, gives the person time to process the idea, and makes it less likely they'll walk out. And if they do, the moment may feel less traumatic or hurtful.

Keep in mind that no matter how carefully you prepare—or how skillfully you facilitate—the meeting can still go poorly. A negative experience could discourage your loved one from speaking with their doctor, delaying care. It may also trigger a spiral into depression or anxiety, or increase their resistance to seeking help. But don't let these possibilities paralyze you. The fact that you're putting in this effort shows your care and commitment. That alone can make a difference.

Bottom line: It's better to try and fall short than to not try at all. If the conversation doesn't go as hoped, give it time. Let the dust settle and try again in a week or a month or more down the road.

Remember, your goal is a positive outcome from this first meeting with your loved one. Rather than leading with "I think you have Alzheimer's," consider a broader, less alarming approach. Focus on other issues—for example, sleep apnea, medication side effects, and alcohol use—that can also affect memory and thinking. You may suggest, "*Why don't we go and get evaluated to see what else could be going on?*"

Avoid saying something like, "Let's rule these other factors out, because you probably have dementia." That kind of framing can leave your loved one thinking, "Well, let's get this terminal diagnosis and be done with it." Instead, focus on reversible causes and the goal of improving brain health. Remind them that, just like muscles, bones, and other internal organs, the brain can return to its more habitual working order with lifestyle interventions and the right support.

If the meeting goes well, your loved one may be willing to confront the reality that something isn't quite right. In fact, it's entirely possible they've already been sensing this themselves. Your loved one may have been thinking for some time, "I don't feel like myself." Many people in the earliest stages of Alzheimer's have these thoughts but keep them private. Hearing their family members and friends voice similar observations can be both painful and validating. It may stir up sadness and vulnerability, too. But with the right tone and support, this conversation can spark courage and resolve. Your loved one may say to themselves, "Well, here are my people. They care. I suppose I should figure this out. I just might feel better as a result."

Suggestions for How to Start the Meeting and What to Say When Tensions Rise

WAYS TO START THE FAMILY MEETING WITH THE PERSON WHO MAY HAVE ALZHEIMER'S

When opening this type of meeting, the primary goals should be:

- Creating safety and trust.
- Focusing on shared care and concern.
- Avoiding confrontation or surprise.

Here are potential ways to start the meeting:

A. Framing the Conversation in a Gentle, Collaborative Way
"We've all been noticing a few things lately, and we wanted to get together because we care about you so much. We just want to talk about how things are going and see how we can support you."

B. Empowering the Person
"We want to hear how you've been feeling and what you've noticed. Your perspective is really important to us."

C. Normalizing the Conversation
"It's natural for all of us, as we get older, to go through changes—sometimes in our bodies, sometimes in our memory. We just wanted to make sure we're all paying attention and thinking together about what's best moving forward."

D. Starting with Shared Stories
"We've been thinking a lot about how things have changed over the years—like how much Dad used to help with [a specific

example]—and we just wanted to talk about what's working well now and where we might need to adjust."

E. Framing the Conversation as a Health Check
"We've always made it a point to check in with each other about health stuff. We wanted to make sure we're doing that now, too—making sure we're all on the same page."

WHEN EMOTIONS RUN HIGH: PHRASES FOR DIFFICULT MOMENTS

When these meetings become emotionally charged, it's critical to:

- De-escalate the moment.
- Return to shared values.
- Acknowledge emotions without escalating.

Here are potential responses and strategies:

A. Acknowledging Emotions
"I can tell this is really upsetting. It's okay to feel that way. None of this is easy, and we're all just trying to figure it out together."

B. Redirecting to Shared Goals
"We all want the same thing here—to make sure everyone is safe, cared for, and heard. Let's try to focus on that."

C. Validating and Slowing Down
"You're right to feel strongly about this. Maybe we're moving too fast right now—let's slow down and really hear each other."

D. Disarming Defensiveness
"This isn't about blaming anyone. It's about understanding what's going on and how we can be the best support for each other."

E. Adjusting the Conversation If Accusations Start Flying

"Let's take a breath. I know everyone is worried, and that comes out in different ways. We're here because we love each other, even when it's hard to talk about these things."

F. Offering a Pause If Needed

"Maybe we can take a short break and come back to this. These are big feelings and it's okay to step away for a minute."

USE THESE RESPONSES AND STRATEGIES WHEN . . .

A. Denial Appears

- *"I understand this might be hard to see right now. It's okay if it feels confusing or surprising."*
- *"None of us are trying to label anything. We just want to talk about what's happening and how we can help."*
- *"We're not saying something is wrong—we're saying we've noticed some changes, and we care enough to check in."*

B. Anger Surfaces

- *"I can see this is upsetting, and that's completely understandable. This isn't easy for anyone."*
- *"Let's take a breath. I know this feels heavy and maybe even unfair, but we're coming from a place of love and concern."*
- *"We're not here to criticize or attack—only to make sure everyone feels supported and safe."*

C. Someone Shuts Down

- *"It seems like this might feel overwhelming. Do you want to take a break and come back to this later?"*
- *"This is a lot to talk about all at once. We can pause if you need some space."*

- *"Even if it's hard to talk right now, I want you to know we're here for you—whenever you're ready."*

D. Accusations Start or Blame Surfaces

- *"I know we all want what's best, even if it doesn't always come out the right way."*
- *"Let's remember we're on the same team—we all love each other."*
- *"This isn't about who's right or wrong—it's about taking care of each other."*

ADDITIONAL FRAMING TIPS

- Use "I" Statements: Keep ownership of observations and feelings
    - ◊ *"I've noticed it's been harder to . . ."*
    - ◊ *"I'm worried because . . ."*
- Avoid Absolutes: Skip words like *always* or *never*, which can escalate defensiveness.

SAMPLE FAMILY MEETING SCRIPTS

Script 1: Opening the First Family Meeting (Without the Person of Concern)
"Thank you all for coming together. I know this isn't an easy conversation, but I've been noticing some changes in Dad's memory and thinking. Mom has seen them, too, and we've been worried. I wanted to start this meeting so we can talk openly, share what we've each noticed, and think about what next steps make sense. I want us to work as a team so we can support each other—and especially Dad—as best we can."

Script 2: Opening the Family Meeting with the Person of Concern

"We wanted to get together today because we love you and we've all noticed some things we wanted to talk about. You're such an important part of this family, and we want to make sure we're supporting you and each other. We've noticed a few changes, and we just want to talk about what you've experienced and what would feel helpful moving forward."

Script 3: Responding to Defensiveness or Anger in the Meeting

"This is hard—I get that. It's hard for all of us, but especially for you. I want you to know we're not trying to tell you what to do or say that something is definitely wrong. We're here because we care about you and we want to figure this out together, at your pace."

Script 4: Pausing When Emotions Overwhelm

"Let's take a moment. I can feel how much this is bringing up for everyone. Maybe we can take a short break, and when we come back, we can talk about what feels most important to you right now."

FINAL TIPS

- Lead with love, not diagnosis.
- Focus on shared goals: safety, support, and connection.
- Use curiosity instead of correction.
- It's okay to pause or reschedule when emotions run too high.

We can never predict how someone will react to difficult news. What you share might make your loved one feel sad, and that's understandable. No one wants to cause pain—and that's natural, too. But it's important to remember that emotions, in and of themselves, are neither good nor bad. They're just part of being human. Sadness or discouragement may be temporary, and in some cases, those feelings are part of what unlocks the door to meaningful care and healing.

What percentage of the time does a family meeting end with a loved one remaining in denial or becoming angry? As far as I know, no formal research has been done on that question. In my opinion, if there's a less-than-ideal outcome, denial and anger are the most likely reactions.

Denial is a logical response. Expect it. It makes sense because many people simply aren't ready to hear what you have to say. Anger, on the other hand, is often how fear shows up. It's a natural emotional defense when someone feels shaken or exposed.

Even if a loved one remains in denial or reacts with anger, try to take it in stride. Don't beat yourself up about it. You've prepared deliberately, approached the conversation sincerely, and taken the courageous first step—for them. You've laid the cornerstone. Sometimes that's all that's needed for the next conversation to go a little better.

Don't mistake a hard reaction for failure. You'll never know if your loved one is ready until you gently break the ice. But if they are, they might be more open to scheduling a primary care visit, completing the cognitive tests, and moving forward with other evaluations.

Here's the way I look at it—it's better to prepare for a tough reaction and be pleasantly surprised if the conversation goes better than expected. If you get a bad reaction, take a step back and stay positive—they've certainly heard you!

The subject is now out in the open. Even if your loved one says you're wrong—or suggests something's wrong with you—the issue has been named, and in time, it will demand attention. That alone is a major hurdle cleared. One thing is certain: The days ahead will be emotional. Give your family, friends, and especially your loved one space to let the idea settle and to process what you've said.

I do not recommend doing what my sister and I did when our mother first shared her suspicions in that family meeting—try to test your loved one yourself. We invited our father—innocently, we thought—to play the numbers game sudoku with us. We shouldn't have done that. First, we weren't memory specialists skilled at administering cognitive assessments.

Second, sudoku, as challenging as it may be, is not a legitimate way to assess someone's thinking abilities. And third, we did it casually, at home, not in a professional setting. Worse still, we sprang it on our father without any real explanation—something I strongly advise against in clinic when working with concerned patients. Even if my father had aced the puzzle, it wouldn't have told us anything meaningful. I hate to admit it, but the fact that he did poorly almost certainly made him feel ashamed. And shame is the last emotion you want your loved one to experience.

I don't remember exactly how my father responded. I do recall asking him to try an easy version of sudoku and being shocked at how much he struggled to grasp its basic rules. I knew how intelligent he was. Seeing his puzzlement and frustration broke my heart. I had hoped to prove my mom wrong. Instead, with each passing minute of watching him falter, the truth sank in deeper and deeper. But whatever happens—and this is important—be present. You can't walk away. You can't turn your back on the loved one you're worried about and say, "Well, that reaction was awful. I'm outta here."

You still have to be present and say, "I'm not going to leave you. I'm not going to force you into anything. I'm here for you. I love you. Let me know what you want to do. I'm here to support you."

That reaffirms what the meeting was hopefully about: your concern, your care, and your love. You're hoping your loved one will earnestly take in what's been said and gradually become more open in the days ahead. It may take time for their initial reaction to soften—and that's okay. What matters is that when they are ready, you'll be there to help them down the path toward the right care—sooner rather than later.

Be clear about your intentions, but don't try to force them. At the same time, don't let yourself be pushed away. A steady presence matters—try saying, "I'm here. Let me know." It may take time. It could be months. But once the seed has been planted in the person's mind, it's not likely to disappear. And if a month passes with no progress, it's okay to tactfully bring it up again. In a conversation you might mention, "I've been doing this reading on such and such. I think this could be helpful." Or you could share with them positive steps you're taking to improve your brain health because you, too, want to stay sharp.

Keep at the forefront of the conversation the reminder that there are many reasons someone's cognitive abilities may change—and not all of them are permanent. Memory loss isn't always due to Alzheimer's. In my practice, I've seen striking improvements in people after stopping a medication that wasn't right for them, treating sleep apnea, or addressing another underlying medical issue.

One of the most meaningful and deeply gratifying moments in memory care is being able to tell someone, "Yes, there are cognitive changes. But I don't believe it's Alzheimer's. I believe it's your poorly controlled diabetes . . . or your depression . . . or your thyroid . . . or a vitamin deficiency." It's a reminder that with answers, improvement is often possible and within reach.

Sometimes when patients realize there's a path forward, they respond with surprise and relief: "Oh, really? I'm willing to come back every month for the next year if it means we can get to the bottom of this!"

In the same vein, on other occasions I've also said, "Let's revisit this in a year, once we've gotten your sleep apnea and depression under control." Then, after repeat cognitive testing, I'll have the privilege of showing them the positive change on a graph: "This is how low your score was before, and now it's up here, back into a normal range. That's because of all your efforts."

Suddenly, they're asking, "So I don't need to see you anymore?"

And my response is, "You could still develop Alzheimer's or Parkinson's in the future—so I may see you again one day. But right now, you're doing great. You don't need to schedule another visit. Congratulations!"

Those are gratifying moments. They may not be the most common outcome, but they happen often enough to offer real hope—especially when someone receives the right medical attention.

Even if your loved one is ultimately diagnosed with Alzheimer's, there is a silver lining. You got a head start. You took early action. Years ago, that might not have made a difference. Today, it does. We now know more about what individuals can do—and what medicine can offer—to help keep the brain healthier for longer and slow the disease's progression. That means the parts you may be fearing most—like the later stages of dementia and possible nursing home placement—can potentially be pushed further into the future. Because of your timely steps, your loved one's medical team now has more time and tools to make a difference.

Finally, keep this in mind—people tend to respond well to a positive approach. One of the reasons I chose to be a geriatrician is that I genuinely enjoy working with older adults. They're often more resilient than younger folks. Tell a twenty-year-old they can't have the corner office on their first day of work or that their vacation request wasn't approved, and there's a decent chance they'll throw a fit and vent about it on social media. Many young people simply haven't yet been tested by life's harder trials.

But someone between fifty-five and eighty-five years old? They've already weathered their fair share of storms. They know what life can throw at them. Their response is more likely to be, "Okay, let's move forward. What can I do? What can you do? What can we do together?"

That's the goal—to work together successfully. Plan ahead so that you, your loved one, and their care team can—united—chart the best course forward.

3

"What Are You Testing Me For?"

HOW TO NAVIGATE THE MEDICAL EVALUATION

Behind-the-Scenes Precharting • Should I See a Geriatrician or Neurologist? • Meet the Doctor's Team—the Neuropsychologist and Social Worker • What the Neuropsychologist Does • The Social Worker's Key Role • Delivering the Diagnosis—and Action Plan

A complete memory evaluation is unlike any other doctor's appointment. This unique visit centers on how you think. We'll test your cognitive and day-to-day abilities for impairment. We'll analyze your mood, personality, lifestyle, and health conditions to assess their potential impact on your symptoms. The goal is to determine if you have Alzheimer's disease or another cause of cognitive impairment.

Most medical appointments are between you and a single provider. A memory evaluation requires a team approach, which may include a bench of experts: a geriatrician or neurologist, a neuropsychologist, a social worker. We also request the involvement of a collateral historian—someone the patient trusts and who knows them well enough to provide accurate information about their history and symptoms. For the purposes of this chapter, I'll refer to this individual (or group) as *family*, though they may be close friends, neighbors, case managers, or members of a faith community.

While the memory evaluation will include cognitive tests and a neurological physical exam, it is geared toward a series of group dialogues with abundant back-and-forth discussion among all parties. Unfortunately, by the time these tests, evaluations, and meetings are over, it's been an exhausting two to four hours. (My staff tells patients and families to bring snacks.) Some medical practices split the evaluation over a number of days. It's helpful to ask the clinic what timeline to expect—whether the evaluation happens in one long visit or over several appointments. If multiple visits are necessary, find out how they're scheduled, which specialties are involved, what each visit is meant to accomplish, how much time typically passes between them, and when to expect a diagnosis and care plan. Regardless of how it's done, a patient and loved ones should leave reassured that they will be well cared for and that the team has established a path forward.

A dementia diagnosis requires hours of expertise from various specialists working together. It may not take a village, but it does take a team. (Remember from chapter 1 that *dementia* is an umbrella term that covers six specific diseases, and only one of them is Alzheimer's.) Most primary care doctors would have a hard time providing this concentrated, in-depth assessment. They often don't know the intricate differences between normal and abnormal aging. The diagnosis requires sifting through many nuances of human behavior. My team and I ask dozens of detailed questions that have, through training and experience with patients, proven to produce reliable answers. Unlike a family doctor, we administer these evaluations every day.

Here is a situation a family doctor might misinterpret. A few years ago, Enid, an eighty-two-year-old woman with four children, came for an evaluation after experiencing what she described as "forgetfulness." Marjorie, one of Enid's children who accompanied her mother to the appointment, told us that Enid was a wonderful chef and had recently stopped cooking. Her mother didn't want to touch a pot or pan, much less wash dishes. Surely there must be something wrong, Marjorie thought, especially since Mom got so grumpy and taciturn whenever the subject of meals came up.

When the neuropsychologist asked Enid in private what was happening, she said, "I don't want to cook anymore. I'm eighty-two, for gosh sakes. I spent my whole life cooking for a family of ungrateful children." That's not an impairment. That's a choice. You must get into those details because Enid would never have admitted such hurtful thoughts in her daughter's presence. The implication of such details is what my team interprets—and at times debates—before making a diagnosis.

My goal is to demystify what happens in these meetings. So, this chapter explores the preplanning (known as precharting) that a geriatrician or neurologist performs before a patient visit, the questions a social worker asks, how a neuropsychologist administers a cognitive evaluation, how we discuss our findings and reach conclusions, and what happens when the doctor meets the patient and his family or loved ones.

NOT ALL STRESS IS THE SAME

Doctors want patients to have the best possible outcomes. It's in our DNA. For me, the work I'm doing in Alzheimer's is literally in my DNA. My dad was the medical director of a rural nursing home that had a dementia unit. When I joined him on weekends, I witnessed how even the most confused and agitated patients would calm down when my dad reached for and held their hands. Such was his gentle touch and nature. My dad's Alzheimer's is also a part of my DNA. I am aware that in the future I, too, may have my hand held in the same way.

Memory clinic patients have more in common than cognitive change. They're stressed, and so are their families. The medical professionals in our field understand that patients who come to us are overwhelmed, and these feelings influence the history they provide and their ability to take cognitive tests.

All stress is not created equal. There is good stress, called *eustress*, like the jitters you feel when preparing for a big trip or exam. Then there is bad stress, which is emotional distress. It's the kind that goes on and on and on. It makes you feel helpless. Like a hamster running on a wheel in a cage, you're trapped in an endless loop. Suffering in a job you hate or seething in traffic can make you physically ill. No wonder humorist Erma Bombeck wrote in one of her syndicated newspaper columns: "Worry is like a rocking chair. It gives you something to do but never gets you anywhere."

By the time a patient comes to my memory clinic, she can be at her wit's end, worn down by the treadmill of anxiety. It's not unusual for families to have spent years obsessing about a loved one's failures and bickering about what to do. As for the patient herself, she has carried an extra burden, ruminating about the meaning and possible causes of her mysterious, intermittent symptoms. In addition to her confusion and fear, she has family and friends offering well-intentioned unsolicited advice.

My goal when patients and families come for a thorough memory evaluation is twofold. I want them to leave with a diagnosis, even if it is not what they want to hear. Knowing the cause of cognitive decline is essential and enables people to move on to the next step in treatment options. After all, Alzheimer's, despite recent advances, remains a terminal illness. But I find that after people meet with me, they almost always, surprisingly, feel relieved.

A POSITIVE WAY FORWARD

That's where my second goal comes in: to give people hope. Once a patient has an answer, they can make plans. Now they can act. I've given them the key to unlock the cage of worry that kept them trapped. After all, the sunlight of knowledge is better than the gloom of fear and doubt.

It's my job to be a truth teller, someone who's going to be honest and explain the diagnosis without equivocating. While I make clear that Alzheimer's is progressive and terminal, I also tell patients—and families—that they can still live a meaningful life, one filled with rich experiences. Today, more than at any other time in history, there is reason for hope because we now have targeted medications that can slow Alzheimer's. It is easier for doctors to inject positivity when they can prescribe a novel drug.

Patients and families often end up smiling and laughing before they leave my office, even though I gave them a dementia diagnosis an hour earlier. Despite the news I bring, I tap into what is meaningful to them. I remind them to cherish what they enjoy, whether it's spending time with grandchildren, playing the ukulele, or watching hummingbirds flitter outside the kitchen window. Giving patients and their families the confidence to live fully, engage with the world, and enjoy the time they have can be therapeutic. Instead of dwelling on a terminal diagnosis, I focus on creating a positive way forward. That's what hope does.

There is always reason to hope, if not for a cure, then for peace of mind. The obstacles ahead are daunting, but with help from your network of healthcare providers, you will no longer be alone. That's one of the reasons dementia organizations have walks and community events. When you gather with others whose situation is like yours, mutual experiences and acceptance, regardless of the outcome, are reassuring.

My dad was in a wheelchair the year I hosted the Alzheimer's Walk in Madison. I could have felt crushed at the sight of the once vibrant man now being pushed by his wife along the designated event route. Instead, my smile mirrored his as we proudly joined others working toward a cure and treatment. Living in the moment does not come easily, but it can change even the toughest of times into something meaningful and unexpected.

GERIATRICIANS VERSUS NEUROLOGISTS: IS THERE A DIFFERENCE?

A memory clinic appointment is usually scheduled following a referral. To make the best use of limited time, prescreening is essential. Patients and families need to be well rested and prepared for what will be a lengthy and tiring day of cognitive testing and discussion. Occasionally, our clinic arranges consultations rather than full memory evaluations. Cognitive testing, a key part of a memory evaluation, is arduous and at times demoralizing. (I've taken these assessments myself and have become frustrated and even panicked, too.) But without these results, a team can't make a definitive diagnosis. Family members often initiate a consultation after struggling to convince their loved one a problem exists.

We educate patients and families about potential causes, modifiable factors, treatment options, and brain health. Most patients return later for the complete series of tests with my neuropsychologist.

In metropolitan areas, consultations with specialists are relatively easy to obtain. In rural settings, primary care doctors, such as those in family and internal medicine, usually do the first screening. The quality of these screenings can vary based on the provider's training, comfort level, and practice style. Family medicine doctors care for the entire family from birth (delivering babies) to death. They have broad knowledge of conditions affecting all age groups. General internists focus on adult health, with expertise in internal organ systems and complex chronic conditions. Both are well equipped to conduct cognitive screenings, especially if they've cared for the patient for years.

Memory specialists, commonly neurologists, geriatricians, or geriatric psychiatrists, utilize their own techniques in conducting the evaluation. Whereas neurologists and geriatricians may be intimately involved in the diagnostic process, geriatric psychiatrists are more focused on addressing the mood and behavioral changes that occur later in the disease. Each specialist has valuable expertise. Some memory specialists, like me, work with a team that evaluates patients together in what's called a memory clinic. Others may see you on their own and will make referrals for cognitive testing later. I'll describe more about the memory clinic approach below, but first, let's address the difference between a neurologist and a geriatrician.

Geriatricians and neurologists are both medical doctors who completed four years of medical school after college. Neurology residents work alongside internists in their first year of training but focus on the brain for the next three years. They learn to diagnose, treat, and manage disorders of the brain and nervous system for all adults aged eighteen and older. Some pursue fellowships and additional specialized training, then focus on conditions such as Alzheimer's and memory disorders. Many others specialize in strokes or multiple sclerosis.

Geriatricians undertake a residency in internal medicine or family medicine, followed by one to three years of fellowship. Geriatricians see patients over sixty-four and are experts in the field of aging, multimorbidity (having more than one chronic health condition), polypharmacy (the management of multiple prescriptions to prevent unwanted interactions), frailty, falling, and cognitive change. They understand how the whole body works in the context of getting older. They usually lead interdisciplinary teams whose members are social workers, nurses, physical therapists, occupational therapists, speech therapists, and others. Most geriatricians provide primary care, but some specialize in fall prevention, hospital or preoperative care, nursing home care, hospice care, and memory care.

I trained in geriatrics, spending a dedicated year working with neurologists and geriatricians in the UW memory program. I was thirty-three years old when I became a full-fledged "memory doctor," after twenty-five years of formal education. I'm proud to work at the Wisconsin Alzheimer's Disease Research Center, one of only thirty-six such institutions in the United States, and the only one led by geriatricians. While the research program doesn't provide clinical care, it is closely associated with the University of Wisconsin's memory clinics. That's where I see patients.

There is, unfortunately, a bias in American medicine that favors neurologists for treating Alzheimer's patients. This is largely due to neurologists' historical involvement in memory evaluations and their specialized focus on brain disorders. However, both neurologists and geriatricians are qualified to assess cognitive complaints. Proceeding with a referral to either specialist is a sound decision. And while not all neurologists and geriatricians have specialized training in memory disorders, they can investigate your symptoms. If possible, your doctor should refer you to a team-based memory clinic to evaluate for Alzheimer's, Lewy body, and other neurodegenerative diseases. Bottom line: Ask the specialist to whom you've been referred to tell you about their background.

PRECHARTING: BEFORE THE PATIENT AND FAMILY VISIT

A new patient, let's call him Jack, has been scheduled for an appointment. Whether your physician is a geriatrician or a neurologist, he or she will go through a process resembling the hypothetical visit presented here.

First, the doctor allocates as much as an hour to review Jack's medical history, the process called precharting. Electronic recordkeeping greatly simplifies sifting through hundreds of archival records. I focus on recent events before Jack's visit, without dismissing the previous decades. I want to concentrate on what prompted the referral. Any doctor will tell you that electronic medical records are a luxury and a curse. No one could study everything in the hundreds of electronic pages, but the computer does make it easier to sift through years of files.

I open a blank note called the "New Assessment Template," which is where I start to record Jack's pertinent details. First, I take note of his age. Why? The older Jack is, the stronger the probability that he has Alzheimer's, vascular disease, or both. Comorbid conditions get a close look. The word *comorbid* sounds scary, but it simply refers to two or more medical diseases that tend to occur together. People with high blood pressure will often have irregular cholesterol panels, too. They aren't necessarily life-threatening. They're just ongoing. Many people sixty-five and older have at least one chronic health condition.

Medical progress never ceases to amaze me. People in their eighties routinely undergo hip replacement surgery with very high success rates. Seniors ranging from Mick Jagger to First Lady Barbara Bush and fitness guru Jack LaLanne all underwent heart valve replacement surgery (in LaLanne's case when he was ninety-five) and continued to live satisfying and active lives. So, it is rare indeed for an older person, even one in seemingly impeccable health, to have no medical issues.

Older patients can live with an average of five to ten comorbidities. Some present with (that's medical lingo for "have" or "appear before me with") as many as fifteen. These can include cardiovascular diseases such as high blood pressure, high cholesterol, diabetes, and heart disease; autoimmune conditions; gastrointestinal issues; vitamin deficiencies; neurological complaints; chronic pain syndromes; glaucoma; osteoporosis; and mental health issues such as depression and anxiety.

Why such a focus on chronic health issues after noting the age of my patient Jack? The presence of high blood pressure, diabetes or prediabetes, obesity, and high cholesterol points doctors in the direction of Alzheimer's or cerebrovascular disease (narrowing of the small blood vessels in the brain). Thyroid issues, mood disorders, chronic pain, and sleep issues such as insomnia, sleep apnea, and restless leg syndrome can all mimic forms of dementia. Fortunately, those chronic conditions can be alleviated, if not reversed.

Jack's daily medications are next on the agenda. Some drugs contribute to cognitive change, especially ones that affect a person's sleep, mood, and mentation (mental activity). If Jack has fifteen health problems, you can be sure he takes multiple prescriptions, over-the-counter drugs, and supplements. Medications that seem benign and cause few side effects in healthy adults can create disturbing symptoms in people with cognitive impairment. Depending on the drug itself—or how it interacts with other medications—there can be serious, even life-threatening complications. Among the most likely suspects are drugs with anticholinergic properties that remove choline from the brain. Choline is neither a vitamin nor a mineral. It's an essential nutrient, a substance that enables communication between brain cells for sufficient memory and attention span.

It turns out that Jack regularly takes an antihistamine. Over-the-counter drugs with anticholinergic properties include many allergy, cold, and sleep preparations, some with the abbreviation PM after the brand name. This term can be misleading. Most of the time it indicates the presence of the ingredient diphenhydramine, commonly known as Benadryl, but it can also mean that a person should only take the drug *post meridiem*, a Latin phrase that means from midday to midnight. For me, the term *PM* is a glaring red flag. Diphenhydramine removes choline from the brain. That's why taking something with PM in its name makes you feel subdued. It suppresses the ability to pay attention. Not surprisingly, that lack of choline could lead to confusion and falls. Studies have linked routine consumption of diphenhydramine (either by itself or in another drug) to an increased risk of cognitive impairment, which might be irreversible.

I see that Jack was prescribed a scopolamine patch because of dizzy spells. This is another red flag. Scopolamine can interact with Benadryl to cause confusion and memory problems. Jack also takes a daily supplement—an herbal medication for "brain health." I sigh. This tells me he has been worried long enough about his memory to seek out nonprescribed "treatment." I make a note of this supplement and will address it, along with the prescription medications, when I speak to Jack. Any supplement that promises to promote "brain health" is misleading the consumer. Companies that make false promises about stimulating brain vitality or reversing Alzheimer's are distorting the truth and providing false hope. Such supplements are not only a waste of money but can also make people's conditions worse by delaying legitimate medical treatment or interacting negatively with other prescribed medications.

But what about supplements in general? The medical community's stance on supplements goes like this: They haven't been studied rigorously to show that they are beneficial. That doesn't mean they are not helpful. It means evidence has *yet to be found* that they are helpful. I sprinkle turmeric in my coffee because its active ingredient curcumin is an anti-inflammatory. So if a patient comes to me and says, "I want to take vitamin D . . . or fish oil . . . or vitamin B complex . . . or turmeric," my response is, "Let's be certain it doesn't interact with your prescriptions, and let's also verify your brand has undergone third-party testing to ensure its purity."

Supplements—Should I Take Them?

Tech entrepreneur Bryan Johnson has become widely known for his intense efforts to slow aging and extend his lifespan. A former Silicon Valley CEO who sold his company to PayPal, Johnson now dedicates his life—and a significant portion of his wealth—to optimizing his biology with the goal of living to age 150. His daily routine includes strict dietary control, rigorous exercise, intensive cancer screening, and taking more than one hundred supplements. These range from common options like zinc, iron, and vitamin C to lesser-known ones such as fisetin (an antioxidant), ubiquinol (for heart health and cancer prevention), and hyaluronic acid (for skin hydration). His longevity quest is the focus of the

Netflix documentary *Don't Die: The Man Who Wants to Live Forever.*

Less-well-heeled people take lots of supplements, too. At the University of Wisconsin–Madison, where I work and teach, I oversee the long-running Wisconsin Registry for Alzheimer's Prevention study, which includes many participants whose parents had Alzheimer's. Many of them take scads of supplements, in some cases up to thirty a day, all in an effort to stave off Alzheimer's and lead longer, healthier lives.

Sometimes my head spins when I think of all the daily pills they take. It sounds crazy, but I can relate. When my dad was first diagnosed, I started taking at least fifteen supplements—turmeric, resveratrol, coffee bean extract, and even broccoli sprout extract—all in a Hail Mary effort to help prevent Alzheimer's. It wasn't rational, but that's what the fear of this disease can do to a family member—even to physicians who work in the field. I was desperate to help my father and, by extension, to stay healthy myself. I hunted the internet and found random information about this one small study in mice or another tiny study of twenty people that supposedly led to a lower risk of Alzheimer's. While I wasn't willing to experiment on my dad, I was for myself—for a short while.

You cling to hope, as Emily Dickinson wrote, "the thing with feathers that perches in the soul—and sings the tunes without the words—and never stops at all." Science is slow, but hope can be constant. People want something *now*, and don't feel they have the time to wait five to seven years for the results of a clinical trial. If the scientific community can't provide them with more options than three to four prescriptions, then it will have to be supplements that loft them to a brighter, sunnier place.

There is, however, a difference between a popular supplement like Prevagen, which has been proven not to work, and others that might make biological, rational sense, like vitamin D, B complex, turmeric, or fish oil. Will any of them stop or prevent Alzheimer's? No, at least so far as anyone knows. But if you're willing to pay for them, they don't interfere with prescription medications, and they don't otherwise harm you, it's up to you.

I never discourage my patients from discussing supplements with me. I want them to be comfortable and honest with me, without feeling embarrassed about what they're considering—because I've been there myself. In fact, I still take six or seven supplements, knowing that the age range from thirty to sixty is a critical window for someone at higher risk for Alzheimer's. The disease's silent, asymptomatic phase can last more than a decade. While definitive proof that supplements prevent Alzheimer's is lacking, similar evidence is missing from clinical trials. Until such data emerges, I'm willing to take the chance that they might help, and at the very least, do no harm.

If you want to take supplements, be sure they are high quality. Read their labels to see if they have been third-party tested. Only take those that are pure, pesticide free, and, ideally, organic.

Taking supplements in a targeted way—specifically to correct documented deficiencies—is a different matter entirely. Deficiencies in B vitamins, particularly B_1 (thiamine), B_6 (pyridoxine), B_9 (folate), and B_{12} (cobalamin), as well as vitamin D, have been linked in studies to cognitive impairments. If lab work confirms that any of these levels are low, then supplementing becomes important, and the dose may need to go beyond what's typically found in a multivitamin to truly correct the deficiency. Still, multivitamins themselves may offer benefit. A Harvard study showed that daily multivitamin use was associated with improved memory performance in older adults, suggesting they may play a modest but helpful role in cognitive health even in the absence of deficiency.

After reviewing Jack's medical history for chronic health issues and medications, the next step is to see if he has a healthcare power of attorney and financial power of attorney. (More on those legal matters in chapter 4.)

SHARING SCANS

Next, any doctor will want to know if Jack has had a brain scan. About half the time, people who see me have either had an MRI (magnetic resonance imaging) or a CT (computed tomography) scan. The question is, when was the scan done? If it was ten years earlier and symptoms started two years ago, that decade-old scan won't identify current problems—though it's still useful to know that an image was done and appeared normal at the time, without structural changes suggestive of brain disease. An image of Jack's brain while he is symptomatic is warranted. I prefer to review an MRI because it gives a detailed view of the brain's structure and vasculature (its blood vessels and how they are arranged), but a CT scan has value, too. If neither has been done, it's likely a neurologist or geriatrician will order an MRI unless it's unobtainable due to a pacemaker or another contraindication (a reason for not having a treatment because it might be harmful).

It turns out that Jack had had a brain scan—an MRI. Why did a doctor order it? Was it because Jack had recurring headaches, or was it due to memory loss? What did the radiologist see? A radiologist usually looks for strokes, brain masses, swelling, bleeding, and the brain's size, as well as for vascular irregularities. Unfortunately, radiologists are unable to read every scan completely. There are too many potential abnormalities to look for. They have many scans to read each day, so most triage each scan by answering the clinical question being asked by the ordering provider. It so happens that Jack had headaches, and his doctor hoped a scan might reveal their cause. In his case, it didn't.

Making the correct diagnosis is all about removing uncertainty. One of the heroes of modern medicine is William Osler, a nineteenth-century Canadian physician who revolutionized the way doctors are educated and how they evaluate patients. "Medicine," he said, "is a science of uncertainty and an art of probability." He wasn't denying the value of certainty, only acknowledging that medicine is rarely absolute. In practice, the aim is to shrink the unknowns, to bring enough clarity to guide the right decisions.

Improving the probability of a correct diagnosis is what precharting is all about. That's why I'll personally review the scan before I meet Jack. First, I want to see how blood vessels in his brain look. When a brain gets insufficient oxygen, it causes white matter hyperintensities (lesions that appear bright white over the gray-looking brain tissue), which is damage to the brain caused by reduced blood flow. Such hyperintensities can support a diagnosis of cerebrovascular disease. Some of these lesions are normal in older people, but after you've seen countless MRIs, it becomes easier to distinguish between the appearance of a healthy brain and one that lacks robust blood flow.

Next, I'll study the size of Jack's hippocampus, the seahorse-shaped, paperclip-sized memory center deep in his brain. A smaller-than-normal appearance supports an Alzheimer's diagnosis. That's because the disease attacks this vital part of the brain's memory storage system. As with many aspects of an Alzheimer's diagnosis, hippocampal atrophy suggests the presence of Alzheimer's but is not a definitive sign. Jack's past and present histories are on display in this three-dimensional image, and it is my job to interpret what it means for his future.

After looking at the scan, I scour Jack's medical record for more information. Viewing the notes from prior visits is like reading his biography. One of the fascinating aspects about being a doctor is that every patient is unique. I get the same joy from exploring my patients' medical lives as a history buff gets from relishing books about ancient Rome or Abraham Lincoln.

BLOOD WORK, SOCIAL HISTORY, AND "DR. SHERLOCK HOLMES"

Blood work gets analyzed next. Has Jack recently had a basic metabolic panel done? That's the standard blood test a doctor orders during a checkup. The panel looks at eight substances in the blood: glucose, calcium, sodium, potassium, carbon dioxide, chloride, and the waste products creatinine and blood urea nitrogen (BUN) that kidneys remove from the blood. I zero in on his liver function, noting inflammation or failure. I look at Jack's blood count—the number of his white and red blood cells and platelets. This will reveal if he is anemic and, if so, whether he's acutely anemic (due to something that suddenly came on) or chronically so. The size of Jack's blood cells could indicate a blood disorder or an as yet unidentified medical disorder. If his MCV (mean corpuscular volume) is greater than one hundred, it might hint at a folate or vitamin B_{12} deficiency. When no explanation is present, it could mean Jack drinks more than he says he does, and chronic overconsumption of alcohol is bad for the brain. Lots of people drink. Unfortunately, too many of those people drink to excess.

Chronic overconsumption of alcohol can cause neurological problems. In retirement some people drink too much because there are fewer demands on their time. They might imbibe because they have taken comfort from studies that show the health benefits from a daily glass of red wine. But more recent findings cast doubt on that theory. While drinking can spark social levity, which is beneficial, alcohol is, in fact, a toxin—a poison.

Twelve percent of seniors binge drink, defined as three or more drinks at a time, according to a recent National Survey on Drug Use and Health. Heavy drinking by seniors is particularly dangerous because older livers process alcohol more slowly, and since older people are more likely to take medications, there's a heightened risk of adverse drug interactions because alcohol impedes the liver's ability to process medications. What's more, drinking every day for decades has a negative impact on the brain. If you are going to drink, whether you are young or old, have only one and don't do so every day.

Now I'm deep in Jack's history. There are more details I want to explore. Put a good geriatrician up against Columbo or Nancy Drew, and he would more than hold his own in any battle of detective wits. My job is to think deeply and view facts with a dispassionate eye. I may not always have a treatment for the causes of someone's cognitive decline, but finding its likely origin can provide some peace of mind and may lead to a more definitive diagnosis.

The rest of Jack's lab results show normal levels of vitamins B_1, B_6, B_{12}, D, and folate, but the amount of the amino acid homocysteine in his blood sample is interesting and could reflect the presence of vascular disease. Smaller blood vessels in the brain are detrimental for brain health. Jack's family history of vascular disease and heart attacks provides important clues, given their impact on the brain. A prior history of cancer is similarly noteworthy because chemotherapy and radiation can cause months of foggy thinking ("chemo brain"), which can be mistaken for Alzheimer's.

All these factors could affect cognition. I'm glad Jack already had the blood work and MRI scan. Today we can concentrate on exploring the meaning and significance of the results.

A different geriatrician or neurologist might see if Jack had other tests, including an electroencephalogram to assess patterns of electrical impulses in his brain. Alzheimer's patients typically have fewer complex signals. Another exam might be a carotid ultrasound, which determines how well blood flows up the neck to the brain. Both are reasonable to order, if the circumstances warrant it.

I use my computer's search function, typing in terms like *memory*, *cognition*, *dementia*, and *mini mental exam*, because for most people who see me, their doctors or other caregivers have utilized one or more of those terms in prior clinic visits. The word *memory* alone usually brings up most of the history I need to review. It's an extensive list of records, including telephone encounters, blood work, and imaging, provided by clinicians who have seen Jack along the way. Comments made about Jack's functional abilities also have value. Has anyone expressed doubts about his safety? Now I input phrases like *safety concern*, *functional impairment*, and *not able to drive*. This brings up comments from occupational and physical therapists.

Let's see . . . what else does the computer record tell me about Jack? A note says eight years ago his wife, Kelsey, expressed worry about his memory. Hmm. That is a long time to wait before something is done. She might be unusually observant, and that's something to keep in mind when we meet. I tap Enter whenever the word *memory* pops up. The further back I go, the more I see comments that state "No memory issues." This gives me license to spend less time reviewing those years.

Ultimately, I want to know what led to Jack's referral. Over the past few years, notes about "memory loss" and "memory concerns" appear with regrettable regularity. Following those are referrals to neurology and geriatrics for unexplained confusion. Eighteen months ago, his primary care doctor noticed Jack's repetitive questioning and difficulty finding the right words. Wait . . . there's an emergency room visit ten months ago. The ER doctor remarked on Jack's poor understanding of his medications—something no one else observed. Six months ago, a social worker made an entry regarding the family's concern about Jack being left home alone—worries they had shared with his primary care provider, who then connected them to the social worker. A physical therapist chimed in just last month that Jack was unable to follow multistep directions.

As I pore over these details, I write in my electronic note: "Four years ago, this symptom was reported . . ." "Two years ago, this memory concern was stated . . ." On my timeline of Jack's history, I write the initial symptom reported, when it started, what else happened around that time, and what Jack's course has been since then. I ask myself, *Has his condition been progressive, stable, better, or fluctuating?*

Let's turn to what the record says about Jack's social history. Is he married, divorced, or widowed? How many children does he have? Do they live nearby? Are they supportive? Does Jack have hired help like a yard service, meal service, or in-home care? What is his level of education—does he have less than a high school degree? Has he attended technical college? Does he have a college or an advanced degree? A PhD, MBA, JD, MD, or degree from a trade school likely means the person experienced lifelong mental stimulation. A career that demands postbachelor education can increase neural networks and provide more resilience against dementia, which slashes like a scythe through synapse connections.

Knowing Jack's schooling helps establish a reference point for his cognitive abilities. The neuropsychologist will delve into this history because it will help her interpret the tests she gives him. Cognitive testing is critical in the evaluation, but even these standardized tests are imperfect and subject to bias. (See the sidebar "A Word of Caution About Cognitive Tests," page 117, for more details.)

What was Jack's vocation? When did he retire and why? Education is important, but so is the work we do throughout life. Both may have an impact on our brain health and resilience to disease. People who've had more education or worked in certain professions may have healthier lifestyles, or they may have formed more neural networks. Or both could be true—no one knows for sure.

I'm ever more curious about Jack. Does he live in a house? How many levels? How many stairs? Did he need to move to a condo for some reason? Who lives with him? If an adult child is living at home, I try to understand the dynamics. Is their presence a source of stress for the patient and spouse? Or did they move back in to offer help? Not all this information will be in his records. The social worker will collect it, but I feel like Sherlock Holmes on the hunt for clues.

The last part of the social history focuses on substance use and abuse. How much Jack drinks, whether he smokes, and what types of recreational drugs he has used throughout his life matter in the evaluation. Like medications, any of these substances could have unforeseen consequences on the brain. People are surprisingly honest about their use of such drugs, like marijuana, but less so about their quantities of consumption. The amount of drinking or drug use a patient reports and what his family says are often different. A patient might admit to having three or maybe four drinks a week, but his family might say, "Oh, no, it's ten a week. Sometimes three a day!" In general, when doctors ask patients about their use of alcohol, we might double—or even triple—the answer we hear.

Moving on in Jack's digital chart, I scroll to see his family history. Did a parent have dementia or Alzheimer's disease? I don't trust such records 100 percent of the time because people can report whatever they want, and medical providers don't usually investigate the difference between Alzheimer's and dementia. But I do want to know what's been reported. That helps gauge a family's level of anxiety or their preconceived ideas before coming to the clinic.

I click Save. My notes are prepped and will load on the networked computer in the room where Jack and his family meet me.

This is my standard precharting practice before a memory evaluation; other physicians may do it differently. Though our processes vary, what we get out of precharting tends to align. By the time I see Jack, I'll know more about him than he might imagine. In some respects, I know Jack better than he knows himself, and our in-person memory evaluation has yet to begin.

ONE VISIT, ONE DIAGNOSIS

If everything is on schedule at the memory clinic, Jack and his family will spend only a few minutes in the waiting room. Jack will go to meet with the neuropsychologist, and his relatives and/or friends will sit separately with our social worker.

Why are these meetings—and then the session with me—conducted in one visit? Why not spread them over a few days or weeks? My program developed this model to reduce burdens and barriers in getting a complete and timely evaluation. If Jack lives hours from a doctor's office, he shouldn't be asked to drive there three times to get a diagnosis he's been worrying about for months or years. My practice is housed in a major university's medical center and treats patients from all over Wisconsin. Few rural areas have such specialized treatment centers.

The clinical program in San Diego where I trained arranged separate visits. The history and physical, also called an H&P, were performed in one visit, followed by a cognitive testing session at a later date with the neuropsychologist. In the final visit, the patient learned the diagnosis and treatment plan. My all-at-once approach is atypical, but I believe there's value in committing to one extended visit and departing with the diagnosis. On the flip side, three hours of talking and testing can tire people out. Patients and families start grumbling among themselves, "Let's get out of here. We're done." Most of the time, though, people are happy with this one-stop diagnosing experience. A practice does have to coordinate a team of people to make such a system work, and we do.

RESPONDING TO THE SOCIAL WORKER: YOU GET OUT WHAT YOU PUT IN

Now the family sits around a table in a private room with our social worker. The term *social worker* can be misunderstood, sometimes conveying a stigma that makes families feel judged or as if something has gone terribly wrong. To some it conjures up images of abandoned children, tenements, and shelters. In the case of older adults, some family members may falsely believe social workers are there to put their loved one in a nursing home. "We don't want to speak to a *caseworker*," family members have said. "There's nothing wrong with our family situation. We're doing fine, thank you very much." My staff are trained to reply, "What we mean by a social worker is a person with a master's degree who understands the needs of families. She is skilled at analyzing interpersonal dynamics and can help families find solutions and resources to challenges that may be ahead." That assistance can range from recommending a cleaning or meal delivery service to offering advice about what to do if your loved one is agitated and yelling. She has a background in counseling and methodically finds answers to questions on daily living. She reassures caregivers and listens to their concerns, which can have a profound impact on how the family implements the new strategies when they leave the clinic.

The social worker's interviews can be challenging, as she must carefully navigate the family's dynamics to gather essential information. At the outset she will want to learn how close each family member is to the loved one and what they understand about his situation. She'll want to learn the family history (e.g., which relatives had cognitive impairment and at what age) and when the loved one first exhibited symptoms. Through the process, she will uncover the details of those symptoms and shed light on changes the family was unaware of.

Understanding social history is a core component of the evaluation. Where does your loved one live? Is he married, divorced, or widowed? Was his partner's death (or his divorce) traumatic? What relationship issues did they have? The social worker will ask for details about the children: where they live, how supportive they are, what their education level and work history is. If the loved one is retired, the social worker will want to know if it was voluntary or forced, what the person does now, and if he has hobbies. The social worker asks about the patient's use of alcohol, drugs, and tobacco. As noted, patients and families often give dramatically different responses to such questions.

Next the social worker turns to the patient's functional history. She starts with the "instrumental activities of daily living," often referred to as IADLs. Reviewing IADLs helps the social worker determine how well the person manages medications, handles finances, makes and keeps appointments, drives, cooks, does household chores, shops, and uses technology. My social worker is more adept at collecting a patient's functional history than I am. Her training includes knowing what to ask, where to inquire more deeply, and when to move on.

The next level of inquiry is about the patient's basic activities of daily living, known as ADLs. Unlike IADLs, which require higher-level thinking and planning, basic ADLs are less cognitively demanding and include fundamental self-care tasks that are essential to getting through the day. The social worker may not need to go into great detail, particularly if the patient is largely independent and functional. However, someone with moderate-stage dementia can experience changes in dressing, personal hygiene and bathing, toileting, walking, or eating. A person with severe dementia will be impaired in all these functions. My team wants to identify these disabilities and determine if they are due to physical limitations, mood, or personality. We'll want to understand the person's baseline ability to determine if the current functional changes truly represent significant decline. If an impairment exists, is it new and due to cognition?

The patient's independence, or lack of it, is essential to map out. The social worker will make this determination based on reports from the family. From that vantage point, the doctor and his team will compare how the person functions today compared to two, five, or ten years ago. Longstanding occasional clumsiness is not an impairment, but because poor coordination and tripping can be signs of motor changes, it's worth exploring. If someone always played the violin poorly, continuing to do so now doesn't qualify as impairment. Being bad at your hobbies is not abnormal and nothing to get strung up over.

The clinical diagnosis will in part be based on the richness of the family's detailed narrative. For example, when a person can't read the medication label on a pill bottle because he is farsighted, he often needs help to take his medications. The social worker will stress in her notes, "Patient's wife needs to organize his medications, but patient knows what each medication is for and when to take them. This is due to poor vision and not a decline in cognition." When children see a parent being unable to use a computer or other electronic devices, they often worry about cognitive decline. However, when the social worker speaks to the spouse, she learns more context and writes in her note, "Patient was never competent with using technology and has always relied on paper calendars and telephone books." Inquiring deeply into reported "deficits" is an area where a primary care provider may struggle. Family members' answers may be nuanced and require deciphering. A social worker knows to ask specific questions that only come from experience.

Safety is inevitably a central topic of discussion with the social worker, often arising because the family came to the clinic with concerns or because safety naturally becomes the primary focus when discussing functional abilities and disabilities. Children often fear the worst. These concerns cover a wide range, from managing medications to falling for financial scams to driving badly. For example, if someone's driving has changed, families rush to judgment and worry about car accidents when that risk may be far down the road. Stovetop fires are also a legitimate concern, but not when the issue at hand is recipe discrepancies and meals not tasting as good. Families may share fears they've never expressed before, like a parent poorly maintaining the home or failing to bathe regularly. These changes might be intentional or unintentional, but there's usually a reason behind them. In these cases, it's important to consider why. For instance, the person may be avoiding the tub because they don't have a step-in shower and struggle to navigate the wall. They may have trouble sequencing the steps needed to bathe. Or they might feel too cold in the bathroom or disconnected from the physical sensation of water.

Other concerns may surface during this conversation as well. Families might reveal worries about their mom forgetting to buy groceries, falling, being incontinent, choking, or forgetting to eat. Every aspect of daily living carries a safety implication that cannot be overlooked. Once these are identified, the social worker can help by offering resources, strategies, or referrals to address the concern and support the family in taking next steps.

Next, the social worker delves into a range of sensitive issues that often occur in dementia, such as wandering, apathy, depression, anxiety, hallucinations, paranoia, suspiciousness, agitation, inappropriate sexual behavior, and other personality changes. Communication changes—such as verbal outbursts, inappropriate comments, or a noticeable decrease in one's social filter—are also important to explore. One critical topic is firearms in the home. If they are present, she may recommend removing them or using gun locks for safety.

The social worker will inquire about sleep patterns and behaviors, such as acting out dreams, restless leg syndrome, or sleep apnea. She will also probe for any issues with vision, hearing, or oral hygiene. This information can help explain cognitive symptoms. For instance, untreated sleep apnea (a disorder causing intermittent breathing pauses and snoring) may lead to forgetfulness or difficulty completing tasks due to sleeplessness. Similarly, if a person acts out dreams, they may have REM sleep behavior disorder, which can be seen in Lewy body disease and not in Alzheimer's.

Focusing on the family's observations, the social worker conducts a targeted cognitive history, especially since patients in later stages of the disease often lack insight into their symptoms. She may ask if the loved one misplaces items more frequently, repeats comments or questions, and forgets details of recent events and conversations. She will explore whether the person struggles with finding words, completing sentences, or keeping track of thoughts, as well as his ability to solve problems. This line of questioning was created by our neuropsychologist and targets key symptoms in each cognitive domain. The social worker is trained to focus on changes from the person's baseline while also recognizing that some of these behaviors may occur in normal aging—the details and context are what matter. Their skill lies in teasing out patterns that reflect typical aging and separating them from those that suggest a progressive condition.

The social worker also addresses legal and end-of-life matters. She poses questions about a designated healthcare or financial power of attorney, a living will, and discussions about dying and death. She'll ask the family about future planning: Where would the person want to live if their condition progresses? Have they considered long-term care options or placed their name on any facility waitlists? Have they toured these places—with or without the patient? Do they hope to remain at home no matter what, and do they understand what services exist to help support that goal, along with the potential costs? She may quiz the family about prior advanced-care planning and offer to assist with these conversations if needed.

Finally, the social worker focuses on the family's needs and well-being, because their health is intimately related to our patient's. Caregiver stress is a significant issue that can lead to burnout. She'll ask open-ended questions in a nonthreatening way. (For practical tips on reducing burnout, visit the Community Resource Finder online, made available by the Alzheimer's Association and AARP, and focus on self-care through exercise, diet, meditation, and other activities.)

At the conclusion of the meeting, the social worker provides recommendations for resources and support. If the patient receives a dementia diagnosis, she will reach out again to share information on caregiver challenges and may arrange a follow-up phone call to answer questions.

THE NEUROPSYCHOLOGIST'S EVALUATION

While the family talks with the social worker, the patient spends time with the neuropsychologist. Like other psychologists, she holds a PhD and provides mental health therapy, but specializes in the "neuro" part. This means she is qualified to administer and interpret cognitive assessments.

Rather than jumping straight into testing, the neuropsychologist begins by collecting a targeted patient history. If the patient is suspected to be early in the disease process, the neuropsychologist focuses on his perspective, thought patterns, and thinking challenges. People who have entered the moderate stage of dementia, conversely, may struggle to provide a complete history of symptoms and day-to-day functioning. Assuming the patient is in the early stages, the neuropsychologist will ask open-ended questions followed by more specific inquiries. For example, she will explore whether the patient is able to recall recent conversations, repeats himself, misplaces items, gets lost, or struggles to find words in conversation. These are the same questions that the social worker is currently asking the family. She also probes mood volatility: *Do you feel depressed, anxious, or worried? How does this impact your thinking ability? Have you ever experienced hallucinations or feelings of paranoia?* To supplement these discussions, the neuropsychologist administers mood-screening forms that measure levels of depression and anxiety.

Sleep is another essential topic, described poetically as "nature's soft nurse" in Shakespeare's *Henry IV, Part II*. The neuropsychologist asks about sleep patterns: *How many hours do you typically sleep? Do you have trouble falling or staying asleep? Do you feel refreshed in the morning?* There will also be questions about sleep apnea, restless leg syndrome, acting out dreams, snoring, and napping. Sleep allows the brain to rinse itself clean of experiences not needed for long-term memory formation. And it's not just experiences that are cleared out during sleep. If a person sleeps poorly, chemicals such as misfolded proteins, metabolic byproducts, and inflammatory molecules that would otherwise dissolve can linger in the brain. Just as stains build up on an unwashed shirt, they eventually affect the mind's fabric. It's believed such accumulation can contribute to the onset of Alzheimer's.

The neuropsychologist will ask questions about motor symptoms such as weakness, falls, dizziness, physical instability, walking ability, and tremors. During her interview, she's making a mental list of potential neurodegenerative conditions, one of which results in the movement disorder called Parkinson's disease. Social history, including academic background, can enhance her understanding of the present situation. Was a learning disability diagnosed during elementary to high school? Did the patient require an IEP (individualized education plan)? How many years of education did the patient have, including his terminal degree (highest academic credential)? This data will help inform the questions and interpretations of the cognitive tests. Besides asking about the patient's professional life, the neuropsychologist also investigates his alcohol, drug, and tobacco use.

While engaging with the patient, the neuropsychologist performs a subtle but crucial task—behavioral observation. She considers a cavalcade of things beyond the patient's appearance and mood: hearing, vision, the rate at which he speaks, his rhythm and tone, his ability to find words and understand directions, his self-insight, how well he walks, if he fidgets while sitting, and, after testing, whether he thinks the cognitive evaluation is valid.

Finally, in a quiet, distraction-free room, the standard battery of cognitive tests begins. There's no clock on the wall, as the patient might later need to reproduce it from memory—placing the numbers and setting the hands to a specific time given by the examiner. If the patient could see the real time, it might influence their response or heighten frustration. There are many valid neuropsychological tests to choose from. Some take hours because they thoroughly test parts (or functions) of the brain. Despite these variations, they have one thing in common: They are far different from the Mini Mental State Examination (MMSE) and cognitive screeners that a general practitioner may offer.

Over the course of more than forty minutes, our neuropsychologist examines every cognitive domain. The testing is valid and rigorous but not overly taxing, striking a balance between detecting issues and avoiding patient exhaustion. Cognitive tests like ours cover all the mental domains that dementia can affect: visual-spatial, language, attention, processing speed, memory (including learning ability and short-term recall), and executive function. Some questions might seem silly or strange. It's not unusual for a patient to chuckle or get frustrated (or both) and ask the neuropsychologist, "What the heck is this all about?"

The questions can seem peculiar because they probe how well a person's brain functions in specific areas. For example, inability to reproduce a simple picture can indicate impairments in visual-spatial construction, an important function of the brain's occipital and parietal lobes. Difficulty learning a list of ten words and recalling them later may hint at issues with the temporal lobe, the location of the memory center known as the hippocampus. One test might be "Draw a clock and put the time at ten past eleven." Another could be "Connect circles labeled as a number or a letter, but alternate between a letter and a number such as A to 1, 1 to B, B to 2, and so forth." A patient's errors could reveal a problem with the frontal lobe, which is responsible for multiple executive functions.

The neuropsychologist's role is challenging. She must compile a wealth of information, swiftly draw conclusions, and present them to our team concisely.

EVERYTHING'S ON THE TABLE: THE MEMORY TEAM MEETS

After the individual meetings with the patient and family, it's time for the whole team to meet. I start by sharing the plethora of details we've learned during precharting. "Jack Jones is seventy-two," I will say. "This is his history . . . This is what's happened to him . . . This is what he's coming in with today . . . His blood work is . . . This is his head scan . . . The family reported this to other healthcare providers . . ."

Next, it's the social worker's turn. "I talked to Jack's daughter Judy, her husband Steve, and his wife Kelsey, and they report . . ." She presents the highlights of Jack's history, functional abilities, and mood and tells us what the family says about his symptoms. She shares interventions she discussed with the family, such as hiring a meal-delivery service, and recommends what she thinks I should emphasize with the patient and his family. She shares other family concerns, like household safety issues and whether the patient should continue to drive.

From this information and my precharting, I already have a sense of whether a person may have dementia—even before I've examined him. If the patient cannot function independently on a day-to-day basis due to his cognitive decline, then it is likely dementia. If, however, the patient is functionally independent, it will either be mild cognitive impairment or normal aging. "Normal aging" doesn't necessarily mean *normal.* It simply means a brain disease is unlikely to be the cause of symptoms. There are still many other organs and health conditions to consider.

The cognitive testing will help us objectively determine how well the brain is functioning. The neuropsychologist summarizes the test results and her assessment. Like the social worker, she recounts her conversation, tells us the patient's insight level, explains what he said about his symptoms, reports his social and family history, and homes in on the history she finds most relevant to someone with a cognitive complaint. But the most critical aspect of her presentation is her interpretation of the patient's test scores, how he behaved during the test, and whether the changes identified on the testing align with his or the family's reported complaints.

After hearing from my colleagues, I propose the diagnosis, explain my reasoning, and then offer a care plan to discuss with the patient and family. "We know Jack's symptoms are the following—X, Y, and Z. Based on what we've learned, Jack has A, B, and C functional impairments, and he has D, E, and F cognitive impairments. This pattern suggests such and such. Jack has mild-stage dementia. I believe his condition is due to Alzheimer's. To confirm the diagnosis, I propose these next steps. In addition, my plan of action includes blood work, future scans, and a referral to this specialist. I'm going to prescribe these medications, and I believe these lifestyle interventions are sensible. Jack also has reversible factors that should be addressed, and this should be his follow-up care."

Our conference lasts twenty to thirty minutes. Only rarely do we disagree about the diagnosis, but on those occasions, we might have a frank back-and-forth. We have worked together for many years and never sugarcoat our disagreements. There's no time for it, and doing so would not serve the patient. "Truth," as the English philosopher John Stuart Mill wrote, "emerges from the clash of adverse ideas."

MY MEETING WITH THE PATIENT AND FAMILY: MORE DETECTIVE WORK AND ACTION-ORIENTED ADVICE

Before I see a family, a staff member sometimes catches me in the hall and says, "Oh, man, they're intense," or "Four or five family members are here. Be ready." But if there is one insight I've gained from doing memory evaluations for nearly a decade, it is to walk in without bias. I usually have a different experience from the rest of the team. Rarely are the visits as intense as I've been led to believe. Conversations can get emotional, particularly when a family is divided and has dug in their heels about turning points in a loved one's life, such as whether the patient should continue to drive or whether a care facility (assisted living, memory care, nursing home) placement is needed. Interacting with any patient and his family in a memory clinic is intellectually and emotionally demanding. It's the first time I've met them, and they often expect me to address countless concerns even before I've shared my diagnosis.

The number of family members in the room can suggest the intensity of the situation. If four or five children and a spouse are present, that usually means there's consensus on severity. They may all want to express themselves about safety and a loved one's abilities. When some say the person should no longer make his own decisions while others feel he's still competent, it can take the wisdom of Solomon—and a fair amount of patience—to reach the best conclusion. Sometimes when the facts are overwhelming, I tell a family that their loved one must not continue to drive. On other occasions, it can be a judgment call, and I try to facilitate that decision. When the patient doesn't believe anything is wrong and doesn't want to be there, such encounters can be frustrating and difficult for everyone.

Many people wonder if physicians sometimes make diagnoses based on first impressions. We all like to think we can sum people up by their posture, eye contact, handshake intensity, or clothing style. In my professional capacity, first appearances are often misleading. If a patient meets me and is in the early stages of Alzheimer's, she can look and act in perfectly normal ways and converse with me for the first few minutes with ease. That's because most of us have well-honed social graces that waltz us like Fred Astaire through brief encounters. Only after I've spent extended time talking to someone and asking complex questions do I realize *Oh, she just said that* or *She's not finishing her sentences* or *Her answer makes no sense.*

But when I enter the clinic room, I do take some first impressions seriously. I ask myself, *Who else is here? Are there children? What about the spouse? Does anyone have an open notebook? Will she have prepared questions? Will she take notes?* Such observations tell me about a patient's level of social and family support.

After I introduce myself, my first goal is to develop rapport. Thanks to my team meeting, I often mention an interesting fact I've learned about the patient or family. My accomplice in this is the social worker, who typically asks family members to tell her a fascinating piece of information about the patient or themselves.

Doctors aren't born with bedside manner. We practice it, sharpening our skills with every patient we meet. I must be engaging, calm, and authoritative, yet friendly. If my news is distressing, I must translate complex technical information to the patient and family in ways that keep them from tumbling down a well of despair. The meaningful information I impart must bring hope, especially about the care plan. Patients and families must not just hear information, they must grasp it and retain it. I need them to be willing to stick with me and my team so they will start to make needed life decisions. If they don't believe in me and in the details I'm sharing, they won't come back. They may not begin to accept the realities I'm setting forth and the care that is required.

So how I present myself is carefully calibrated. I often find myself thinking about my family's experience with my father. As traumatic as that was, it was the proverbial blessing in disguise. The experience of having lived alongside someone with Alzheimer's gave me more empathy and compassion for those going through the same experience. It made me a better person—and a better caregiver. From time to time, I tell families about my father, decisions my mother made, and how we all lived through the experience. And, yes, it is a trying period, one that leaves no emotion untouched. A doctor's bedside manner is a learned way of being—a performance, if you will. Sometimes that bedside manner comes from life's bruises and is more heartfelt than a patient may realize.

After trying to establish rapport with everyone in the room, I review the visit, saying, "Jack, you met with the neuropsychologist and took tests, and your family met with the social worker, who asked questions similar to ones you answered. My team and I are building a three-dimensional picture of who you are and what you've been through. Those are crucial factors in figuring out what's happening. While you were waiting for me, my team and I put our heads together to figure out what's going on and what we can do." Then I perform a brief physical exam. I listen to the heart and carotid arteries, check cranial nerves, and assess the patient's movement and coordination to look for features of Parkinson's disease. This only takes five to ten minutes.

Then I say, "I'd like to review your thinking test with you. Do you have questions before I begin? How do you feel you did?" I show the patient and his family a graph created by the neuropsychologist that depicts the results. This visual aid is incredibly useful. It's hard to argue with a picture, though some patients do. "This is the range considered to be normal, acceptable, or anticipated based on your age," I will say. "Age is the only factor we controlled for. Your results are compared to those of healthy people from the community who took the same test." The graph is based on the principles of the bell curve. Such curves show standard deviations in a population like one that depicts the height of adult women or weight of men in a certain age range. In such a bell curve, most people fall in the middle. The results trail off at both ends because, for example, only a few women are very tall or very short.

"We are graphing five different parts of the brain," I'll add. "We'll go over everything together. I'll explain how each test shows up in the graph. For example, this part is based on the XYZ test. Your score was such and such. Because it was a low score, you might be experiencing these symptoms." Or I might say, "A score of X suggests these impairments. That means your brain is working, but not as well as it should. What's going on is more than just aging. Something else is happening. You have these impairments and these symptoms but are doing well in these other areas. We're going to leverage your strengths to keep you doing your best and closely watch for any future changes."

It's time to put the pieces together for the patient. "You have these symptoms and these functional changes, and I see these impairments in your thinking test results. To me, this means you meet the criteria for dementia." I define both mild cognitive impairment (MCI) and dementia so the patient and family know what each means. (Recall that Alzheimer's causes MCI and dementia, and MCI precedes dementia but doesn't always progress to it.) I make clear that MCI and dementia are not names of a disease but conditions used to describe symptoms and stages of cognitive change.

This leads to a conversation about the root cause of the symptoms. "Before we get to what we should do, it's my job to search for the underlying cause of your dementia. I may not be able to provide a definitive diagnosis, but that won't be for a lack of trying." The tests we have offer us a glimmer of the vast potential of our brains, but alongside that brilliance is this prodigious lack of knowledge of what we don't understand and can't fix, which is almost shameful in the twenty-first century. We don't have the needed tools to identify the major brain diseases causing dementia, nor do we have disease-modifying therapies to alter their course—except in the case of Alzheimer's, which has both. However, in this new world of artificial intelligence, advancement that used to take decades might now only be years away. Until then, I tell patients, "We know the most common brain diseases and the typical symptoms and findings that result from them. They are the ones that could be affecting you. We need to consider all of them, even though we're limited in what we can treat."

I always say the words *Alzheimer's disease* because the patient and family are thinking about it. I either say "I think this could be Alzheimer's disease, but we need to do more to see if that's the precise issue" or "I don't believe it's Alzheimer's for these reasons." Then I go into other factors contributing to the mild cognitive impairment or dementia, or I admit we don't yet know what is causing the symptoms and need to investigate further.

I'll summarize by saying, "Jack, your diagnosis is dementia, most likely due to Alzheimer's disease." I include other factors that could be contributing to his symptoms, a consideration that applies to nearly all patients. It's usually not just one condition causing symptoms but myriad factors, some of them treatable. The list can be long and overwhelming, which is why I write them down for the patient and family. Because the conversation is vital to their understanding of the big picture, I say, "I'm also worried about vascular changes in your brain, as well as your medications, sleep apnea, anxiety, and lack of activity. I'm going to write all this out for you, but I want you to hear and absorb these details so I can answer your questions."

At this point, some patients react with shock and disbelief. They turn pale and appear shaken. Others will be distressed but not surprised. I try to give the diagnosis early in our meeting so we can spend most of our time together talking about positive, constructive plans. Families will ask questions about what they're going to do now. I am always prepared for this and have a care plan ready to share. I start by saying I want to order blood work, an MRI, and a biomarker test that may show byproducts of Alzheimer's in the blood, in spinal fluid, or on positron emission tomography (PET) brain scans. Then I'll talk about medications and end by suggesting referrals and certain evidence-based lifestyle interventions.

I like to end, if I can, with action-oriented advice. I want families and patients to recognize that there is much within their control. Providing them with step-by-step actions they can take, which may include new activities or simple adjustments to medications, routines, habits, and their environment, can be empowering and is foundational for the patient's future needs. Typically, I discuss sleep, exercise, and mental stimulation, all of which are lifestyle interventions a patient and their family can take ownership of. At some point, families begin to chime in and suggest ways to boost social engagement and reduce stress. I love their participation. We are, after all, on the same team. Diet is hard for most people to modify, so I mention the importance of eating healthy whole foods and ask patients, "What's one food you're eating regularly that you probably should limit?" Change can only happen when patients and families drive the plan. Our team will follow up with them in a few months, but these habit changes start at home.

Patients and families may still be afraid, and sad, but they can leave my clinic committed to a plan and fully supported by a team. The patient may still be in shock from hearing the diagnosis, but the anxiety tied to not knowing whether something was wrong, or if they had Alzheimer's, has begun to lift. They're calmer. They're thinking, *Okay, good. Finally, after all this time, we know what's going on. We can do something.* I tell them to see my nurse practitioner for follow-up in a few months and note that we'll repeat certain tests in a year or two. A full battery of cognitive tests is not needed again if a patient has dementia. The testing is meant to identify cognitive impairment. At the dementia stage, longer testing can be demoralizing to a patient, reminding him of inabilities he has already accepted. To me, repeating such tests will not change my management, and doing so feels cruel. How the patient feels and the functional changes the family observes provide more meaningful information.

After I explain this to patients and families, the patient is usually grateful, but the family often has a new category of questions. They'll ask, "How will we know when Mom has progressed from the mild to the moderate stage?" I remind them that our memory team will continue to see them regularly. The information we gather at these shorter visits will guide the care and answer their questions. While it may be risky to end a long family meeting with open-ended questions, I do so anyway. I ask, "What does this diagnosis mean to you?" "How are you interpreting everything I said?" and "Do you have any other questions?" My visit has taken anywhere from forty-five to eighty-five minutes. Before parting with the patient and his family, I type a take-home summary, which lets them know they can call our social worker or our nurses with questions.

Despite spending hours on evaluation, sometimes our team cannot diagnose the specific cause of a memory ailment—and that's frustrating for the patient, their family, and my team. For example, a retired engineer named Godfrey saw me three years in a row. Though his test scores were normal, he reported horrible memory loss and other cognitive problems. Perhaps because he was an engineer, he wanted a concrete answer grounded in a physical problem. I didn't have one and told him, "I don't see anything that looks like Alzheimer's. Your MRI brain scan doesn't show vascular issues. You don't have a movement disorder that looks like Parkinson's disease or Lewy body disease." I could identify nothing physically wrong. He was certain he had a brain disease and wanted me to confirm it. While I understood his desire to be validated, his symptoms were real, so I looked beyond neurodegenerative conditions to the personal issues that were causing him anguish. I said, "Your anxiety is high. It could be driving your symptoms or at least exacerbating normal age-related changes." That's not what he wanted to hear, but his anxiety was something he could work to control, and having a sense of empowerment can help lead to positive outcomes.

A Word of Caution About Cognitive Tests

Arithmetic tests in elementary school are black and white. Either you know what 8 × 7 equals or you don't. Get enough multiplication problems wrong, and you won't get a gold star.

Many tests in medicine are that way, too. There's no disputing that an X-ray will show broken bones or that an eye exam reveals whether someone needs glasses.

On the other hand, cognitive tests for dementia can have many shades of gray. This is true whether the test is the short, thirty-question type administered in a few minutes by a general practitioner or a multipart battery of quizzes overseen by a neuropsychologist that takes most of an hour to complete. Cognitive screening tests have limited value beyond identifying *possible* cognitive impairment. They were not designed to diagnose mild cognitive impairment or dementia. They simply don't probe deeply enough, and many patients who have passed such brief quizzes with flying colors have come to me and performed poorly when required to focus at great length on a multitude of tests. The opposite situation is also seen, with patients performing poorly on these brief thinking tests but scoring in the average to superior range on the more difficult lengthy exams.

Even so, patients and their loved ones can understandably be wary of accepting the results of longer tests at face value. There are sound reasons why such exams administered by a skilled neuropsychologist could give misleading results. Maybe the patient had a bad night of sleep, is on a mind-numbing medication, or is nervous. Perhaps the patient had no rapport with the tester. A common oversight in testing older adults relates to communication. If the patient can't hear well or English isn't his first language, this can negatively—and falsely—impact results.

One important caveat to note about cognitive tests that most people, including healthcare providers, don't recognize is cultural bias. Many tests were developed decades ago, and their creators devised them relying on a small number of people, almost all of whom were white. Normal cultural cues and responses for someone in rural Minnesota in 1950 may be very different from what is typical today in Miami, Florida. In addition, many cognitive tests fail to take into account that people with different levels of education might perform differently without it representing a deficiency. It is not easy or straightforward to determine what is normal for an individual based on a set of scores from a group of people with different backgrounds and life experiences.

That's not all. The brain is a very complicated organ, and even an hour-long test may be too brief to provide a comprehensive assessment. A lengthy test might, for example, have only two tasks focused on the brain's executive function, which governs multitasking and problem-solving. Anyone who's anxious or hasn't slept well might get those two sections wrong and thus be mistakenly deemed to have executive dysfunction when that's not the case. Cognitive testing must balance thoroughness with efficiency, and so each part (or domain) of the brain can only be checked so much.

As a patient or caregiver, how should you regard the imperfectness of cognitive tests? I recommend that you approach the results as you would any important medical finding: with discernment. Does this result align with all the other evidence, including your own observations and report? In general, the longer the testing, the better, because it means more parts of the brain are examined and more tasks were used to determine the conclusion. If the test was given by a neuropsychologist and reviewed by a memory specialist, it is highly likely they interpreted its results correctly. Neuropsychologists are trained to administer these tests. They understand how they were created—as well as their possible flaws—and they have interpreted hundreds of patients' test results. The doctor has likely cared for many other patients with cognitive impairment and has developed good instincts in differentiating normal from abnormal aging. Equally important, he is evaluating the neuropsychologist's conclusions alongside information from the patient's medical record, family report, and the social worker's input.

Despite its limitations, cognitive testing must be done to receive a proper memory evaluation. It's valuable to go into the post-testing discussion with your eyes and ears open, recognizing that your performance does not define you, or even diagnose you. If you believe the test results do not reflect what is happening, then talk with your doctor. You can ask for a repeat test in the future. Depending on the type of test—like brief cognitive screening tools—you may be able to repeat it in as little as three to four months.

In fact, sometimes it takes multiple tests to get a reliable answer. That's because performance can be influenced by untreated, reversible conditions—such as sleep apnea, vitamin deficiencies, depression, or thyroid disorders—as well as temporary factors like fatigue, anxiety, pain, or poor sleep. If any of these factors are present, they may detract from a patient's true cognitive ability. It's also important to remember that some individuals begin with very high cognitive function, so a test result that appears "average" could actually represent a meaningful decline for them. Repeat testing helps to confirm patterns over time and distinguish between a bad day, a high baseline, and a true progressive change—something more reflective of disease. Medicare covers testing with a neuropsychologist once a year, which may mean waiting, but this also gives you time to address reversible factors like sleep apnea or medication side effects. Even though it may take time, and multiple appointments, to get a diagnosis, don't wait to address your brain health (see chapter 5 for more details).

DOCTOR'S HONESTY IS THE BEST POLICY

Families are usually glad that the problem they've worried about has a name and that they can go home with a plan. It's powerful to have a diagnosis. It enables people to take much-needed (and sometimes delayed) next steps. Opening the door to action is therapeutic.

There is no question that people can go into denial when hearing an Alzheimer's diagnosis. Some will say, "No, no, that can't be true." The later a person is in the disease, the more likely it is he will have lost the insight to understand what's happening to him. He will have reached the point where he might not understand the information or even the words people say. At some point, not recognizing what is lost can be seen as a gift to the person with dementia. He doesn't need to suffer by comparing himself to the way he used to be. Instead, it is the family that grieves the absence of the person they once knew.

Denial is a powerful reaction, one that may even lessen the shock of receiving traumatic news. Just as my sister and I refused to believe my mom when she first shared her concerns, my dad also went into denial. When a doctor told him he had Alzheimer's, he replied, "No, I don't have Alzheimer's." The doctor had to say several times, "No. You do have Alzheimer's. You do have Alzheimer's." Granted, the doctor wasn't 100 percent correct at that point, because he didn't truly know if it was Alzheimer's. As it turned out, an autopsy showed that my father suffered from something common—mixed dementia. My father was in the earliest stage of dementia, possibly still MCI. Nonetheless, my mom recorded that doctor's visit. The next day she played it again for my dad to be sure he would remember what he had been told.

To sum up, your doctor must be honest about the diagnosis. If she thinks the diagnosis is dementia or the symptoms are caused by Alzheimer's, she must say it. She must make sure it sinks in and makes sense. She must be firm. It's much easier for a doctor to avoid using the word *Alzheimer's* or *dementia*. Some might take the easy path by saying "You have some memory changes" and letting it go at that. It's hard to tell a patient he likely has Alzheimer's disease, but those words must be said.

It's challenging for most primary care doctors to speak that frankly, which is one reason they don't do in-depth memory evaluations. I've had many patients whose primary care doctor dismissed worries about their memory. Here's an example of what happens. After three years of reporting symptoms and having them dismissed, the person returns for an annual wellness visit. This time his daughter comes along. "There's something wrong," she insists. "You have to do more." That forces the primary care doctor to make a referral to me for a full evaluation. My team ends up finding multiple factors causing the memory loss. Let me be clear: The primary care doctor is not malicious or incompetent (at least the overwhelming majority are not). But they lack the knowledge, training, or experience to discuss these matters to the degree that patients and families rightfully expect.

Health conditions can run the gamut from minor to life threatening. Dementia is a devastating disease that changes a person's life forever. Ask any patient living with a brain disorder or their family, and they'll tell you the same thing. A diagnosis must be certain, requiring a methodical and comprehensive evaluation. Primary care doctors can often recognize and even diagnose mild cognitive impairment or dementia. Still, confirmation—and the diagnosis of Alzheimer's or another brain disease—would ideally come from a memory specialist, not be left to a compassionate but underresourced primary care doctor.

Even memory specialists can have difficulty telling a patient he has Alzheimer's. We're giving a patient what is called "a terminal diagnosis." It is the equivalent of saying, "You have terminal cancer." Nobody wants to deliver that news. We want the best for people, so it's hard to do. Your doctor must have a policy of being honest yet kind and firm. If that's not what he demands of himself every day, he will let down his patients and himself. As Benjamin Franklin said, "Half the truth is often a great lie."

4

"My World Has Fallen Apart"

HAVE FAITH—YOU WILL BUILD A NEW LIFE AFTER THE DIAGNOSIS

Denial, Grief, and Adjustment • Treating Other Health Conditions in the Context of Alzheimer's • #1 Task? Getting a Healthcare Power of Attorney • Update Wills, Trusts, and Financial Powers of Attorney • Be Careful Picking the Right Agent • Setting Daily Routines and Establishing Health Habits

Shell-shocked. That's not an unusual state to find yourself in after receiving a diagnosis of Alzheimer's disease.

The body's physiological response is fight, flight, or freeze. The brain perceives all acute stress as life-threatening. Whether you stumble onto a black bear and her cub or you're being told you have a terminal disease, the brain doesn't differentiate between physical and existential danger. To your brain, a diagnosis of Alzheimer's disease is a perceived threat to your existence. It will force you to choose a course of action, consciously or not. Fighting might sound like the most heroic and noble decision. Who doesn't admire the champion who bests every opponent?

But Alzheimer's is not an adversary that can be overpowered and outmaneuvered. Success doesn't come from force—it comes from preparation and endurance. Avoiding the diagnosis or fleeing from its implications and prognosis is an understandable impulse. Many try. But no one outruns the eventual declines of a neurodegenerative condition. The changes will come.

When I speak with patients and their families, I advocate for fighting *and* running, but in a different context. Not as reactions to the diagnosis itself but as tools for living with it. As you'll learn in the next chapter, lifestyle habits are foundational for brain health and overall memory care. For now, don't freeze. Instead, pause and catch your breath.

"Worrying about the past or the future isn't productive," wrote self-help author Harvey Mackay. "Stop and take a breath and ask yourself what you can do right now to succeed." In other words, it's okay to sit with your feelings and absorb your new reality; just don't stay there too long. Take control of your response and become mindful of how you inhale and exhale. This will have an immediate effect on the stress in your body. Deep breathing has remarkable powers beyond giving your lungs more of the beneficial oxygen they need. It lessens feelings of anxiety and depression, lowers blood pressure, slows your heartbeat, and calms your nervous system. These effects are real, measurable, and available to you at any moment.

So whether you're reading this in a bookstore, a doctor's waiting room, or your own home, put the book down for a second. Close your eyes and take a few slow, deep breaths. You will feel better, more relaxed, and more in control—even under the most difficult circumstances, such as learning a diagnosis of Alzheimer's.

The week before my mother told my sister and me that our dad was ill, she told her own family. As she described it, her mother and three sisters were all sitting around the kitchen table in their family home, visiting and catching up. Then, abruptly, Mom blurted it out—Moe, my dad, had a memory problem.

Her mother was a hospice nurse. Her youngest sister was an infection control nurse. The oldest sibling was a social worker. Only her identical twin, Kathryn, didn't work in healthcare. As a family law attorney, she often saw situations from a different perspective.

Mom told me later that everyone at the table listened patiently to her evidence. They reassured her it was probably just stress, nothing to worry about. All except Kathryn. She waited for the chorus of comfort to end, and then concluded by saying, "This is a situation that needs immediate attention, and I'm going to set up an appointment with a colleague to discuss next steps." And that's exactly what she did.

Everyone at that kitchen table helped my mom in their own way. But while most offered sympathy, which she definitely needed, her twin gave her what no one else did: honesty and directness. I call this truth telling. It's not easy. However, change can't begin without acknowledgment.

This chapter is about taking back control—by compiling a comprehensive list of routines and strategies that will build a balanced framework for living. Let this new landscape house your castle, a fortress whose sturdy walls, strong roof, and solid foundation will shelter you from any medical and emotional storms ahead. Your action plan will replace anxiety and uncertainty about the future by helping you live with the disease without being defined by it.

In the following pages, I'll walk you through essential strategies for living well with Alzheimer's. These include adapting to a medical care regimen, facing legal considerations, developing healthy routines, and caring for the caregiver.

Start by carving out a space dedicated to mind and body practices such as yoga, tai chi, or qigong, to name a few. Stretch and walk, ideally in nature. You can find guided instructions on the internet, through community centers, or in books and videos at your local library.

I start my own day with deep breathing and the yoga sequence "Salutation to the Sun," all of which I practice in five minutes. It grounds and energizes me. Healthcare providers like myself recommend these types of habits as forms of preventative medicine because they can boost the immune system, reduce stress hormones, and keep you healthy. Depending on the exercise, they can also help with balance, which becomes a significant concern for people as they age.

So inhale deeply, and let's begin.

GETTING THE DIAGNOSIS—THE SHOCK OF KNOWING

There is a nearly universal reaction to receiving bad news—disbelief. Whether it is losing someone you love or receiving a poor prognosis, these experiences usher in a time of tumultuous change. Grieving is commonplace, widely shared yet intimate and completely normal.

For those navigating this terrain, I often recommend the groundbreaking 1969 book *On Death and Dying* by Swiss American psychiatrist Elisabeth Kübler-Ross. While the stages of denial, anger, bargaining, depression, and acceptance that she outlines are a necessary part of adjusting to traumatic events, grief is as individual as the person experiencing it. How we respond to and live with that grief differs significantly, dictated by individual circumstances.

Learning of my father's illness transformed my life. At the time, I had completed my medical training and was happily working as a hospitalist at Kaiser Permanente in San Diego. My wife and I were planning to build a life there—we were even eyeing a house in Bird Rock, a coastal neighborhood we loved. Despite wanting to stay in sunny California, we made the decision to relocate two thousand miles northeast to Wisconsin. We both had to say goodbye to friends and change our careers in the ensuing years. I became a caregiver to both my parents, went back into training, and eventually started working as a memory specialist. My grief became a pilgrimage, transforming who I was and my life's mission.

The sorrow I've shouldered hasn't made my work easier, but it has made it far more meaningful. My father's ethereal presence is illuminated in my patients, and my sweet mother's perseverance in their spouses, partners, and family members. Aside from the "street cred" my loss has given me, families recognize that I speak with a wisdom that comes from more than textbooks. These are lived experiences they, too, will come to know.

Insights into Alzheimer's rarely arrive all at once—they accumulate gradually through trial and error and a desire to do better. At times it felt like I was walking in the dark, grasping for answers that were nearby but still unseen. Advancements in brain health and science have come a long way but were not prevalent during those difficult years when my dad was losing his grip on reality. As families, we often learn not through grand revelations but through each other—the shared stories, stumbles, and steady resilience of those who've walked this road before. In the words of

Isaac Newton, "If I have seen further, it is by standing on the shoulders of giants." Here, those giants are everyday people—caregivers and loved ones—who teach us how to adapt and move forward.

As both a recipient and bearer of bad news, I am precise about my word choice, cadence, and body language when delivering diagnoses to patients. I know how vulnerable and exposed one feels to be on the receiving end of these details. The information I share can be jarring, made worse when expressed poorly. There can be physical reactions like ringing in the ears, unfocused or tunnel-like vision, and the sense that time has frozen. Most people, especially families, anticipate what I'm about to say. They're not shocked; they're validated. Some individuals, however, are caught off guard, and my words land like an earthquake. Their world is shaken, with the ground shifting beneath them.

When I was an intern in San Diego in 2010, I had my own deer-in-the-headlights moment. My supervising physician asked me to lance a lesion on the thigh of a patient with HIV. Before starting the procedure, I injected the painkiller lidocaine to numb the surrounding area. While pushing in the syringe, a mist of red blood suddenly spurted up, blanketing my face, eyes, and nose. These areas are a direct pathway to the bloodstream, the very routes through which the virus could take root in my body.

My vision blurred and my heart pounded. I could barely hear anything beyond the roaring sound in my ears. Seeing my shock, the patient, whose viral load (amount of virus in the blood) was low, began to comfort me. In a rare reversal of roles, he assured me I would be fine and told me not to worry.

The senior doctor immediately sent me for blood tests and then home to my wife, who was equally distressed. We had to wait two weeks for the test results. Years later, I suffered a bout of pneumonia and had to be rechecked for HIV. Lung infections are rare in people under forty, so they wanted to rule it out as a potential cause for weakened immunity. Once again, the wait seemed interminable. I had now dodged the proverbial bullet—twice—but the experience left an indelible imprint.

That moment gave me a glimpse into the raw fear that comes with hearing potentially life-changing news—the kind that knocks the wind out of you. It was a lesson in emotional whiplash: the immediate sense of doom, the uncertainty, the fragile hope that follows. Years later, I would revisit these feelings with my own father's diagnosis. That event marked a pivotal chapter in my life's story, encompassing two distinct phases: before and after his diagnosis. I carry that understanding with me into the exam room. It allows me to meet my patients and their families not only as a physician but as someone who has felt the floor drop out beneath him—and who remembers what it means to try to rebuild afterward.

One question I often ask patients and families after giving the diagnosis is, "What does this mean to you?" Their responses reveal the deeper emotional impact this information has on them. Some say, "What does this mean? I already knew I had this. My mom had it and gave up, and I'm gonna fight it." Others respond with, "My life is over" or "At least I'm old." My staff and I always address these grim reactions early, before they have a chance to percolate and fester. After all, life is what we make of it. There are tools, techniques, and drugs that help with disease progression, but mindset matters just as much.

Controlling one's attitude and maintaining a positive outlook is crucial for physical and emotional well-being. A hopeful mindset in the face of this disease is not easy, and I don't pretend otherwise. Still, I've seen firsthand that focusing on what's good in each day—even small moments of connection, purpose, or enjoyment—can offer real benefits. My patients who hold onto gratitude or a sense of meaning seem to carry a kind of resilience that others do not. And that mindset, while hard-earned, is worth striving for. It doesn't deny the difficulty of the diagnosis—but it does shape how a person chooses to live with it. And that, in itself, can make all the difference.

We each come to express grief differently through our own set of anticipatory expectations and life philosophies. When a diagnosis catches you off guard, denial is a predictable response. Doubt and anger usually follow. The loss of a future once envisioned and carefully planned for is neither fair nor just. It's wretched to start over under compromised circumstances. Even the most reasonable plans—like traveling in retirement—suddenly seem daunting.

My family traversed the globe starting when I was in kindergarten. In 2007, we traveled to Peru to climb Machu Picchu. Unfortunately, I developed high-altitude pulmonary edema (fluid in my lungs) in the middle of the night, midway up the mountain range. My dad, who always traveled with a stethoscope, diagnosed my condition and initiated a complicated rescue. Down the mountain we went, the whole family packed into an ambulance. I spent three days in and out of a hyperbaric chamber, my dad a constant companion.

But after his Alzheimer's diagnosis, all but the most essential travel stopped. I've made many mistakes along the way, but the one I regret most is not continuing with the hobby he loved most of all right after his diagnosis, when he was most capable of travel. Don't let that chance pass you by.

AFTER THE DIAGNOSIS—COMING TO TERMS WITH THE TRUTH

Patients in the early stages also mourn anticipated loss of identity, fearing that the person they are today will simply fade away. At some point, though, I see people accept their new reality. Gradually opening up and sharing details of the disease is therapeutic for them. It builds support by allowing others to become involved.

In my clinical experience, patients who have confided in family and friends tend to be more optimistic about what lies ahead. They have faith that they will continue to be a productive member of their family and community. Not everyone, however, is able to come to terms with the prognosis. Some people squander precious time stewing in their anger and resentment about how unfair life can be. I feel for these patients. We all must eventually grapple with these existential questions.

Caregivers have shared with me that they are ashamed of the resentment they feel toward their spouse or parent. It's more common than most people realize. Statistically, spousal caregivers are at a higher risk of developing cognitive problems later in life compared to nonspousal partners. That is why our clinic counsels caregivers separately during appointments, offering programs and advice to help them maintain their own health. Some support groups even provide two separate meeting rooms for their programs. That way caregivers have an opportunity to vent, share, and provide encouragement to one another while their loved one is engaged in supervised activities in the other room. Because dementia worsens over a span of years, it takes a tremendous emotional and physical toll on the healthy spouse or children who are involved with the caregiving. Support for caregivers, through counseling, respite, and assistance at home, is absolutely essential.

My mother was an avid beekeeper. One day I was visiting my dad on a day when she was harvesting honey. Dad and I were watching out the window when we saw her suddenly drop the frame she was holding and make a mad dash for the house. She burst through the door, her bee suit half-hanging off, screaming as she ran for the shower. My mom—a stoic German woman—does not scream. Needless to say, my dad and I were frightened.

The ER doctor stopped counting at fifty stingers. Fortunately, my mom wasn't allergic to bees and had never been stung like this before. Although she didn't go into anaphylactic shock, she was completely drained. A neighbor had come over to stay with my dad while we were gone, but it quickly became clear that we needed more help—for both my parents.

From the hospital, we called hospice and explained what had happened. Our primary goal was to see if my dad could be admitted to their facility for a short stay while mom recovered. Discussing respite was the first time I saw her—my mom, the caregiver—break down and cry. She had been carrying the weight of her world and my dad's on her shoulders. And that day in the ER, she finally felt it.

Later that night, as I drove home, I felt a different kind of weight. It was the weight of disappointment. I was angry at myself for not having had a respite plan for my mother. Here I was, a geriatric fellow becoming an expert in caring for older adults, particularly those with dementia and their caregiver, and I missed this fundamental step of establishing a backup plan in case the primary caregiver becomes ill. *Selfish* and *shortsighted* were the kinder words I used to berate myself.

I now use my mom's bee story as a teaching moment for physicians in training and the families I work with. Always have a backup plan for the primary caregiver. For any number of reasons, she may need respite—and she deserves it. Plan ahead so she has the space to recharge, and so the loved one with dementia continues to receive care without disruption.

One of the benefits of hospice is the flexibility it offers in adapting care. Despite our last-minute scrambling, my family was able to arrange respite support even though we ended up not using it. My mom responded positively to the anti-inflammatory drug prednisone and insisted on staying with my dad, against my recommendation.

We cannot plan for every situation, but we can learn from others who have come before us. When it comes to caregiving, developing contingency plans to avoid a crisis is worth its weight in gold.

Families often enter the bargaining or negotiating stage of grief by searching for magical cures, like supplements that promise to improve memory or reverse Alzheimer's. Believe me, I lived that myself.

At one point, I requested and reviewed all my father's lab results. His vitamin D levels came back low, and that mild irregularity became my "silver bullet." I clung to the hope that a remedy of high doses of cholecalciferol (vitamin D_3) supplementation would somehow reverse his course. While insufficient vitamin D can cause cognitive changes, it is highly unlikely to cause dementia. But I didn't know that then. I was in my second year of residency, grasping for anything that might make a difference.

I googled every intervention I could find to counteract vitamin D deficiency, hanging on to that slender reed of hope. Eventually, I realized I was chasing a solution that didn't exist. Searching for meaningful treatment, even if it doesn't yet exist, is not a waste of time. It is a labor of love and part of grieving.

Just like my immediate reaction during my HIV scare, patients at first go through uncertainty and fear that creates a kind of numbness—a cottony sensation in the brain, like the way your mouth feels after a dentist injects a local anesthetic into the gums. Not talking and needing a quiet space are natural responses to a long day of memory testing. The diagnosis takes time to sink in, and that's okay. Communication is important—but not necessarily during the car ride home or even later that evening.

LIVING WITH THE DIAGNOSIS—A NEW KIND OF MEDICINE

Adapting to the care plan will become a central part of life. Everything medically related will be influenced by the overarching importance of memory care. This changes priorities for patients and reframes goals for all healthcare providers.

A common phrase used by doctors to contextualize a patient issue is "in the setting of . . ." These four words personalize the patient's situation and clarify why a recommendation may—or may not—be appropriate.

For example, my patient Otto is being admitted into the hospital with pneumonia. At first glance, many providers might think this is inappropriate and he could be managed at home with oral antibiotics. However, when I talk to my colleagues about his case, I say, "My patient Otto has pneumonia *in the setting of* poorly controlled diabetes and a history of liver failure requiring transplant, and he is now taking multiple immunosuppressive medications requiring hospital-level treatment for A, B, and C." A common condition like pneumonia is no longer straightforward in the context of other serious, chronic health problems.

Cognitive impairment, particularly dementia, is one of the most serious, complex chronic health conditions a person can face. Consequently, cognitive care becomes the medical framework around which all services will revolve. Memory care effectively becomes *primary care*, because a patient's osteoarthritis, eczema, and even metabolic disease likely are not as fundamental as memory loss.

The ability to think clearly ranks high when weighed against other medical disorders. If you had to choose between slightly higher blood pressure and slightly lower cognition, most people—physicians and patients alike—would prioritize thinking ability, so long as the trade-off is deemed acceptable to the patient and his doctor.

Let me be clear: Each ailment is worthy of medical attention. Your primary care providers and specialists will address them. But for someone living with Alzheimer's, all care considerations center around what's best for the brain.

At my clinic, our nurse practitioners see patients every two to four months. They routinely order blood tests to assess for vitamin deficiencies, thyroid abnormalities, cholesterol ranges, and blood sugar levels. During the visit, they'll check vital signs like blood pressure and weight and look for any changes in the neurological exam. Sometimes they'll request a brain scan to see if there's additional atrophy or blood vessel change.

However, the most important aspect of their care is talking to the patient and family about changes in cognition, daily function, mood, behavior, and brain-healthy habits. Family observations are seminal in recognizing disease progression, making it prudent to incorporate family in each visit.

Once all the information is collected, the nurse practitioners will propose small adjustments to align with the patient's stated goals and review the medication list—not only to ensure the patient is taking what's prescribed but also to eliminate anything that's no longer needed.

If a patient has mild cognitive impairment, they're still functionally independent and won't need many clinic services. Patients and families require varying degrees of reassurance and support. Some don't reach out until they confront a situation they can't handle, whereas others call with questions every month. Our medical staff, especially the nurses and social workers, reinforce the treatment plan as often as needed. Families learn to tap into the collective wisdom of our interdisciplinary team. What feels scary and unfamiliar to them is not new to us. Sadly, we've seen their situation more times than we can count, but the blessing is we can share what has worked for others. That's why my clinic's motto is simple: "We're here. Call anytime."

People with mild cognitive impairment may become frustrated with their fluctuating symptoms, but many will have several years—or more—of independent living ahead of them. They might struggle with tasks like managing medications or remembering appointments, but with the right systems in place, they can continue to live a full, mostly uninterrupted life.

During office visits, phone calls, or chart messages, our clinic offers practical alternatives for most of the challenging situations patients and families encounter. A common example is handling daily medication. In the early stages, patients may be able to take their prescriptions and supplements at appropriate doses and times, but when that's no longer feasible, we recommend a pillbox. To preserve as much independence as possible, patients can organize their own pillbox under supervision or, to be more diplomatic, observation. Over time, however, family or friends will need to take over this responsibility. Alternatively, many pharmacies offer medication packaging services for a fee, which can ease the burden on both the patient and their caregivers. As the disease progresses and the patient's abilities decline, reminders and oversight are essential to ensure medications are taken reliably. For patients living alone, we may recommend a pillbox with an alarm that beeps with the next scheduled dose. Not every suggestion will work, but our team has a nearly endless list of ideas—most learned directly from other patients and families over the past thirty years.

One frequently addressed concern is incontinence of both stool and urine. This is a delicate subject for many people, but our team addresses it with as much sensitivity and finesse as possible. After all, adult diapers are sold in every grocery store—not because everyone has dementia but because accidents happen, even without it. Normalizing the situation allows for open conversation and maintaining dignity. Toward the later stages of Alzheimer's, incontinence is almost a certainty. That's why we discuss early how to be prepared and to never be embarrassed asking a question that may seem impolite. Shame has no place in memory care.

When my sister Maggie came home to visit Dad the autumn before he died, she took him into the bathroom. Mom had him on a routine schedule to avoid changing his Depends too frequently. Skin dampened with caustic urine can eventually break down and lead to bedsores.

I heard Mom say, "I'll take Dad," but Maggie insisted. She helped him lower his Depends, and before she knew what was happening, urine sprayed all over the toilet and wall. Dad was fine, but Mom was furious about the mess, and Maggie was speechless.

We all had a good chuckle about Maggie, the family practice doctor, who couldn't manage a stream of urine. Our house was filled with laughter that afternoon, not humiliation or embarrassment.

Over time, the focus of medical care will change because when someone has Alzheimer's, other conditions begin to matter less. Quality of life drives decision-making. Steve, a patient of mine, had been a lifelong skier, winning trophies in college competitions. When he developed chronic knee pain, he consulted with an orthopedic specialist. The surgeon told him he could operate on the knee to replace the joint, but Steve asked him, "Will the operation and the anesthesia make my Alzheimer's worse? If it does, I'm not sure alleviating the pain is worth the trade-off." Doctors admire patients who weigh the pros and cons of medical decisions.

Everyone involved—patients, families, geriatricians, surgeons, and other specialists—should ask this of any proposed medical procedure: "Could this accelerate cognitive change? Might it hasten the timeline for dying from dementia?" The bottom line is that people can live with other medical issues, but they can't live without their brains. Anesthesia, wide variations in blood pressure during surgery, or surgical complications can worsen cognition afterward.

Existing medications must be reconciled in the context of Alzheimer's. Doctors and patients need to be mindful of anything with anticholinergic properties, a substance that can slow thinking. (For more on this, see page 92.) Drugs like gabapentin, an often-prescribed medication sold under various brand names to treat nerve pain, can also sedate the brain. In this respect, gabapentin is like alcohol. Other common prescription remedies with similar brain-slowing effects are those in the benzodiazepine family, commonly used to treat anxiety. Even over-the-counter allergy medications can have a malign effect on a vulnerable brain. One reason a patient might prefer a geriatrician to a neurologist is the geriatrician's expertise in medication management—knowing what each drug is for, when to consider a lower dose, and when it may be best to avoid the medication altogether.

Diabetes care provides a good example of how the presence of Alzheimer's can influence other medical decisions. One of the key tools in diabetes management is the hemoglobin A1c test (HbA1c), which estimates blood glucose (sugar) levels over the previous few months. A normal HbA1c value is less than 5.8, while anything above 6.4 indicates diabetes. Typically, a doctor aims to lower that score, potentially through an injection of insulin, to around 7. However, for those with Alzheimer's dementia, a more relaxed target of 8 is often used in clinical practice.

Although diabetes is a serious and potentially life-threatening condition, its management in dementia care must be more holistic. In the later stages of dementia, administering injections often requires a caregiver's involvement—a task that may prove unrealistic for an exhausted or overwhelmed spouse or child already juggling the patient's daily needs. Injections can also be distressing for patients who no longer fully understand their health or the purpose of the treatment. Repeated needle use may provoke fear and diminish their quality of life. In such cases, doctors may opt for a more compassionate solution, such as prescribing pills. While less effective, oral medications still help manage blood sugars while prioritizing the patient's comfort and overall well-being.

Cancer screenings should be viewed the same way. For adult men, the PSA (prostate-specific antigen) test for prostate cancer is typically part of routine blood work during a checkup. But because most prostate cancers grow very slowly, it's fair to ask—why test at all? Indeed, many doctors have stopped ordering it for this reason. It's not unusual for men in their nineties to die of unrelated causes while harboring prostate cancer that never caused symptoms or spread beyond the prostate. For someone diagnosed with dementia in their sixties or seventies, it is far more likely that they will die from that—not prostate cancer.

By the same token, many of my female patients in their sixties and older have come to me saying they no longer feel the need for an annual mammogram. That could also be reasonable. Small lumps, however, when detected during screening, are easily removed. While such tumors may not be fatal, they can become uncomfortable, and removal might be done for palliative rather than curative reasons. Some patients have also said they're finished with colonoscopies. That decision is more complicated, because colon cancer can come on quickly and be devastating. Again, as with diabetes, when someone has Alzheimer's, we must consider how traumatic the test may be and whether it's worth pursuing.

Many patients are not used to hearing doctors say, "It's okay *not* to do XYZ." We live in a culture where the expectation is that you must do all available screenings. But once a diagnosis of Alzheimer's (or any form of dementia) has been made, all decisions about testing should be made in the context of that diagnosis. I'm intentionally saying *dementia*, not mild cognitive impairment, because if it's still early in the disease process, it makes sense to perform cancer screenings. However, for someone with progressive, later-stage dementia, it's reasonable for a patient to say, "I'm done. I'm not doing the colonoscopy, the mammogram, or the prostate exam again. I'm no longer worried about those conditions."

To some degree, this has to do with the evolution of how society views doctors. My patients grew up in the era of impeccable TV doctors such as Dr. Kildare, *Star Trek*'s Dr. McCoy, and the beloved Marcus Welby, MD, whose show ranked number one in the Nielsen ratings in 1970. Back then, people believed physicians knew everything and could do anything, even perform open-heart surgery on a Vulcan during a space battle. Doctors were treated with that kind of reverence.

Next came the era when patients viewed doctors as cogs and sprockets in a colossal multistate hospital system—tools of a corporate conglomerate. As a result, doctors—fortunately, in my view—instead of being alarmed that they were no longer seen as the hand of God, thought instead, *You know what? I'm a consultant with knowledge and training. People want my opinion, but I don't dictate their lives. I offer my best advice, and patients can make their own informed decisions.* That's a healthier partnership based on mutual respect.

So, as you go forward, consider each treatment plan carefully. Nothing is written in stone or handed down from the mountaintop. If you trust your doctor's recommendations, then proceed knowing you're making an informed decision that works best for you. If, however, what you are being told seems off-kilter, discuss it with the doctor. Finally, if you find yourself consistently at odds with your doctor's approach, it may be time to find another physician.

LEGAL NEXT STEPS

The famed inventor, writer, and Founding Father Benjamin Franklin supposedly said, "By failing to prepare, you are preparing to fail." He learned this lesson from hard experience. Few people think of Franklin as a healer, but he played an influential role in medical debates of his time, especially on the issue of smallpox immunization. To his dying day, he regretted his role as a young man on his older brother's newspaper, the *New England Courant*. Back then the paper raged against what was then a bizarre, controversial practice. But years later, following the death of Franklin's son Francis from smallpox, he editorialized in his own newspaper, the *Pennsylvania Gazette,* in favor of immunization. Not only did he publicly change his stance but he backed his beliefs in favor of inoculations by presenting statistics—then a newfangled science.

Just as Franklin gathered statistics to support his beliefs, it makes sense to prepare thoughtfully for legal issues near the end of life—and to document them with the guidance of an attorney. Legal matters that arise from an Alzheimer's or dementia diagnosis can be complicated and time-consuming. Despite how daunting they are, they must be faced. Few people want to talk about dying and the logistics that follow. But consider this: If you don't address your affairs in advance, your family will have to do so in addition to grieving your death. By failing to prepare, you are shifting this burden onto them. Act now for their benefit, not yours.

An attorney who specializes in elder law can explain your options for protecting assets and making provisions for the future. Look for someone certified by the National Elder Law Foundation (NELF) or trained specifically in the legal rights of older adults. The field continues to evolve, so ask any prospective attorney to describe their experience in elder law.

(Note: I am not a lawyer, and nothing in this section should be interpreted as legal advice.)

The legal process becomes more complicated as the disease progresses. A diagnosis of Alzheimer's does not necessarily mean that a person lacks the mental capacity to make medical or legal decisions. In the more advanced stages, when capacity becomes questionable, the healthcare power of attorney (HCPOA) document can be activated. Activation means the form has been signed by the required medical professionals following an assessment. Until that point, the document does not grant anyone authority; legal medical decision-making remains with the individual.

However, most people living with mild cognitive impairment and mild-stage dementia retain their ability to decide health, legal, and financial matters. Whenever possible, decisions about the future should be determined by the individual.

It is better to conduct advance-care and legal planning with your loved one while their cognitive abilities are intact and before any legal or financial deadlines have been breached. Medicaid, for example, has a look-back window for finances, with each state having a different time period. (*Look-back* means Medicaid will review financial records for several years prior to an application.) My family charted dates of legal importance on a five-year calendar.

There are four (or five) key legal documents that patients and their loved ones need to consider having in place as the disease progresses: (1) a healthcare power of attorney (HCPOA); (2) a living will; (3) a financial power of attorney; (4) a will and/or trust. Let's briefly review each one.

HEALTHCARE POWER OF ATTORNEY (HCPOA)

All adults, regardless of their age or health status, should have an HCPOA. This essential document governs your medical care while you are alive. Your doctor will prioritize having the HCPOA in place because it designates who would make medical decisions when you cannot (i.e., when you're incapacitated), including when you're hospitalized or critically ill. This legal agreement also lists specific wishes about your care, though this can also be outlined in more detail in a separate living will. By contrast, wills (last will and testament) and trusts determine what happens after death. Your family will want to ensure that one or both of these is in place so that your assets are handled according to your preferences.

Frequently, patients come to the hospital after a devastating accident, stroke, or other sudden health crisis. If they do not have an HCPOA, the medical professionals have no notion of what your loved one (the patient) wants. The only way they can make such determinations without an HCPOA is by asking questions of people who are now in crisis.

I have witnessed situations where families do not know a patient's wishes, and this causes the patient undue stress and the family needless suffering. Ultimately, an HCPOA is about who you trust to make medical decisions on your behalf, the types of care desired, and an acceptable end-of-life strategy.

The healthcare power of attorney is a legally binding document that appoints an agent (and backup agent) to make decisions about your healthcare if you cannot. You are giving someone the legal authority to act on your behalf, including scheduling medical appointments, consenting to surgery, or arranging nursing home placement. Life-altering decisions can be made under the authority of the HCPOA, so it is critical for agents to understand a patient's wishes and approach to healthcare. If a specific situation has not been discussed in advance, the HCPOA must rely on what's known as substituted judgment—that is, basing their decision on what the patient likely would have wanted. This is easier said than done. Interpreting a patient's values and preferences should not be done lightly. The HCPOA must be trusted to do what is right for the patient, even if the agent personally disagrees with the decision.

Laws vary by state regarding HCPOAs, and many now offer a standardized form for this purpose. The problem with "one-size-fits-all" documents is that they may restrict your ability to express specific wishes. No matter where you reside, you can always create a new HCPOA if your circumstances or preferences change. Each new version invalidates the last. Keep in mind, your appointed agent may one day end up making life-and-death decisions for you.

When drafting your HCPOA, it's wise to begin thinking about your present and prospective living arrangement. Do you want to move closer to family? If so, which child, sibling, or relative makes the most sense? Or would you prefer to remain in your current community? In that case, you will need to decide between in-home services and care facilities (e.g., senior communities, assisted-living facilities, or nursing homes). Most communities provide a range of support networks, and each should be considered carefully, especially for those living alone. It is better to build your support system early, before a crisis demands it.

The HCPOA is a static document—it does not easily allow for changes, though it can be supplanted by a new one. That's why some preferences, like where you want to live, are best handled through open conversation rather than formal documentation. Including overly specific details in the legal form could restrict your family's flexibility to act in your best interest if circumstances change.

The terms *healthcare power of attorney*, *living will*, and *advanced directive* are sometimes used interchangeably, but they guarantee different protections. A living will outlines the specific medical interventions you do and do not approve to keep you alive, particularly when your heart or lungs stop working. More specifically, it can detail decisions about cardiopulmonary resuscitation (CPR), tube feeding, dialysis, mechanical ventilation, acceptable forms of comfort care, and organ donation. Living wills may also include instructions on general treatments, such as the use of intravenous fluids or antibiotics. While a living will spells out care choices, it does not assign a decision-maker for you, unlike an HCPOA.

Advanced directive is the umbrella term used to include legal documents that provide instructions for medical care, which go into effect when a person cannot make their own decisions. HCPOAs and living wills fall within this category. Frequently, healthcare providers will mistakenly use the expression *advanced directive* to imply that a patient has chosen a do not resuscitate (DNR) order. This narrow and incomplete view should be avoided—it does a disservice to both the patient and family.

FINANCIAL POWER OF ATTORNEY

A financial power of attorney, also known as a durable power of attorney, gives your chosen agent decision-making authority over your financial, legal, and business interests. As with HCPOAs, these documents can either be limited or broad in scope, so be cautious when using a ready-made state form. The power of attorney gives the person you select, sometimes referred to as an *attorney-in-fact*, agency to act on your behalf. This person is not your lawyer; rather, the designation grants them legal authority in your state or jurisdiction. It is another term for *fiduciary*, meaning a person you have entrusted with legal and ethical responsibilities to act in your best interest and to perform duties in a manner as designed by you.

The existence of an HCPOA or financial power of attorney (POA) does not mean you can no longer make decisions for yourself. These documents are typically put in place for potential future use, becoming active only if and when you're no longer able to make informed choices on your own, though some financial POAs are written to take effect immediately upon signing.

For medical decisions, two healthcare providers are generally needed to sign a certificate of incapacity. Depending on the state, this could be a physician (an MD or DO, a doctor of osteopathic medicine), nurse practitioner, or psychologist. Interestingly, only one provider is required to reverse the power of attorney activation (called *deactivation*), a rare occurrence in dementia cases.

Financial POAs follow a different process, and in many cases, no formal declaration of incapacity is required. In some states, an attorney can help activate the document by notifying financial institutions or third parties of the agent's authority.

Once you have formalized a power of attorney, share the document with your financial institutions. You may also choose to add the agent to your accounts as a representative, which is different from naming them as a joint owner. Some institutions may require you to complete their own internal authorization forms before recognizing the POA.

The consequences of not having a healthcare or financial power of attorney can be devastating. Without them, loved ones may be forced to go to court to prove that a person with Alzheimer's is legally incompetent. Besides being a traumatic, time-consuming, and expensive ordeal, decision-making power would be assigned by a judge. The court could select a guardian ad litem (for the purpose of legal action) who is neither a family member nor a friend to make impartial decisions without anyone else's input. This situation should be avoided if at all possible.

No one enjoys spending money on legal fees, but the cost of completing these forms incorrectly is much greater. Ensuring your healthcare instructions are followed and your finances are directed by you is worth the expense. Generic forms, while convenient, may overlook critical legal requirements—such as having the document notarized or signed in the presence of witnesses—that vary by state. A court may not uphold documents that fail to meet all legal requirements and could declare them invalid.

In some cases, completing an HCPOA can be done at no cost. Many healthcare institutions offer this service through trained social workers or care coordinators, and using your state's official HCPOA form is often the best route. Your medical provider can direct you to in-house staff who are familiar with the legal and logistical details. Once you have completed the form, be sure to share a copy with your healthcare institution so it's available in your medical record. I also encourage families to take photos of their healthcare legal documents with their smartphones so they have them at their fingertips should they ever be at a hospital that doesn't already have their loved one's records.

Just as important as completing the forms are the conversations that go with it. A helpful approach is to reflect on real-life examples—"Remember when Uncle Charlie was sick and chose X? What would you want in that situation?" Asking your loved one what they value most in their health and finances can be a powerful guide for future decision-making.

The bottom line? To quote Charles Dickens, "The law is a ass." In British parlance when he wrote *Oliver Twist*, he was referring to a donkey, not a part of the body. Frankly, either meaning works. If that quote is insufficiently chastening, consider this Chinese proverb: Avoid law courts in life as you would hell in death. The message is clear: Protect yourself and your loved ones by getting the best legal advice you can when it comes to healthcare and financial powers of attorney.

WILLS AND TRUSTS

Having a proper will or trust in place will alleviate a number of problems at death. When a person dies without a will—known as *intestate* in legalese—state laws determine how assets are distributed and debts are paid. Typically, the surviving spouse and children take precedence over other parties, but this may not always be the case. However, relying on statutes (laws) means the state, instead of you, decides how your estate will be disbursed. It's far better to clearly express your wishes in a will or trust and pay the legal fees up front than to leave matters up to the government.

But what is a trust? Aren't those only for very wealthy people? That's a myth. A trust is a legal arrangement that allows a third party, called a trustee, to hold and manage assets on behalf of someone else. It creates a simple and straightforward inventory of holdings, but it will trigger a separate tax return, so it's best to consult with an accountant or financial institution when setting one up. A trust basically works hand in glove with a will. Both can be used to dispose of your estate, but a trust offers added benefits. Trusts help you bypass probate, which is a time-consuming and bureaucratic court process. By avoiding probate, your affairs are kept private rather than becoming part of the public record. You'll also save on the legal fees of going through this clerical court process, which can add up to thousands, and assets will be distributed more efficiently. This matters because probate can drag on for months or even years while your family waits to access your funds, which they may need sooner.

In addition to their advantages after you die, trusts can also support you while you're still alive and managing your assets. In some circumstances, a trust can even reduce estate taxes. On the other hand, it may also require annual reviews and come with administrative expenses. Keep in mind that having a trust does not inherently mean you have a financial power of attorney in place, so it's important to understand the specifics of your trust to ensure you know what additional steps may be necessary. As with HCPOAs and financial powers of attorney, consult with an attorney to determine what's best for your situation.

Not having a financial power of attorney is a gamble. So is going without a trust or will. If you were to have a stroke next week, your spouse or children might be unable to access your checking, savings, and investment accounts. They could be left unable to pay your mortgage or manage basic monthly expenses. These legal documents not only prevent such negative outcomes but can also protect against fraud. If a trusted loved one or agent has access to financial accounts, they can keep an eye on them and watch for suspicious activity or scams.

Lastly, proceeds from life insurance policies, retirement plans, and investment accounts will go directly to the listed beneficiaries. Remember to periodically review the people designated on each document and keep them up to date. These assets will be distributed according to the named beneficiaries, even if your will or trust says otherwise.

ADVANCE CARE PLANNING

"We [your loved ones] can't do what you want if we don't know what that is," says the organization Honoring Choices, based in La Crosse, Wisconsin. It doesn't get much more straightforward than that. Honoring Choices provides information and a stepwise plan to help people articulate, verbally and in writing, their preferences for future care. Programs like this may also offer patients and families the option to engage in advance care planning (ACP) meetings to navigate these conversations.

An ACP session is a semistructured encounter with a professional facilitator that sketches out your future medical care before finalizing legal documents such as HCPOA, financial POA, wills, and trusts with an attorney. Often the facilitator is a social worker or someone with supportive counseling experience who is well versed in healthcare and familiar with the basics of estate planning. They have specialized training to navigate difficult conversations between patients and families with empathy and in a nonjudgmental fashion.

During ACP meetings, patients and families may go over advanced directives, living wills, and HCPOAs, discussing in detail the patient's wishes for care, especially during the dying process. While they may address financial POAs, wills, and trusts, an attorney is still required to draft, formalize, and register any legal documents initiated through the session.

Estate and elder law attorneys can execute HCPOAs, but they are likely not as knowledgeable about specific medical situations where the topics of tube feeding, certain medications, and chest compressions are discussed. In contrast, the ACP facilitators are better equipped to guide patients and families through these complex scenarios. They will likely refer patients back to their primary care provider, especially for discussions on code status or DNR orders. While the facilitator can cover these topics, the PCP is best positioned to explain the medical risks and outcomes in depth and to complete the necessary documentation.

Emotional outbursts in the ACP meetings that I've attended run the gamut—from shouting matches to silent sobs. This is especially true when patients express their wish to not be resuscitated or to have life support withdrawn; such declarations can be unsettling for spouses and children to hear. Yet most sessions do conclude with tenderness and affection, restoring my faith in the resilience of family ties.

Even if you don't live in Wisconsin, where Honoring Choices is based, the organization has a national network that extends to nine other states, and similar programs may exist in your area. I recommend visiting the website honoringchoices.org for its commonsense advice.

WHO DO YOU TRUST TO BE YOUR AGENT?

I recently had a fascinating experience with a patient and her husband, both of whom had mild cognitive impairment. We talked about driving safety, firearms, assisted living, stress, and financial management. I asked them who was in their "circle of trust." They said they trusted their son completely and had already given him access to their investment accounts. He had even met with their accountant and financial adviser, but there was a catch. They didn't want to give their son financial power of attorney.

When I asked why, their answer caught me a little off guard. "We want him here," they said. "But we don't want him telling us what to do, and we don't want him judging how we live."

"That's perfectly understandable," I replied. I suggested they consider having a family meeting and saying, "We're worried, son. Would you be willing to help? But there are a couple of boundaries—like our day-to-day decisions and lifestyle—that we are not willing to budge on."

In every family there will be nuances in how financial, health, or legal matters are handled. In many cases, all it takes is a frank but low-key conversation around the kitchen table. Take a deep breath and have those talks. You will likely be glad you did. One honest conversation can get ahead of years of worry.

How do you go about selecting an agent you can count on to carry out your wishes? Remember—you want that person to think the way *you* do and honor *your* desires. Let's say you have two children—Emily lives down the street, and Patrick lives across the country. If you generally see eye to eye with Emily and spend time with her regularly, she's likely your best choice. Even if Emily isn't a perfect choice, she may still be the better fit, especially if you and Patrick rarely communicate or struggle to get along.

Patients and families often ask me for advice about who they should choose as an agent. Because every family is different, there's no one-size-fits-all solution. The person you pick should be someone who would make the choices you would make—who knows how you view healthcare, how you want to live going forward, and how you want to die. A spouse is often the first choice to serve as the agent, but what if he or she is in poor health?

In my experience, proximity to the loved one, along with the quality of the relationship, often turns out to be the deciding factor. The nearby child is usually the one taking the parent to medical appointments, shopping for groceries, and either overseeing or providing home care. Yet that child may be less in tune with the parent than a more thoughtful, and possibly more capable, sibling who lives farther away. Whether the nearby child becomes the agent for legal or healthcare matters is ultimately the patient's decision, but when it comes to daily life, the local child is almost always the de facto decision-maker.

What I often see in my practice when a patient has several children is that one may be smart and caring but lives far away, and with the best of intentions, he upsets an existing care plan. Sometimes he has better ideas than the nearby primary caregiver, but when a geographically far-off yet well-meaning child swoops in from the airport with ideas and plans that are dramatically different, this one-man sibling tornado can create a lot of upset. While some of his suggestions may be reasonable and heartfelt, he isn't living in the home, and his suggestions often turn out to be impracticable in the face of day-to-day life.

For me, the bottom line is this: When it comes to Alzheimer's caregiving, you've got to go with what works. If you face this type of "swoop-down" management from afar, remember—that family member is making suggestions because they love their parent and want to help. And if you happen to be the "child from California," as I sometimes call such family members from where I sit in Wisconsin, remember who is shouldering the day-to-day burden of care. Try to approach the situation with compassion—for your parent and for the sibling managing the hard, unglamorous parts of caregiving. The last thing either child should want to do is unnecessarily upset a parent who has Alzheimer's. Mom will likely be unable to adjudicate disputes the way she did when you were fighting over G.I. Joes or Barbies. Be an adult. As I wrote in the beginning of this chapter, take a deep breath. Maybe take ten.

Confronting caregiving for a parent with a long-term illness can bring out the best—and worst—in families. Sometimes two siblings are involved who never got along, and there's only so much a doctor or social worker can do to resolve such conflict. In such cases, we may suggest family counseling. Sometimes it helps. Sadly, in many cases, it doesn't. One tactic my social worker uses is to bring two battling children together in the same room with their parent. She gets everyone talking, and sometimes, when the right questions are asked and the room feels safe, they start to open up to other perspectives.

One last point—I recommend having an alternate agent (or agents) on your HCPOAs and financial powers of attorney, in case your primary choice is ever unable to serve. Life happens. The first-named person may pass away, become incapacitated, or simply no longer feel up to the responsibility. By the same token, if you signed your HCPOA or other legal documents years ago, now is a good time to review them. Make sure your agent is still willing and able to carry out your wishes.

If I had to sum up this section in two words, they would be "invest early." If you already have a will (and possibly a trust), an HCPOA, and a financial power of attorney, great. Take a moment to revisit them and confirm they're still current. If you haven't yet explored these documents, don't wait for the "right" time. The best time to act isn't tomorrow. It's now.

Supporting Emotional Well-Being After Diagnosis

Moving forward after a diagnosis of cognitive impairment starts with one essential step: embracing where you are. From that place of understanding, it becomes possible to develop strategies for living meaningfully—with clarity, intention, and joy. For one person, that might mean learning how to paint; for another, it could mean taking cooking lessons, improving gardening skills, doing woodworking, or practicing flower arranging. The trick is to find the activity that helps calm your soul, lift your spirits, and challenge your brain.

Having this positive attitude is rooted in acceptance and purposeful adaptation, and it lies at the heart of the work I do alongside my colleague Dr. Adrienne Johnson, a health psychologist at the UW Health Geriatric Memory Clinics. Together, we've seen firsthand that emotional resilience is as important as medical treatment in helping patients chart a fulfilling path ahead.

To meet this need, Dr. Johnson launched a specialty psychotherapy clinic in UW Health's geriatric memory clinical program. It offers short-term, evidence-based support for individuals with mild cognitive impairment or mild dementia, conditions that carry an increased risk of anxiety and depression yet often go untreated in terms of mental healthcare.

Patients referred to the clinic receive care through acceptance and commitment therapy (ACT), an approach that is rooted in mindfulness, values, and behavior change. Many studies have supported its effectiveness in treating anxiety, depression, and medical comorbidities (the presence of two or more diseases in a patient). ACT helps patients build psychological flexibility and find ways to engage meaningfully with their lives, even as they face the uncertainty of a progressive disease.

The therapy is highly personalized. Sessions are shaped by each individual's concerns and priorities, and care partners are encouraged to attend. Common themes include grief over loss of independence, difficulty communicating with loved ones, changes in identity, and fear about the future. Patients are taught tools to accept difficult thoughts and feelings and to take meaningful, positive action anchored in their own deeply held values.

One of the most empowering concepts in ACT is adaptability. Older adults have often spent their lives adjusting to major transitions—marriage, parenting, careers, retirement. When patients are encouraged to view this diagnosis as another life transition, they often rediscover their capacity to adapt. By focusing on what they can control—how they spend their time, how they connect with others, how they live their values—they find purpose and peace in the present.

Connect with your doctor, talk with available therapists, and recognize you're stronger than you know. Instead of rebelling against what you cannot change, accept it. It may seem illogical, but this recognition creates inner peace, resilience, and feelings of self-control.

GOOD HABITS, GOOD ROUTINES—GOOD RESULTS

"How do you know what stage of Alzheimer's my mom is in? What criteria are you using, and how will we know she's progressing?" Families understandably want to know where their loved one falls on the continuum of decline and what tomorrow might look like. Unfortunately, doctors are surprisingly poor at prognosticating, and the clinical scales available are far from precise.

The scientific literature sets forth either three broad stages (mild, moderate, severe) or seven more detailed levels (ranging from early and mild to late and severe). The terminology can be confusing—and often feels restrictive to families witnessing far more than what is described at each phase. Staging, however, remains a valuable tool for planning.

Many people find comfort in knowing that they're still early in the progression of the disease, with symptoms that are relatively mild. But they will need to juxtapose that current reality against more severe developments that lie ahead, which few people want to hear about. At every stage, one principle holds true: Establishing routines that become second nature—habits for both patient and caregiver—goes a long way. Familiar patterns provide stability, reduce stress, and can ease transitions as the disease progresses.

All of us, whether we are adults or children, benefit from keeping to a schedule. People with Alzheimer's are no exception. Daily routines help reduce the stress and anxiety someone with MCI or dementia might experience. Regular activities create structure and add purpose to daily life. These pleasant activities reduce agitation and lead to balanced emotions and contentment.

Remember that the brain, through entrainment, discussed in chapter 1, has the ability to cement routines into the cerebral cortex. This happens by strengthening neural networks so that the same ones fire together with less effort each time. Repeated behaviors, even those that don't require conscious thought, like eating and drinking, walking, singing, brushing teeth, and using the toilet on a schedule, can continue to be performed with modifications as the disease advances.

When creating routines, consider your loved one's interests and strengths, the time of day he's at his best, and how he once organized his day. Here are some categories for habit formation that might spark ideas: meals (helping with preparation), creative activities (painting or making music), physical movement (going for walks), chores (helping around the house or yard), spiritual practices (going to church or daily mass), shopping, and socializing with neighbors. Caring for a pet or plant or helping someone else in a manageable way can also provide daily structure. People benefit from having a sense of purpose and often take joy in being helpful to others—even in small ways.

I recommend waking up and going to bed at consistent times for everyone, especially caregivers. As toy inventor E. Joseph Cossman said, "The best bridge between despair and hope is a good night's sleep."

On average it takes 66 days for a new behavior to become a habit, but the range is wide—from 18 to 254 days—depending on the circumstances and person. Some people have a head start on consistent bedtimes or a morning routine. The key is regularity. Habits should not be arbitrarily applied to how you are feeling in the moment. The longer you persist, the more deeply it becomes ingrained in long-term memory, even in the face of Alzheimer's.

Power of Habit: Routines Strengthen the Brain

A toothbrush is small, but the impact of using one is huge. Behind this daily ritual lies the potential to reconnect a person to his day—and to himself. In the end, the path to brain health may be as humble as a habit repeated with care.

"Habits as simple as brushing your teeth at the same time each morning can help your brain adapt to changes from cognitive impairment," says occupational therapist Dr. Gordon Giles. Few tools are as accessible and undervalued as habit, according to Giles, who is a professor emeritus at Samuel Merritt University in Oakland, California.

In my conversation with him, he made the case that habits and routines are more than behavioral conveniences—they are neurological interventions. Especially for individuals with mild cognitive impairment (MCI) or early-stage dementia, routines offer structure, predictability, and—most important—opportunity for neural reinforcement.

When behaviors are repeated consistently, they become automatic. This frees up mental energy for higher-order thinking and decision-making. Automaticity, says Giles, isn't just efficiency—it's resilience.

One habit he recommends is planning mealtimes. Eating meals at the same time each day provides rhythmic structure, minimizes the burden of decision-making, and helps orient a person to time and sequence. Over time, even small, predictable routines like this become anchors that steady the day.

Repetition creates structure, and structure becomes

familiarity—a crucial factor for people with cognitive impairment who may struggle with novelty or unpredictability. Routines also reduce decision fatigue, minimize confusion, and promote self-efficacy.

One of the best things about this approach is its accessibility. Habits require no prescriptions or high-tech devices—just the gentle force of consistency.

Giles's perspective is shaped by a philosophy of aging and adaptation known as selection, optimization, and compensation. "Everyone adapts," he says. "I'm sixty-seven, and I don't run up hills anymore. I've optimized what I can do. I still lift weights. I hike. I ride my bike. I do things that let me keep living the way I want." This mindset—choosing what matters most, doing it as well as you can, and compensating where needed—is a cornerstone of his approach, especially in the context of memory loss. For example, selecting one consistent time for a daily phone call, optimizing it with a quiet space, and compensating with a calendar reminder makes that connection sustainable.

Giles also reminds us that "motivation isn't always necessary for learning. By making the process rewarding and consistent—like afternoon walks with hats for shade—habitual patterns emerge almost naturally." This insight is especially relevant in dementia care, where repeated action, not internal drive, often yields lasting routine.

Technology, often seen as either a crutch or a complication, is for Giles a practical ally. "I use alarms on my phone. I automate bill payments. I set routines that reinforce behavior." For those with memory issues, smartphones and smart home devices can serve as reliable cues. When used consistently, these external prompts fade as internal habits form—solid, silent, and sustaining. And while newer tech helps, many older adults are already deeply attuned to the rhythms of traditional routines—like watching the evening news or *Jeopardy!* Tying a new habit to an old one, such as walking around the block before a favorite show, can make the new behavior easier to remember and reinforce.

Dr. Giles reframes habit from mundane repetition to meaningful therapy. Routines are miniature acts of self-organization and identity preservation. They offer structure when cognition falters, empower autonomy when memory fades, and enable a sense of continuity that is both psychological and biological.

Of course, setting routines is only part of the equation. Just as important is coming to terms with your diagnosis and learning to live with confidence and follow-through. Even when the reality feels daunting, recognizing what's happening can make it easier to live with greater consistency and stability. (See sidebar on page 149: "Supporting Emotional Well-Being After Diagnosis.")

In some families, a parent with Alzheimer's may live with one child for a few weeks and then stay with another family member for a few more. While well intentioned, this is not ideal because it interferes with the formation of habits. The parent is going to forget important details or become confused. Houses and families are different. Transitioning from one home to another is going to be a hard adjustment. Anytime a routine or environment changes, it creates anxiety for someone with Alzheimer's. They feel on edge and become more forgetful or disoriented. They might lash out in frustration. It's not unusual for an adult child in this situation to call my practice and say, "Mom's so confused." That's because the family keeps moving her every two weeks. Of course she's going to feel uneasy and less secure. Habits and routines ground us, making all of us feel safe. They're comforting.

If you're not walking or exercising every day, you're failing to support your brain. If you're eating ultra-processed meals instead of whole foods, your brain is not getting the nutrients it needs. When I was in high school and college, I played tennis all the time; my hero was Andre Agassi, who was once the world's number one tennis champion. In 1992, Agassi, now in his mid-fifties, confessed to *Sports Illustrated* his love for Taco Bell and junk food. Since then he's reformed his diet and starts his days with hot lemon water. It is never too late to make progress. Go slowly. No one has to run a marathon right out of the gate or try to crush the competition at Wimbledon. If you expect silver cup results overnight, you're setting yourself up for disappointment. Slow and steady wins the race.

Some people with Alzheimer's are sedentary. They lounge in front of a computer or watch TV all day. This isn't surprising given that the Centers for Disease Control and Prevention (CDC) reported 25 percent of U.S. adults are physically inactive. That's true of many caregivers as well. Stress is tiring and habitual, and that is a recipe for the formation and continuation of bad habits. But even for someone who's been inactive for most of their life—a "lifetime couch potato"—movement is still possible. We can create new habits one small step at a time.

For people who don't like to move, start with something that feels natural or necessary. Ask them to help with light household chores. Get them to go up and down stairs by asking for help bringing items to the kitchen, laundry, or dining table. Encourage errands that involve walking—like returning library books, grabbing the groceries from the car, or browsing a big-box store. A pet can be a helpful motivator, especially if the person feels responsible for its care. Others may respond better if movement is connected to something they enjoy: going to a favorite place, socializing, or getting a (hopefully healthy) treat.

You can also turn movement into moments of purpose: watering plants, setting the table, folding towels, or checking the weather outside. For some, music can be a powerful tool—try turning on a favorite song and inviting them to sway, tap, or dance. Even sitting exercises, like marching in place from a chair or stretching to a rhythm, can help build momentum.

For motivated individuals, make a plan, schedule your week in advance, and say to yourself, *I'm going to walk this far, even if it's just going to the mailbox or around the block*. Write down what you do each day. When walking around the block becomes too easy, challenge yourself to go farther. Other tricks to building good habits include doing them at the same time every day and associating them with special clothes such as dazzling yellow running shoes only used for exercise. The key is to keep it simple, relevant, and repetitive—and to celebrate small wins. Motivation may not come first; often, it follows action.

What about existing bad habits like drinking and smoking, both of which harm brain health and can worsen Alzheimer's? In the best circumstances, everyone in the household who smokes stops, and everyone who drinks either quits or limits their use of alcohol. The same is true of eating excessive amounts of candy, other sweets, and junk food. Use the diagnosis of Alzheimer's or cognitive impairment as a motivator to improve the health of everyone in the household. If you deny a person with Alzheimer's access to liquor, sometimes they will forget they ever drank.

By the same token, people with Alzheimer's may forget to eat, which can interfere with sleep, cause dizziness and falls, negatively affect mood, and lead to difficulty recovering from even minor illnesses. Keeping healthy foods well stocked and leaving easy-to-eat, wholesome options visible on the counter can help encourage better choices throughout the day. Serving healthy food on a regular schedule supports their nutrition and benefits everyone at the table. (For more on healthy habits, see the next chapter.)

OPTIMIZE HEALTH, DON'T JUST MANAGE IT

When someone is diagnosed with cognitive impairment, it's vital not only to develop routines but also to optimize their other medical conditions. That means doing more than just accepting "okay" blood sugar, blood pressure, or cholesterol levels. It means aiming for the *best possible control* of chronic conditions with as few side effects as possible.

That means addressing every chronic ailment with intention—glucose, cholesterol, blood pressure, weight, kidney function, thyroid balance, inflammation, mental health, and anything related to the cardiovascular system. All these factors influence cognitive function, and all deserve attention. At the same time, your doctor will also take a hard look at your medications. Are they still necessary? Is each drug being used at the *lowest effective dose*? Do your supplements make sense?

With lifestyle changes, appropriate medications, and close medical follow-ups, the status of a chronic disease can often be improved, sometimes reversed. It might mean working with a health coach, dietitian, or personal trainer, or even getting a second opinion. It's worth it.

Take blood pressure, for example. In dementia care, doctors often allow higher-than-normal levels—a practice called *permissive hypertension*—to avoid the risks of dizziness and falls from low blood pressure. That concern is valid, but it must be weighed against the evidence that links uncontrolled high blood pressure with faster cognitive decline. The goal should be the *lowest blood pressure a person can safely tolerate.* If changes are necessary, they should start with lifestyle modifications and then add medications when needed.

The same issue arises in diabetes care. People with cognitive impairment are often permitted to run higher blood sugars to avoid hypoglycemia. While caution is understandable, poorly controlled diabetes can worsen cognitive function. That's why it's important to be proactive—safely bringing HbA1c levels down, starting with diet and exercise and supported by medications when appropriate.

In short, seeking a safe but optimal target is better than complacently doing nothing. Cognitive health depends on systemic health. It's not enough to just tread water—your doctor should be helping patients with Alzheimer's *thrive.*

Mrs. Chin Remembers—Explore the World Around You

Don't lock yourself inside. Do things you and your loved one always wanted to do. These can be adventures, not just trips to the grocery store.

About a year after Moe was diagnosed, we flew from Madison, Wisconsin, to San Francisco for a family wedding. Moe did very well. I was probably more hesitant to go than anyone else. My children encouraged me to make the trip.

It wasn't totally easy either. It was winter. Our flight was canceled, and we had to come back home and wait for the next day's flight. Anytime you change the routine of someone with cognitive problems, it adds to their stress, which makes life more stressful for the person taking care of them.

So, we had to go to the airport twice. When we got there the second time, Moe was congenial, just as he had always been until close to the end. I sat next to him at the gate. He struck up a conversation with the gentleman on his other side, telling a nice story about when he saw patients. Five minutes later, he told the same anecdote. The man Moe was talking to got that look on his face like "I just heard that." I didn't say anything, because that would have embarrassed my husband. He didn't know he'd repeated himself—and there was no reason he needed to.

I admit traveling was harder than it used to be, but Moe was still in fine shape. I didn't feel that he had any problems. He could go to the bathroom by himself. He could be left alone. There were many things he was capable of doing.

I'm always amazed by people who don't do things with their loved one, though I empathize with their hesitation. You could always change your mind, change your plan, or do something else. The point is, you don't want to be homebound. Dementia takes a long time between diagnosis and death. That would be a long time to not do anything. A long time.

There is meaning in each day, so take action. Live a little. Don't hesitate. You can always turn around.

EVERYONE NEEDS SUPPORT

Social connections save lives. Research shows that seniors who have adequate social support have less cognitive decline than those who are solitary. Social isolation does not cause Alzheimer's, but studies have found that a lack of meaningful interactions with people heightens the risk of dementia. And today, with more people living far from family members, and our world increasingly busy and modern, one in four older Americans reports loneliness. It's not just those with Alzheimer's who need social stimulation, but their caregivers can also suffer from feeling isolated, a characteristic that induces stress and leads to depression.

Who are your people? Are you married? Do you have children? Extended family? Close friends? Do you have a pet who is your loyal companion? Are you involved with any organizations or social service programs—a church, synagogue, or a local civic or hobby group? If the answer to some (or all) of these questions is no, don't despair. A place where you can go to start building community is your local Alzheimer's organization or senior center. Your doctor and Area Agency on Aging will also have ideas.

Sharing your diagnosis with family, friends, and neighbors is an important step in creating a support network. You may be surprised at how they respond; people's compassion and generosity can spontaneously emerge when given the opportunity. One of my nurses told me that when members of her church "shared the peace" (greeted each other) during the Sunday service, a man who had just been diagnosed with mild cognitive impairment told the news to every person with whom he shook hands. She found that remarkable—and his bravery paid off. Members of the congregation approached him and his wife to learn how they could help.

So don't let old-fashioned notions hold you back. Being the strong, silent type may work in the movies, but in real life when people share their needs and reach out, more often than not, others will respond with kindness. By allowing yourself to be vulnerable, you show strength of character, which in turn opens the door for others to step up and offer genuine help.

Unfortunately, old friends can fade away. They may not want to see the decline that ensues or be reminded of what the future could hold for them. Whatever their reasons, they stop calling or inviting you to gatherings, and you slowly drift apart. Greg and Sandy, who lived directly across the road from my parents, were different. They were invaluable. When my dad could no longer move from the bed to the wheelchair, Greg came over to lift and transfer him. This went on for months.

Don't waste energy on resentment if longtime friends disappear. Others may emerge just when you need them most. Sometimes, stoic politeness keeps people at a distance—they worry that reaching out would feel like an intrusion into your difficult circumstances. Once informed, they may surprise you with their willingness to help.

When these folks show up, let them know how they can help and where you want space. It's okay to be specific and to draw boundaries. One person might drop by on Thursday afternoons or help with the yard. Another might enjoy going for walks or cooking the occasional meal. Or maybe you simply need someone to stay with your loved one once a month so you can get a haircut, or every Friday morning so you can have coffee with a friend. You'll never know unless you put yourself out there.

Sometimes it helps to bring a loved one to a doctor's appointment, especially if they haven't been intimately involved. They may not realize how serious the situation is or what the needs are now and in the future. You can sign a release of information form to authorize any individual you choose to speak with the doctor or medical team outside of clinic visits. Important medical information usually needs to be conveyed more than once, and in different settings. Often the child or friend will say, "Oh, I didn't realize the situation was this severe." The power of information is that it leads to action; in healthcare, it leads to interventions and support. The catch is that you have to inform loved ones and involve them.

Unfortunately, people with MCI and dementia often become isolated. This happens more often in rural areas where services are less available and driving is necessary. Isolation leads not only to loneliness but also to negative health outcomes like depression, anxiety, physical inactivity, unhealthy diet, and disrupted sleep. Services like home-delivered meals, pharmacy-prepackaged medications, in-home companion care, or help with indoor and outdoor chores can improve people's health and well-being. Whatever your social situation, don't hesitate to contact your doctor's office. This is an emotional process, and a medical assistant, nurse, or social worker will reinforce messages the doctor has given and provide ways to implement change.

Finally, if you are a caregiver, friend, or relative, respect the autonomy of a person with Alzheimer's. They should make their own decisions so far as it is practical and safe. People have the right to make decisions, even if it's not the "correct choice" or one we think they should make. You and I are free to make poor choices without anyone calling us out on it or stepping in.

Just because a person has dementia doesn't mean we should think, *You can't do that, and we're going to make you do it our way.* Forcing someone against their preferences will only lead to resistance and struggle. Instead, if a certain behavior is preferable, try to plant a seed by talking about it periodically and explaining how it could benefit them. It is not threatening or controlling to say every once in a while, "You know, it might be helpful for you to have some company in your house." One day the message might land, and when it does, you can be there to provide help with the next steps.

When I was in my final year of college and applying to medical schools, I told my parents I was considering my state school, the University of Wisconsin School of Medicine and Public Health, where I had been offered a scholarship. I had also been accepted to programs in other states, and during a family brunch, Erin—who would later become my wife—and I announced that I was leaning toward either Brown University or Oregon Health Sciences University. I was eager to live in a coastal city, and frankly, it didn't matter which coast. My dad was immediately congratulatory, but my mom's response was more pointed. "We will not be funding that," she said. I looked at her with exasperation and replied, "You told me you'd honor my decision." Without missing a beat, she retorted, "That was because I assumed you'd make the right one."

Although I was angry at the time, I'm now grateful for my mother's strong conviction. Staying in Wisconsin gave me four more years with my father—before his diagnosis—while he was in the prime of his life. Sometimes a little flexibility—along with a willingness to adapt and listen—can have its virtues and lead to unexpected gifts.

Memory care also relies on clear communication, though ideally in a more tactful way than my mom's verdict on my medical school deliberation. Patients and families need all the information, but it needs to be delivered gradually and at their pace. The medical team's role is to provide guidance and remain available for support. Families can do the same: honoring dignity by allowing personal decision-making, even when choices are imperfect. And if a decision becomes unsafe, they can step in with support and suggest alternatives.

For caregivers, it's helpful to ask yourself, *What does my mom (or dad or spouse) want?* And be honest—sometimes you know exactly what they want, even if it's not what you think they should want. The goal is to act in accordance with their values, not your own preferences. It's important to reflect on the situation and your role. You may not agree with the outcome, but keeping your loved one at the center of care is key. For example, years before one of my patients developed dementia, she made a down payment and completed everything necessary to move into a superb senior living community. The facility consisted of graduated housing from fully independent to round-the-clock nursing care. One of its best aspects was its location around the corner from where her children lived. Yet when her Alzheimer's progressed, she lost all interest in leaving the condominium where she had moved in with a son. Her decision was to stay put. Though it caused strife among her children and hardship for the child she lived with, her children respected her choice. She passed away in accordance with her long-standing desire to die at home in her own bed. She was her own person, and she decided how she wanted to live—and end—her life. Her wishes were upheld by those who loved her. That's how it should be, when possible.

Growing up, I became familiar early on with Frank Lloyd Wright, a fellow Wisconsin native and renowned architect known for designing buildings in harmony with their surroundings. Harmony, in this sense, is about balance and unity—an agreement in action that withstands even harsh challenges. Let this principle guide your relationships, especially with a loved one who has Alzheimer's. As Wright once said, "The longer I live, the more beautiful life becomes."

You won't always agree on everything, but seeking harmony—rather than control—can carry you through the hardest days.

5

"Yes, You Can Live the Good Life"

BUILD STRONG HABITS, REDUCE RISK, AND SLOW PROGRESSION

Set Reasonable Goals • Why Walking Works • "Keystone Habits" • The Red Wine Myth • MIND Diet Saves Money • Healthy Gut Ecosystem for Brain Health • Soothing Sleep Tips • Can Crosswords Help? • The Deafness-Dementia Connection

Stability is the victory.

Let me explain. I recently diagnosed an eighty-two-year-old carpenter named Randolph with mild cognitive impairment. We discussed the benefits of healthy diet choices and daily exercise (intentional movement to get his heart rate elevated and keep it up for a period of time). No more soda and cookies throughout the day. Additionally, I asked him to replace his naps on the couch with a walk outside. As I spoke, I noticed his wife's eyes had fixed on me. Her emphatic nodding was the affirmation I was looking for to help Randolph construct these new habits.

He had spent his life framing houses, designing custom interiors, and creating handcrafted furniture in his fully equipped basement workshop. He thrived on hard work, and he knew the satisfaction of a job well done. He listened and was quiet during most of our visit. His pursed lips and serious expression mirrored his wife's. As he left, in a voice so low I could barely hear him, he said, "I'll see what I can do."

A year later, Randolph and his wife were excited to see me. He was walking every day and no longer ate junk food or drank soda. As an added benefit, he had almost entirely stopped drinking beer and eating red meat. My referral to a sleep clinic led to a diagnosis of obstructive sleep apnea and a prescription for a CPAP (continuous positive airway pressure) machine. It now greatly reduced the moments during the night when his breathing stopped, disrupted his rest, and interfered with his brain's health. After a few months of adjustments, Randolph was sleeping better and no longer felt the need to nap during the day.

The latest cognitive test scores showed improvement. Mild cognitive impairment was still present, but his disease progression was halted. Despite still having symptoms, Randolph was deservedly proud because his medical condition had stabilized due to his dedication. He had worked on himself, polishing his behavior just as he had for many years transformed rough wood into beautiful, strong furniture. For him, stability was indeed a victory. His resolve impressed me. With the encouragement of his wife, he had made so many positive transformations that even I was pleasantly surprised by his dogged determination. His actions, not his words, spoke volumes.

Randolph's story is not an exception. During the course of a month, I see at least a handful of returning patients who have improved their circumstances. Many have stopped drinking and quit smoking because they are pressed into action by the fear of dementia. It may sound strange to say it, but that prognosis can be a powerful incentive to improve one's life, health, and well-being.

* * *

As Dr. Benjamin Spock famously advised new parents, "You know more than you think you do." It's the same for older people, even those who have received a life-changing diagnosis. Most people know what they need to do, but what they struggle with is *how* to do it, *how* to get started.

Talking about brain health—and acting on those discussions—represents a meaningful, person-centric mindset to ward off dementia and reduce the fear and stigma that surround it. People with proven Alzheimer's proteins in their brain will still benefit from lifestyle interventions. By building resiliency in the brain, people can forestall or delay symptoms associated with dementia. This buffer against decline, created by healthy lifestyle habits, has additional benefits that can be appreciated immediately, too.

A few decades ago, an Alzheimer's diagnosis meant that a person had about eight years to live with limited established treatments. Some patients described devastating experiences of being given a curt (and deeply hurtful) "Get your affairs in order" command from a doctor following their diagnosis. Behind closed doors, people in the medical profession called this "diagnose and then adios." Thankfully, such days are gone—or at least on their way out. We now have a host of options and opportunities, thanks to advances in science. This chapter will delve into implementing those new brain-healthy habits and demonstrating how we are slowing Alzheimer's progression.

REPAIRING THE MIND'S WEB

The Lancet, one of the world's most prestigious medical journals, created a multidisciplinary international commission on dementia prevention. These leading experts developed and categorized fourteen *modifiable* risk factors that could prevent or delay up to *45 percent* of all dementia cases. Growing old is a certainty, but it turns out there are dozens of ways to cut the risk for cognitive impairment.

Fourteen Alzheimer's Risk Factors

From a population standpoint, nearly half of all cases of dementia could be prevented by addressing these fourteen lifestyle factors:

EARLY LIFE

1. Less education

MIDLIFE

2. Hearing loss
3. High blood pressure
4. High LDL cholesterol
5. Diabetes
6. Obesity
7. Physical inactivity
8. Depression
9. Smoking
10. Alcohol use
11. Traumatic brain injury

LATE LIFE

12. Social isolation
13. Vision loss
14. Air pollution

Some of the potential harmful variables are no surprise—diabetes, high blood pressure, obesity, smoking, drinking too much alcohol, and physical inactivity. Living a healthy life clearly makes a difference. While lifelong habits are best, it's never too late to start. Newly adopted changes can still deliver meaningful benefits, even in older adulthood. Exercise, in particular, plays a major role in staving off dementia.

The commission agreed that, in mid-to-late life, depression, social isolation, and even air pollution also contributed to risk. Soot, smoke, and other airborne toxins may enter the bloodstream and interfere with cognition—possibly through inflammation and oxidative stress—but they may also impair the blood vessels' ability to clear waste from the brain. Such debris includes amyloid and tau, which are normally present in the brain but appear in great excess in Alzheimer's cases.

The Lancet's commission of experts concluded that in early life, addressing lower educational attainment levels—by extending years of schooling and improving the quality of instruction—could reduce dementia cases by 5 percent. Rigorous learning at any age, however, creates more neural networks and thus more backup systems in the brain.

Think of the brain's physiological network as being like a spiderweb. Every axon or dendrite is like a thread of silk, and every place where they meet is a neuron. Just as each spiral in the web performs a specific function, so does the brain's neural network. Consider how often the wind wrecks a spiderweb and the next day a fully functional replacement has materialized.

I'd like to apply that webbing regeneration ability to brain health. "Some scientists believe a spider's mind radiates out through the strands of its web beyond the limits of its body . . . it's a map of the spider's memories," according to the PBS documentary *Is a Spider's Web a Part of Its Mind?* Our latest Alzheimer's research suggests that, like the spider, we also have the ability not just to rewire parts of our brain but also to influence and improve our overall health through mechanisms such as exercise and the gut microbiome. By making small, consistent changes, we can repair and rebuild our own web of life, habit by habit. The more we study the connections between the gut, diet, exercise, inflammation, mitochondrial health, and brain health, the closer we come to a breakthrough in understanding how the body can adapt, compensate, and even repair itself.

SET REASONABLE GOALS

An optimal level of health cannot be accomplished immediately, but over time small steps can make a difference. Hundreds of books offer diet and exercise advice. This book's goal is simply to *nudge* you toward making changes in your life and get you feeling better and closer to your optimal self. You don't need to throw out everything in your refrigerator or run a marathon tomorrow.

It's okay to enjoy yourself and not be perfect. The meaning of life is not to vow to religiously adopt three hundred new behaviors and live by a checklist, stopwatch, and scorecard. Do what you can by setting reasonable goals. Work at it. Your utmost priority should be to enjoy your life, your family, and your passions. Don't beat yourself up if you fail to meet an imaginary expectation. No one can master all the good habits covered below, but anyone can try.

Creating brain-healthy habits is a gradual process that requires patience, persistence, and kindness toward oneself. It's important to focus on one habit at a time and use specific plans to reduce barriers to success. Whether it's sleeping in your workout clothes or waking up and putting on stylish Lululemon apparel to encourage early-morning exercise, small steps can make a big difference. Even something as simple as setting a consistent sleep schedule can lead to significant improvements in brain health. By remaining mindful of the purpose behind these efforts and continuously moving forward, you can make meaningful strides toward protecting your mind. This strategy is for anyone who wants to lead a healthy life, not just for those with a medical condition.

BE THE TURTLE, NOT THE HARE

How do you start? Make *one* modification. That's it. Your health journey of a thousand miles begins with a single step. Maybe it's a five-minute walk after you eat to lower your blood sugar level. Do that for a week, then for ten minutes every day, then fifteen, and then say to yourself, *What's next? Is there another change—maybe dropping a highly processed food like Hostess Cupcakes or Oreos from my diet?*

If you don't eat that packaged sugary food before your walk, your muscles will feed off the sugar already in your system, which is why your blood sugar remains lower and less goes into your fat cells. But if you do eat that sweet factory food before walking, it will take greater effort for the body to burn the additional sugar consumed, and it may not be able to compensate. That will lead to blood sugar and insulin spikes, fat storage, and increased inflammation.

Gradually build on what you've achieved and extend what is already working. Don't try to do everything at once or be a superhero. Slow changes win the proverbial race just as Aesop's turtle did. After steady, gradual effort, you will be surprised by what you've changed, who you've become, and how good you feel.

Key to this transformation is not just the actions of habit change but the right mindset. Willpower alone will not suffice. Accept your present baseline and feel no shame about it. Love who you are today. Maybe it will take you longer than you thought to achieve a certain goal. That's okay, because small progress is still progress, and temporary setbacks are just that—temporary. That mentality of losing twenty pounds in a month is for the birds. Be that tortoise, and you might instead achieve that goal in a year, or maybe you'll only lose five or ten pounds, and that's okay, too.

Remember—a person diagnosed with mild cognitive impairment from a brain disease like Alzheimer's could stay in that stage for many years. During that period, she will gradually decline and develop more cognitive symptoms. It will require more effort daily to stay functionally independent. By creating and living with new healthy habits, she creates a buffer, giving herself more time to live her present life. For her, what could have been three years of mild cognitive impairment can become five years.

Beneficial practices strengthen cognitive reserve just as ten rubber bands are stronger than one. Every new habit you add is like wrapping around another rubber band that reinforces your health. Even in older age—and even if you live with cognitive impairment—you continue, albeit slowly, to generate new brain cells. At the cellular level, lifestyle changes can have three major impacts: neurogenesis, the creation of new neurons; synaptogenesis, the formation of new synapses (the connections between neurons); and epigenetic modification, changes in a gene's activity level but not its genetic code. Conversely, unhealthy behaviors and environmental exposures can lead to the opposite outcomes—fewer neurons, fewer new synapses, and less healthy cells.

I care for adults in a unique period of their lives. While humans are aging from the moment they're born, the term takes on a different meaning in our sixth and seventh decades of life. It fascinates me that although growing older is a universal experience, people have vastly different expectations of what life will be like when they are old. If a person's expectations are unrealistic or too rigid, they risk setting themselves up for disappointment. My patients have taught me that activities in life become more meaningful as they start to slip away. If you put off until tomorrow what you could improve today, you will miss this opportunity of becoming something better—more fit and healthier—because every delay can be a setback that will keep you from a higher level of functioning and enjoyment down the road. When young people strain a muscle, it takes a relatively short time to bounce back. When you are in the geriatric range, it takes longer, and sometimes a full recovery is unattainable. Brain health, heart health, and physical health are all connected. They need your attention right now! This is not an emergency; it's a priority.

There's a wonderful line from the song "Nick of Time" by musician Bonnie Raitt—"Life gets mighty precious when there's less of it to waste." The underlying importance of a healthy lifestyle is twofold—it allows one to maintain their abilities for a little longer, thus making it possible to enjoy life a little bit more.

Fear is a powerful motivator, too, and it changes the lives of caregivers. As a hospitalist (doctor caring for patients in the hospital), I stood at many bedside deaths. Some were "codes" (emergencies such as cardiac arrests), where a team of healthcare professionals worked methodically to keep a patient alive. Other times I was there to bear witness to a life that was no longer able to sustain itself. The act of dying is an immense phenomenon because there is frequently some form of struggle, a letting go. (For more on the dying process, see chapter 9.) Death itself is the body's final release of energy. Why not use that life force now while you have it?

STACK THOSE HABITS

It's almost insulting for doctors to say, "Lose weight, exercise, eat healthy." What patients need is an honest plan that demonstrates how to do it and to understand why you should care. There's growing agreement that something called *habit stacking* works.

This expression refers to the practice of linking a new habit to an existing one, making each change a "small win." James Clear popularized this concept in his book *Atomic Habits*. It builds on the work of Charles Duhigg, whose 2012 book *The Power of Habit* explores the "habit loop" of cue, routine, and reward, a model that helps explain how habits form and change. (Both authors owe much to B. F. Skinner, who won a Nobel Prize for his work on behavioral psychology. His research found that positive reinforcement makes it more likely that new habits will be cemented in a person's long-term behavior.)

Duhigg writes that these little victories "have enormous power, an influence disproportionate to the accomplishments of the victories themselves . . . small wins fuel transformative changes by leveraging tiny advantages into patterns that convince people that bigger achievements are within reach." His framework serves as a cornerstone for understanding behavior change and lays the groundwork for strategies like habit stacking.

Once you develop a new behavior, it's easier to adopt the next one and so forth. If you feel better because you're no longer drinking, you become motivated to start exercising; perhaps by walking every day, your mood improves, and then you're more willing to modify your diet. A positive shift can have ripple effects leading to changes that would not have happened on their own.

Willpower plays a role in behavioral change, too, but the white-knuckle approach of staring down a plate of chocolate chip cookies typically only works for a little while. As a long-term plan, it is literally a sugary recipe for disaster. That's why offbeat fad diets don't work—not just because they're unrealistic but because they're often too rigid to stick with. Nobody can sustain a lifestyle that doesn't allow room for flexibility, pleasure, or real life.

A better approach is to change your environment. Instead of keeping dumbbells or exercise equipment in a drafty, dusty, out-of-the-way part of the house, put them in the den or living room where you spend most of your time. Instead of keeping sweets in the drawer, buy a bowlful of fresh, crisp apples and enjoy their beauty and scent as you draw them down for snacks throughout the week. Exercise in clothes that make you feel comfortable and excited to do the work, not just the dreary, tattered duds you hesitate to throw away. Instead of mindlessly scrolling through time-sucking phone apps, delete them. By casting out temptation you make it easier to strengthen your willpower and become successful.

THE CHIN UP! METHOD

Brain health is based on ways to prevent disease and live longer with an intact mind. I've always been fascinated by Super Agers, a term coined by Northwestern University researchers in 2008 for people in their eighties and beyond who have the mental and physical capabilities of folks thirty years younger. Evidence reveals that as a subgroup they eat well, exercise regularly, drink in moderation, and maintain a healthy weight. This varies, of course—they're not perfect, but over the course of years they maintain their routines.

The precise mechanism that keeps them biologically young is still a mystery. I once met a 102-year-old retired urologist. (He was celebrating his twentieth wedding anniversary with his 99-year-old wife.) His mind was sharp as a scalpel, and though he got around with a walker and electric scooter, his physical condition was superb—for his age. He told me there were a couple of secrets to living a long life. "Treat your mind and body like the treasures they are," he said, and, with a wink, he added, "Be lucky, and pick the right parents." It could be that people like him have an evolutionarily enhanced disposition thanks to their genes. Alas, there's no magic formula, like drinking carrot juice every day, for aging. While we have yet to find the recipe for the Super Agers' secret sauce, they remain credible role models for us to emulate.

There are plenty of protocols and plans Super Agers may be using to get fit and stay healthy. Some may follow the system called BE MORE as a part of AARP's Six Pillars of Brain Health program. BE MORE stands for Be Social, Engage Your Brain, Manage Stress, Ongoing Exercise, Restorative Sleep, and Eat Right. Others may follow a different protocol. Some may have no system at all. I recommend having some framework to help you stay organized.

My personal acronym, CHIN UP!, keeps me energized. It's both my name and my north star. Like my patients, friends, and family, I can also succumb to disheartenment. I worry about early-onset Alzheimer's and whether I'll follow my dad's experience. Have I protected my family if I have to retire at an early age? Am I utilizing all the advice on healthy living? But then I say to myself, *Chin up, Nate, seize the day. Make a difference while you can for yourself and others. You don't know what tomorrow will bring. It could be Alzheimer's. It could be cancer. It could be a car running a red light or any one of a thousand things.*

For those who meditate, a mantra keeps you focused. Choose your own and have a bit of fun with it. CHIN UP! keeps me positive and reminds me of my heritage, behaviors that are meaningful to me, and ones I encourage others to follow for brain health.

CHIN UP! stands for:

Choose Calmness
Hone Your Healthy Habits
Improve Sleep
Nurture Relationships
Uplift Your Intellect
Protect Your Senses
(To emphasize the acronym's positive spirit, I put an exclamation point at the end!)

"Aging," as the late rock star David Bowie supposedly said, "is an extraordinary process whereby you become the person you always should have been." And that's something to get excited about. Without further ado, here's my advice for creating your own extraordinary process for developing habits and behaviors that boost brain health.

CHOOSE CALMNESS

Our brains are, in a way, dumb. The parts of the brain that activate when playing the piano are the identical ones that go to work when a person imagines playing the piano. The brain is unable to differentiate between what's real and what's perceived. That's why therapists address fear of spiders by showing their patients photos of the eight-legged creepers.

Beliefs are important and can drive success or failure in most areas of life; that's why repetitive negative thinking is so detrimental. When you believe you are incompetent or incapable of completing a task, that sentiment cascades down through the chemical and electrical pathways of the brain, right through to your toes. You become sluggish. Your limbs respond slowly to movement, and they might tremble in hesitancy. That's not a good start. You must sincerely desire to change habits for new ways of thought and action to become ingrained in your heart and mind.

I know there is an "Age of Aquarius" philosophy that contends that if the message you send out to the universe is "I am content" or "I am miserable," it will come back in similar form. What I observe through the work I do is that that message isn't sent out. Instead, it is internalized. Contentment equals peace and calm. Consider the words of Japanese novelist Haruki Murakami: "Pain is inevitable. Suffering is optional."

The mental web of chronic stress is often overlooked and can have significant negative impacts on overall health, particularly brain health. While acute stress serves an evolutionary purpose (i.e., fleeing a saber-toothed tiger), chronic stress can lead to persistently elevated levels of the hormone cortisol, which can be harmful. High cortisol levels are associated with anxiety, depression, weakened immune function, heart disease, high blood pressure, and high blood sugar, among other issues. Chronic stress can also affect the brain. Studies have shown that soaring cortisol levels are linked to poorer memory, impaired visual perception, and a reduction in brain volume. Think of high cortisol levels like caffeine—too much makes you jittery and cranky. You can monitor caffeine by not having that third cup of coffee, but cortisol is your body's chemical response to what you're thinking and feeling, which is much harder to control.

Many of my patients deny having stress because they're retired. They presume that their work was the one true stressor in their lives. But when I invite them to share what keeps them up at night, they start talking about the price of eggs, world politics, or how their children are raising their grandchildren. Woes caused by stress have some people tangled in knots, but they're so used to it, they think worrying is actually *normal.*

Choosing calmness is meditative and soothing. It means deciding to be more aware of how you feel, acknowledging the presence of stress, and making a conscious effort to reduce its impact by taking time to seek a relaxed state of being. Instead of letting stress control you, you control it. Practices like mindfulness meditation, yoga, and deep breathing exercises can all help mitigate the harmful impact of repetitive negative thinking. Mindfulness frees the brain for more positive thoughts.

Mindfulness is one of those terms that's become fairly mainstream in recent years, especially among younger generations and healthcare professionals. But for many older adults—particularly those now facing memory changes—it can still sound like a New Age concept. At its core, though, mindfulness simply means choosing to bring awareness to the present moment with a quality of kindness in your attention, according to Dr. Vincent Minichiello, my colleague at the University of Wisconsin School of Medicine and Public Health. You stop what you are doing to take a moment for yourself. This mindful attention might be a simple pause, a breath, or an extended practice done sitting or lying down, standing, or walking.

"The key point to remember is that out of this pause, whatever form that pause takes or however long it lasts, you start to see in a different light your relationship to yourself and those around you. By being aware of this relationship, you might respond to yourself or others in a way that is healthy as well as compassionate," says Minichiello.

Some of the characteristics of being mindful include patience, trust, having a beginner's mind (approaching each moment with curiosity, openness, and without assumptions, as if for the first time), and being nonjudgmental, which means training yourself not to have an opinion about everything. One of the wisest works ever written is the Serenity Prayer, whose authorship is attributed to the twentieth-century American theologian Reinhold Niebuhr—"God grant me the serenity to accept the things I cannot change, the courage to change the things I can, and the wisdom to know the difference." Yes, the price of eggs is high, but since you have no control over it, what's the point in obsessing? The same is true with countless other issues in life.

Another quote I find just as relevant—perhaps even more so in daily caregiving—is comedian Craig Ferguson's Three-Question Rule: "Does this need to be said? Does this need to be said now? Does this need to be said now by me?" While the Serenity Prayer helps cultivate inner peace, Ferguson's rule is a practical tool for building emotional intelligence. It can prevent unnecessary arguments, help caregivers regulate their own reactions, and encourage more thoughtful, respectful communication with someone who may be struggling. Pausing to reflect before speaking is not about silence—it's about intention. For loved ones of people with cognitive impairment, these questions can be the difference between conflict and connection.

MRIs reveal that during periods of mindfulness or meditation, the prefrontal cortex, which regulates thoughts, actions, and emotions, is more activated. Similarly, the left anterior cerebral cortex, which plays a strong role in decision-making, also shows increased functioning. At least one study found that devoted meditators have a thicker cerebral cortex, which indicates that meditation increases one's attention span. Some studies suggest that meditation leads to lower cortisol levels in the bloodstream, thus leading to less stress or inflammation, especially in the brain.

Countless local classes, online programs, apps, books, and articles offer mindfulness tips. An ideal place to start would be with books by Dr. Jon Kabat-Zinn, a professor emeritus at the University of Massachusetts Medical School, who created the Stress Reduction Clinic and the Center for Mindfulness in Medicine, Health Care, and Society there. His best-known work is *Wherever You Go, There You Are: Mindfulness Meditation in Everyday Life.*

"You can't stop the waves," wrote Kabat-Zinn. "But you can learn to surf." Translation: There are many things you can't control, such as a diagnosis of Alzheimer's, but you can learn to master how you react to bad news, setbacks, and distressing events. Doing so doesn't require going to a yoga studio, stretchy clothes, or incense. Being mindful can be as simple as sitting in a quiet place in a straight chair for a minute or five minutes once a day and breathing slowly to empty your mind of thoughts while thinking *In. Out.* or even thinking the words *Chin Up!* to yourself. Try doing this behind the wheel of your car while stopped in traffic—it's better than getting angry!

Box breathing is one quick and easy way to manage stress and anxiety. Here's how to do it—stand up straight or sit up straight in a chair. Close your eyes. Slowly inhale through your nose while counting to four. Hold for four. Then exhale through your nose or mouth while again counting to four. Now hold your breath while counting to four. Then repeat. Navy SEALs use it to stay calm. If it works for them, it can work for you.

HONE YOUR HEALTHY HABITS

Exercise

When I learned my father's diagnosis, my immediate reaction was to begin to run three to six miles every day, and I followed this routine religiously. Running wasn't new to me—I'd been on the cross-country team my freshman year of high school and enjoyed running during college and medical school. Eventually, once I renewed the habit, I began training for a marathon in San Diego. Over time, I adjusted to my own aging. At age forty, I started lifting weights to maintain muscle mass, as well as biking and rowing. These days, I walk on an incline. It protects my joints and gets my heart rate up. I walk after eating, just five minutes with my dog, because doing so, even for a short while, has been shown to moderate blood sugars.

There are two lessons from my experience. First, in regard to exercise, along with everything in life, adjust to changing circumstances, such as age, but always seek the same goal—continuous improvement. Second, do what is right for you.

Exercise is personal. It can't be some rigid plan prescribed by me or any doctor. It's unhelpful when a physician only says, "You should exercise every day. Get in 150 minutes a week." Upon hearing that, most people think—how does that relate to me? Does the doctor understand my life or what my limitations are? Instead, doctors should ask patients and loved ones questions like, "What activities do *you* enjoy doing?" And if they don't ask, you should feel empowered to speak up and share what you enjoy—because that's the key to making it stick. If you like to walk, then walk. If you prefer swimming, dive in. And if you like to dance, wonderful, move the couch back. Whether it's square dancing or plié-ing at the barre, dancing requires strong concentration and enhances memory. We can't all be guests on *Dancing with the Stars*, but when it comes to exercise, we all need to stay on our toes.

Above all else—get moving. The health benefits of regular exercise of any type are well known. It helps control weight, lowers the risk of cardiovascular disease, makes bones and muscles stronger, boosts self-esteem, promotes better sleep, and creates a better sex life through increased energy. Of course, it also improves cognitive functioning.

The problem is many people hate the chore of exercise but love the enjoyment of physical activity. And let's be frank—some older people can't work out the way they did when they were younger. Moderately vigorous aerobic activity should be your goal, but you need to start where you are comfortable and work toward ratcheting up your efforts, regardless of whether you're walking, swimming, lifting weights, or doing something else.

There are so many reasons people don't and can't exercise, and I want to acknowledge that. I know how challenging it can be to make time to exercise, especially if you have let that habit lapse since you were younger. For example, if walking is an issue for you, consider using an arm crank instead. (It's like a bicycle whose pedals you work with your hands, but you use it while sitting.) If a physical limitation keeps you from going to a yoga class, do chair yoga while watching a video on YouTube. Many gyms also have Sit and Be Fit classes, water aerobics, or other classes designed for seniors. Check out your local resale shop; you might be surprised by how much gently used exercise equipment is there waiting for a second life.

Any activity is better than none. If you like to play golf, don't take a cart. If you must use a cart, walk as much as you can between greens. Not a golfer? Walk the perimeter of a course near you in the late afternoon. There are always ways to move more while still being safe and reasonable. Are you a gardener? Dig the holes for plant placement with gusto. Try to keep your heartbeat up as much as possible during the entire activity. Weed the garden intensely without letting up so that your heart pumps hard for five or ten minutes straight before you rest. Any master gardener will tell you that cultivating a plot of land is a *labor* of love.

What's the best exercise? If you're a swimmer, hooray for you. Swimming might win the gold medal among all types of exercise. It gives all muscles a stellar workout with no wear and tear on the joints. Of course, the downside is you must go to a pool, and swimming does lack the social aspect of many other forms of exercise. One of my patients with mild cognitive impairment loved to go to the YMCA at dawn three days a week to swim—even in her mid-eighties. Later, after she stopped driving, she walked instead.

We humans are literally born to walk, having evolved to be bipedal (walking on two feet). Other than birds, few species get around as we do. Research shows that regular sustained walks have countless benefits.

Walking with someone else outdoors boosts the benefits by creating social connectedness along with enjoying the inherent beauty of the natural world. (The Japanese call this sort of getting back to nature *Shinrin-yoku*—forest bathing, a term coined in an ad campaign, not by an ancient philosopher.) Like a warm bath, walking on a sunny day does wonders for the soul and leaves one feeling physically and spiritually refreshed. Plus, you need the vitamin D that sunlight provides for free.

If you want a famous role model for walking, Beethoven loved to stroll in nature. He is believed to have said, "How happy I am to be able to walk among the shrubs, the trees, the woods, the grass, and the rocks!"

The best-known American walker might be President Harry Truman, who took thirty- to forty-minute power walks most mornings on Pennsylvania Avenue. His constitutionals, as they were called, continued into his seventies and were so brisk that Secret Service agents supposedly had to hustle to keep up. Truman knew that when it came to making decisions about exercise, only he could get himself up before dawn to hit the pavement. Let "Give 'em Hell" Harry be your role model. The buck stops with you.

One way to measure the intensity of any exercise is the "Talk Test." If you're exercising and can easily chat with a friend, that's a low-intensity workout. If you can talk but not sing, that means you're at moderate intensity, but if you can only get out a few words at a time, that signals high-intensity exercise.

While moderate aerobic intensity is what you're aiming for, there's nothing wrong with high intensity, either. For an extra challenge, wear soft padded weights while you're walking. I now wear a weighted vest while walking at an incline on the treadmill and it's made an incredible difference without the knee strain running once caused.

The CDC recommends 150 to 300 minutes of weekly moderate aerobic activity. Meanwhile, the American Heart Association says people only need 150 minutes a week of moderate-intensity exercise. Who's right? That's not a debate I want to wade into. The point is, we all need to get our heart rates up. That could be thirty minutes a day, five days a week. Maybe you start with ten minutes a day and work up. Or maybe it's a strenuous one-hour workout three times a week. Start where you feel comfortable. Keep trying to increase the intensity of your exercise. And remember, as you become physically fitter, you need to exert more effort to get your heart rate up. This is why training is never static.

Engaging in aerobic exercise means reaching 70 to 80 percent of one's maximum heart rate, and doing so has been shown to improve episodic memory and executive function. Both are linked to increased brain glucose metabolism, particularly in the prefrontal cortex, which is responsible for higher-order cognitive processes like decision-making, problem-solving, and attention. Those with higher cardiorespiratory fitness tend to have larger brain volumes, particularly in the hippocampus, the region crucial for memory formation, and less amyloid protein in the brain. This doesn't mean exercise causes greater brain volume or reduced amyloid, but there is some relationship between them.

Exercise, notably weight training, has an added benefit for older people. Beginning in our thirties, we lose muscle mass as we age, as much as 5 percent every decade. Unless you exercise, especially via strength training, you can lose 30 percent of your muscle mass by age seventy. That increases the risk of osteoporosis, falls, and injuries. So, you should address your strength and balance just as you address your cardiovascular system via exercise. There's little value to having a strong heart and lungs if you lack strong muscles and bones to get around. To top it off, there is evidence that weightlifting, to some degree, benefits brain health.

As a starting point, set realistic goals that reflect your current fitness level. You don't want to get injured. Start slow and increase the intensity or duration over time. You don't need to set a personal record, but you do need to move and do so regularly. Studies show that walking between four and seven thousand steps a day can reduce your risk of death of *any cause.*

Consider this final thought—there's no better advice than what Irish brain researcher Shane O'Mara offers in his book *In Praise of Walking*—"You don't get old until you stop walking, and you don't stop walking because you're old."

Stop Smoking

Smoking shrinks blood vessels in the brain, making smokers *70 percent* more likely to develop dementia. People who smoke are at greater risk of dying and developing cancer in general. Constantly inhaling superheated, chemical-laced tobacco smoke damages your body from head to toe. Google "lungs of a cigarette smoker" to see how black as soot the lungs appear. It's hard to imagine a person is breathing comfortably with lungs so scarred.

There is good news. Within twenty minutes of quitting, a smoker's blood pressure drops. Within twenty-four hours, the risk of a heart attack decreases, and it falls by one-half within a year. The probability of having a stroke becomes similar to a nonsmoker's within five years, and the likelihood of having a heart attack becomes the same as a nonsmoker's within fifteen years. In this case, time really does seem to heal all wounds.

Your brain also benefits from smoking cessation. Within three years of quitting, the risk of developing dementia is similar to that of someone who has never smoked. Research shows that within eight years of quitting, a person's chance of developing Alzheimer's disease specifically is comparable to someone who's never smoked. This is true even as we age, not just when we're young.

The key is to stop smoking, and facts alone are not going to motivate someone to make that decision. Most smokers know their habit is unhealthy. Quitting is not a matter of intelligence or willpower. Most smokers need help, and they should have every resource available to them. Here are some general ideas to consider: First, make a list of reasons why you want to quit and a list of what triggers your need to smoke. "To know thyself is the beginning of wisdom," said Socrates. You are your strongest ally and your biggest opponent. Second, seek the aid of a spouse, child, or friend in your efforts. Surround yourself with a community of support. Don't do this alone. Third, quitting cold turkey doesn't work for everyone, and there are more pharmacological ways to help people than before. Talk to your primary care provider about your desire to quit. She can discuss options with you, including nicotine replacement therapy, such as nicotine patches, gum, or lozenges, or prescription medications. Fourth, try cognitive behavioral techniques like choosing a quit day, having a plan for the days following your quit day, and developing backup plans for when you encounter your triggers.

If you still don't feel motivated to start the conversation, consider how jaw-droppingly expensive cigarettes are. If you smoke a pack a day, the money you spend on one year's worth of cigarettes could buy you an inexpensive used car, a weeklong Caribbean cruise for two people including airfare, many months' worth of groceries, or a year's in-state tuition for a grandchild at a less expensive state university.

For many people, quitting takes time and multiple attempts. The first few weeks can be the hardest. When you stop or reach your milestones to cessation, reward yourself with something special. Going through this immensely helpful life change will benefit you in every way.

For more, call 1-800-QUIT-NOW, a free national smoking-cessation quitline that offers coaching.

The best smoking habit is the habit of being smoke-free.

You can do it.

Avoid Alcohol

The true health benefits of alcohol, specifically in mild to moderate amounts, remain a deeply debated topic in the scientific field. Decades ago, researchers became intrigued by the "French paradox"—the observation that French people, despite eating food rich in saturated fats, had lower rates of heart disease. Some proposed that drinking red wine with meals provided a protective effect. Studies suggested that resveratrol, an antioxidant polyphenol compound in red wine, might relax blood vessels, lower blood pressure, reduce low-density lipoprotein (LDL) cholesterol, and reduce inflammation. However, more recent research has questioned the conclusion that moderate amounts of alcohol are "heart healthy." New findings indicate that even low levels of alcohol consumption may increase the risk of cardiovascular disease.

Alcohol is deeply embedded in cultures worldwide, serving as a nearly universal social lubricant. However, socializing and having a good time do not require drinking. Eliminating beer, wine, and spirits from one's diet can bring immediate benefits. Even individuals in the early stages of cognitive decline may notice improved mental sharpness, better sleep, and reduced late-night snacking. Increased energy levels and better overall well-being are additional advantages of abstinence.

Alcohol, in all its forms, is a neurotoxin. It acts as a depressant, slowing brain function and impairing judgment. It seemingly lifts you up while its ultimate actual effect is to lower your mood and cognitive function. Occasional consumption allows the brain to recover, but chronic, excessive use has been associated with an increased risk of dementia. Decades of daily drinking can take a lasting toll on brain health.

Researchers continue to debate whether moderate alcohol consumption contributes to Alzheimer's disease risk. Although no definitive conclusions have been reached, the medical problems caused by alcohol are truly sobering and so worrisome that any prudent person should avoid drinking. Alcohol negatively influences numerous systems in the body, including the heart, pancreas, bones, and immune system. It also impacts the liver, which metabolizes medications. Since liver function declines with age and older adults are more likely to take prescription or over-the-counter medications, the interaction between alcohol and drug metabolism presents another compelling reason to limit consumption. As if that's not enough, studies now confirm alcohol is the third most common reversible cause of many cancers.

For seniors, drinking carries much higher risks than for young adults. Besides worsening memory issues and mood disorders, alcohol makes diabetes, high blood pressure, and cardiovascular disease harder to control. Drinking also increases the risk of falls. The problem of falling has become so alarming *The Wall Street Journal* in 2024 called it an "epidemic." Every year, more than 25 percent of Americans over the age of sixty-five fall. Each year such slips result in 1.2 million hospital stays and 41,000 deaths. Undoubtedly, alcohol use and abuse play a role in this crisis. Moreover, given that 90 percent of seniors take some form of medication or supplement, the potential for harmful drug interactions further underscores the dangers of drinking.

Why might epidemiological studies be wrong when they suggest low to moderate alcohol use is healthy? The answer I hear most is that while alcohol can facilitate social interaction, it is the social engagement itself—not the alcohol—that contributes to well-being.

Many studies have limitations simply because it's impossible to account for every variable or see the whole picture from limited data. Some failed to consider the impact of other contributing factors such as socioeconomic status, one's neighborhood, home, or other living conditions, and personal health behaviors like diet, exercise, and sleep. For example, people who drink lightly may also have better access to healthcare and fewer chronic health conditions. Another common research error, called *selection bias,* can also distort results. Nondrinkers in these studies may include former heavy drinkers or individuals with existing health problems that prevent alcohol use, making the group appear less healthy regardless of alcohol consumption. Then there's *reverse causation*, a flaw that often trips up observational studies. Some nondrinkers may abstain because of poor health, which would naturally place them at higher risk for the outcome being studied. Lastly, there's *measurement error.* Because these studies are not randomized controlled trials in which all variables are tightly controlled, alcohol consumption is determined by self-reporting, which can be subject to recall bias and underreporting.

Ideally, people would choose not to drink. For those who do consume alcohol, moderation is key. I ask my patients to consume one drink per day, fewer than four days per week. For those with cognitive complaints, I strongly advocate for no alcohol until the symptoms resolve.

Reducing alcohol intake—or avoiding it altogether—can significantly improve physical and cognitive health. If you don't drink, there is no reason to start. For those who do, cutting back can be one of the most impactful steps toward a healthier life.

Eat Right

Changing what we eat is hard. Food is personal. It's cultural. In many ways it symbolizes love, comfort, and tradition. During my first year of residency, I gained twenty pounds, not just because I ate too much but because I wasn't managing stress in a healthy way. With little free time during the day, I consumed whatever was in front of me, usually the free pizza during lectures. I wasn't even tasting my food, let alone enjoying it. Food is more than just macronutrients to fuel our bodies, which is why changing eating habits isn't as simple as just deciding to "eat better."

Healthy food can also be expensive and not always readily available. For people with cognitive impairment, the steps involved in cooking can become a minefield to maneuver, and for busy caregivers, preparing well-balanced meals regularly can be a challenge.

To complicate matters, the sheer number of diets out there is overwhelming—and each one seems to come with its own set of "expert" opinions. You could try Atkins, Ornish, keto, Paleo, a juice cleanse, Weight Watchers, the South Beach Diet, gluten-free, Nutrisystem, or the ice cream diet. You might believe I made up the last one, but it's real, and probably a rocky road for anyone who tries it. There are dozens more, each with its own catchy angle and miraculous yet simple approach. I'm not judging those who try them, I've tried my fair share, too.

The truth is that most people simply cannot adhere to the strict eating regimens that diets impose. These plans rely on willpower to succeed, and when that inevitably fades, people eat the so-called forbidden food, feel guilty, and move on to the next trend touted in magazines, on TV, and on the internet. Unfortunately, these diet fads don't address the deeper issues behind our relationships with food, nor do they provide long-term strategies for sustainable change.

In my practice, I encourage patients to focus on small, practical lifestyle modifications rather than drastic menu overhauls. It's been my experience that people won't change what they eat just because a doctor tells them, "You should have a Mediterranean diet. Here's a three-page printout. Good luck!" Early in my career, I thought I could make a difference that way, but my patients taught me how naïve that approach ultimately was. Even with scientific explanations and a strong rationale, most patients left my clinic understanding that they should change their eating patterns but also knowing they wouldn't.

Dietary change must come from the patient and his family. They, not the physician, should drive this behavior change. As they would to quit smoking, a person must have the belief that change is beneficial and the desire to follow through. Without wanting to sincerely make the change, it either won't happen or won't last. Some are motivated by facts, others by fear, and for some of my patients, it's the encouragement of their spouse. Whatever the reason, I use that inspiration and encourage what I call *reverse habit stacking* (losing one bad habit leads to the desire to shed the next) to build small victories.

Ask yourself—what is one food you eat regularly that you know you probably shouldn't? Everyone has a guilty pleasure—some dessert, processed meat, or salty, crunchy snack they know they should cut back on or stop buying. As with taking up walking or cutting back on drinking, once a person removes one unhealthy item from their diet, it often becomes easier to make additional modifications. The benefits multiply with a cascade of positive changes, especially if the family joins in. After the first item is axed and the new habit formed, a second item can be chosen, and a new cycle begins.

At the same time, ask yourself another equally important question: What's one healthy food you genuinely love? Double down on that. Eat it more often. I've never heard a dietitian warn someone against a daily salad, a handful of nuts, or having too many vegetables. Eventually, those nourishing choices begin to crowd out the old ones—and the new diet emerges organically, not by force.

Despite my skepticism toward rigid diets, I do believe in the benefits of the Mediterranean diet and its close relative, the MIND (Mediterranean-DASH Intervention for Neurodegenerative Delay) diet. They are both delicious, relatively affordable, and widely recognized for their numerous health benefits, particularly in reducing markers of inflammation, lowering the rates of heart disease and diabetes, and aiding in weight loss.

Both diets emphasize fruits, vegetables (especially dark green, leafy ones), whole grains, fish, berries, nuts, and olive oil while limiting red meat and processed foods. I also recommend avoiding foods high in salt and beverages high in sugar like juices and soda. In fact, for many of my patients, the first step is eliminating soda altogether. The ultimate goal is to consume only coffee, tea, and water, avoiding liquid calories entirely.

Researchers at Rush University in Chicago created the MIND diet with low-salt and antioxidant-rich foods. Research on its effects has shown that it provides significant cognitive benefits. According to one study, participants who adhered most strictly to it had a 53 percent reduced risk of developing Alzheimer's disease. Even those who moderately followed the diet saw a 35 percent reduced risk. Notably, those in the highest adherence group had brains that appeared, on average, seven years younger than those of participants who followed the diet the least.

I follow the MIND diet, though I'm not a fanatic about it. I take a flexible approach, adhering to suggestions found in a range of diets while always being mindful about how much sugar and salt I consume. You could call my diet the "Pick-and-Choose" diet. In my home, with a three- and a six-year-old, we keep sugary foods to a minimum, and that means no soda or fruit juices. (I'm not always that popular with my kids.) We love berries of all types but eat them in moderation. We rarely have ultra-processed desserts except for the occasional treat from Trader Joe's. We avoid white bread in favor of ancient grains. Last but not least, pretzels are completely banned. I'm incapable of just having one or a handful, so they simply can't be in the pantry.

The MIND diet can be tough for some people to follow. It allows fried foods and seafood no more than once a week, less than an ounce of whole-fat cheese a week, no more than a pat of butter a day, and three servings of red meat a week. "I think everybody will be a little bit different in what is a challenge for them," admits the diet's co-creator Martha Clare Morris, a professor of epidemiology at Rush University. What's nice about the MIND diet is you don't have to be perfect at it, unlike the Mediterranean diet, which tends to show results only with stricter adherence. If you follow the MIND diet even moderately, you will still benefit from it, as studies have shown.

The MIND Diet—a Practical Approach to Brain Health

It's hard to know what diet is best for your health, especially your brain. One week the headlines praise a Mediterranean approach; the next, they warn about carbs or tout a new superfood. For those trying to reduce their risk of cognitive decline, the mixed messages can be frustrating. Currently the MIND diet stands out as a reasonable, research-supported framework that emphasizes whole foods, moderation, and long-term brain health. Each one of us has a wonderful opportunity, every day, to take charge of the foods we eat.

The MIND diet is a combination of the Mediterranean and DASH (Dietary Approaches to Stop Hypertension) diets, two well-known and heart-healthy diets. But it goes a step further by targeting foods specifically associated with cognitive protection. Developed by researchers at Rush University, the MIND diet zeroes in on nutrients and food patterns thought to support brain structure and function, including those linked to reduced Alzheimer's pathology.

At its core, the MIND diet promotes regular eating of green leafy vegetables, other vegetables, berries (especially blueberries), nuts, whole grains, fish, beans, poultry, and olive oil. A glass of wine a day is permitted, though not required, and is the one item I would discourage. These foods are rich in antioxidants, healthy fats, fiber, and polyphenols—all compounds thought to play a role in reducing inflammation and oxidative stress in the brain.

This diet does have one drawback. It recommends limiting foods that may contribute to vascular and neurodegenerative harm, such as red meats, full-fat cheese, butter and margarine, fried or fast food, pastries, and sweets. As someone from Wisconsin, I consciously choose to ignore the recommended limitation on cheese. After all, you can't be perfect—and the studies show you don't need to be.

The question, of course, is whether this diet works. A number of observational studies suggest it does. Higher MIND diet adherence has been associated with significantly lower Alzheimer's pathology—specifically lower levels of amyloid and tau tangles—in the autopsied brains of participants from the Rush Memory and Aging Project. Even after adjusting for age, education, and genetic risk (like APOE 4 status—the most common and strongest genetic risk factor for late-onset Alzheimer's disease), the association held. Those who ate more green leafy vegetables in particular had fewer signs of Alzheimer's in their brains. Another study from the same group of people found that individuals with high MIND scores maintained better cognition and experienced slower cognitive decline, even when their brains showed evidence of disease. This suggests what researchers call "cognitive resilience"—the ability to function well despite the presence of the disease.

Larger population-based studies support these findings. In another study, which followed more than fourteen thousand people, higher MIND diet adherence was associated with lower risk of developing cognitive impairment over time, particularly among women. What's more, a 2023 meta-analysis pooled data from eleven studies and also found that individuals in the highest MIND diet adherence group had a 17 percent lower risk of dementia compared to those who failed to stick closely to the diet.

To be clear, the evidence is imperfect. A recent three-year randomized controlled trial of older adults with a family history of dementia found no significant differences in cognitive outcomes between those who followed the diet and those who did not. Both groups, however, improved slightly, perhaps because all participants received nutritional counseling and limited their calorie intake. The study's authors noted that longer studies or studies starting earlier in life may be needed to detect more definitive cognitive benefits.

Still, what makes the MIND diet appealing is its practicality. It does not require strict elimination of entire food groups. It does not demand calorie counting or complicated rules. Adherence need not be rigidly followed to be beneficial. Several studies have shown that even moderate adherence is associated with cognitive benefits. In other words, small changes matter. I try to follow it myself as much as I can, knowing that consistency—not perfection—is what counts.

Eating by the Clock?

Beyond food choices, meal timing may also play a role in health. Ideally, everyone should avoid eating two to three hours before bed. (See sidebar on page 191 for more on fasting.) If you're feeling ambitious, you might combine changes in your diet with a modified form of fasting called time-restricted eating, in which you limit eating and drinking to a six- or eight-hour window every day. Fasting isn't new. People have practiced it for centuries, and it plays a major role in present-day Judaism, Islam, and, to a lesser degree, Christianity, though fasting during Lent was once a standard practice.

A great deal of recent research in humans and animals has explored the impact of various types of fasting not just on obesity but also on cardiovascular disease, diabetes, cancer, asthma, arthritis, recovery from surgery and injury, and neurodegenerative disorders such as Alzheimer's. The findings are promising, but up to this point doctors rarely suggest to patients that they fast for sixteen to eighteen hours a day. A big hurdle to overcome is the deeply ingrained habit of taking three meals a day—plus snacks! But if you think about it, fasting and human evolution (as well as animal evolution) go hand in hand. Our caveman ancestors did not wake up and grab their morning brontoburger from a refrigerator. They had to hunt for it, and if prey was scarce, they did without.

I've practiced intermittent fasting for over a decade. It started when I was a resident and had no time for breakfast. I also wanted to lose the twenty pounds I'd gained during my intern year, and this strategy helped. I grabbed coffee when I could and rarely ate before lunch. (Yes, intermittent fasting does allow one to drink water and coffee, so long as the coffee contains no cream or sweetener. In fact, a recent study of two hundred thousand coffee drinkers found that they have a lower risk of developing Alzheimer's but only if they drink it black.) My experience with skipping breakfast and only eating from noon to 6 PM is that I feel more energized and clearheaded throughout the day.

Should you consider such fasting to promote cognitive health? I believe it's worth considering, but the research is still evolving. More important, each person is different, and what works for one person may not for another. If you're interested in fasting, talk to your doctor and someone who's done it. To be safe, start with shorter fasting periods and then extend them if all goes well.

Are Keto and Fasting Safe?

Some people explore variations beyond the MIND framework, such as intermittent fasting or ketogenic-style eating. Both have gained attention for their potential benefits to the body and brain and may complement the MIND diet when applied thoughtfully.

Intermittent fasting focuses on when you eat rather than what you consume. Common patterns include daily time-restricted meals (such as sixteen hours fasting, eight hours eating), alternate-day fasting, or eating five hundred calories two to three days per week. Research suggests that fasting triggers beneficial cellular processes like autophagy (removal of damaged cells), enhances insulin sensitivity, and may reduce neuroinflammation. Several studies—including a 2024 randomized trial published in *Cell Metabolism*—have linked fasting with improvements in executive function and memory in older adults at risk for cognitive decline. Animal studies and emerging human data also suggest the increased presence of brain-derived neurotrophic factor (BDNF), a molecule associated with learning, memory, and neuroplasticity.

The ketogenic diet, by contrast, is high in fat, moderate in protein, and very low in carbohydrates. It promotes a metabolic state called ketosis, in which the brain uses ketones instead of glucose as fuel. This shift appears to have neuroprotective effects. In research studies of adults with mild cognitive impairment and Alzheimer's disease, a ketogenic diet was associated with improved memory and attention, likely due to enhanced mitochondrial function, reduced oxidative stress, and stabilization of brain metabolism. Another trial reported improved daily functioning and quality of life in Alzheimer's patients following a ketogenic intervention.

While a strict keto diet may not align fully with MIND's emphasis on fruits, legumes, and whole grains, some hybrid approaches incorporate the neuroprotective elements of both—for example, a person might emphasize olive oil, fish, and non-starchy vegetables while reducing sugars and refined carbs.

These approaches aren't for everyone. People with diabetes, low body weight, disordered eating, or certain medical conditions should consult a healthcare provider before starting any diet. There is no one-size-fits-all approach. The value lies in personalization—choosing what works for your biology, your lifestyle, and what is sustainable for you over the long term.

In practice, someone might follow the MIND diet for its food choices and eat within a daily eight-hour window to gain fasting benefits, or a person might emphasize fat-based brain fuels like nuts, fish, and olive oil to promote mild ketosis. Others may adopt a few core MIND principles and stop there.

What matters most is building a way of eating that supports your goals, your values, and your brain.

Given rising food prices, following the MIND and Mediterranean diets may actually be more affordable than regularly purchasing steaks, potato chips, imported beer, and soda. (Did you know that a twelve-ounce can of regular Coke contains nearly three-and-a-half *tablespoons* of sugar? Yikes!) Either diet allows you to reallocate what you would have spent on junk food and processed meat and put those hard-earned dollars toward healthier foods. One study found that the Mediterranean diet could save a family of four about $1,500 a year.

The key is to start small. Make modest changes in your diet, beginning with foods you feel guilty about eating. As with easing into an exercise program, you will be surprised and pleased by how good you feel physically and mentally if you make healthy diet modifications—and build on them. If the MIND diet appeals to you, don't try to obey its every suggestion, but follow it as much as you can with the goal of making continuous, sustainable improvements. Be kind to yourself—no diet should feel like a punishment.

One final tip—when grocery shopping, steer your shopping cart clear of the grocery store's center aisles where ultra-processed foods lurk like nutritional vultures for the unwary. Such laboratory-created foods include sodas, ready-made frozen meals, super-sugary cereals, and salty snacks. Just read their unpronounceable ingredients—the artificial flavorings, hydrogenated oils, chemical preservatives and colorings, and high-fructose syrups that are light-years from the plants they were created from. If nature made your food, good, but if a factory did, beware.

Nine Commonsense Diet Guidelines

Rigid diets are too hard for most people to follow. Instead, I encourage all my patients to find the balance that's right for them—a healthy balance. Here are nine guidelines.

1. Focus on eating more plant-based whole foods instead of ultra-processed foods. In other words, shop the perimeter of the grocery store, not its aisles where most factory-made foods are shelved.
2. Avoid fast foods and prepackaged meals.
3. Make protein a priority and keep carbs, such as bread, in their proper place. Choose healthy fats like olive oil, nuts,

and avocados, while limiting trans fats and being mindful of saturated fats, which affect people differently.

4. Eat the rainbow by including vegetables of all colors in meals every day.
5. Minimize the amount of red meat and processed meat you eat. Instead, eat more lean meats and fish.
6. Use smaller plates to decrease portion sizes, and avoid second helpings.
7. Drink more water and shun sugary sodas and juices.
8. Read product labels to make sure you're not eating foods with hidden sugars.
9. Protect your gut by staying away from foods that harm its ecosystem of microorganisms.

Be Kind to Your Gut Microbiome

There's a little-known connection between diet, nutrition, and digestion—the gut microbiome and how it affects the brain. This environment of microorganisms consists of millions of bacteria, fungi, protozoa, archaea, and viruses in the stomach and upper and lower intestines. All these factors strongly influence the overall function of our digestive tracts because of their vital role in processing nutrients, proteins, vitamins, and minerals.

What's fascinating—and what some might find a little weird—about these armies of minuscule helpers is their impact on far-flung aspects of our life, from our mood to how well we sleep. All bodily systems are connected in many ways, so it shouldn't be surprising that what happens in digestion affects our brains.

In 2017, researchers at the University of Wisconsin compared people who had Alzheimer's to those who did not. They found that people with dementia had startling differences in their microbiome. "One of those differences was less diversity, fewer kinds of bugs in the gut in Alzheimer's patients. There actually seems to be really early relationships between what we see in the gut and what we see in the brain," says Dr. Barbara Bendlin, a senior author of the study and a professor of geriatrics and gerontology and deputy director at UW's Center for Health Disparities Research. Other factors such as medications a person takes and where a person lives can affect gut health, so the mechanisms behind this gut-brain relationship remain unclear.

Declining gut microbiome diversity also happens naturally as people age and is seen in type 2 diabetes, obesity, and diseases affecting the intestinal tract. So it makes sense that one would want to have a flourishing gut ecosystem like those found in jungles, forests, and oceans, whose species diversity confers countless environmental benefits.

Gut health can also impact the brain via gut inflammation, a trend that tends to increase with age. If there's inflammation in the gut, it could stimulate increased inflammation elsewhere. Abnormal levels of gut inflammation lead to a condition called "leaky gut," in which the intestinal barrier weakens and toxins and bacteria enter the bloodstream, causing systemic inflammation in the body and brain. While inflammation is part of the body's defense system, chronic inflammation is increasingly regarded as a key factor not just in Alzheimer's but also in cancer, cardiovascular disease, and other illnesses.

Eating fruits, vegetables, and fiber promotes the increased growth of healthier gut bacteria, and those, in turn, lower inflammation. If the gut microbiome were a garden, you would nurture it with daily care—feeding it nutrients that help it flourish, not the toxins that make it wither. For a happier gut, avoid sugar, processed foods, and other foods discouraged in the MIND and Mediterranean diets.

Prescription drugs and other medications, especially antibiotics, can throw the gut microbiome out of kilter, too. Beware of taking them unless their use is essential.

Some people swear by probiotic and prebiotic supplements. Probiotics are live microorganisms, primarily bacteria, that provide health benefits when consumed in high enough quantities. Prebiotics, however, are the nondigestible fibers and compounds that act as food for the gut bacteria, nourishing them to grow and function. Quality matters: A top-tier probiotic should be strain specific, stable through the end of its shelf life, include sufficient CFUs (colony-forming units), and be clinically tested for safety and efficacy, while high-quality prebiotics deliver clinically effective doses of well-researched fibers like inulin and FOS and undergo purity testing.

Because the bacteria in probiotics pass through the digestive system in a few days to a few weeks, they don't colonize the gut. This means a person would need to regularly consume supplements to maintain the benefits of the probiotics. While this is feasible for some, an alternative would be to consume probiotic-rich foods, such as yogurt, sauerkraut, kimchi, pickles, tempeh, certain cheeses, and kombucha. Prebiotic-rich foods are typically high in fiber and include bananas, whole grains, onions, leeks, asparagus, apples, berries, lentils, chickpeas, almonds, and seaweed. Combining prebiotics with probiotics can lead to enhanced gut health, as well as flavorful meals. In general, the more diverse your diet is, the better off your brain and gut will be.

IMPROVE SLEEP

I've always loved to sleep. It's the treasure we give ourselves at the end of every day. During the first year of my children's lives, I was obsessed with their sleep. I did everything I could to ensure they slept well. While my wife was pregnant, I read countless books on sleep techniques. I even read research papers to learn the latest in the field. I talked to other parents to learn from their experiences—what worked, what didn't. At the clinic, I cornered my sleep medicine colleagues to ask questions that kept me up at night. I wanted to be as informed as possible because I knew sleep was important—not just for my children but for me, too.

Once my boys were born, I studied their sleep patterns. I tracked what led to good and bad naps, timed their sleep cycles, and analyzed what contributed to long, deep sleep. My eldest slept like a dream, logging twelve hours straight each night by the time he was eight weeks old, and he took two- or three-hour naps. My second son, well, let's just say he had different plans.

Through my children, I learned two universal truths. First, sleep is a habit—it can be trained and shaped by everything happening before and after it. Second, as anyone (parent or not) can attest, sleep determines how you feel and what you're willing to do the next day. A bad night's sleep can make you irritable and sluggish. Tossing and turning might mean skipping the gym or giving in to that doughnut at the office. Too little sleep can shorten one's patience, increasing the likelihood of snapping at someone you love. On the flip side, is there anything better than waking up feeling refreshed? Don't we, as adults, deserve the same care invested into our sleep that we put into our children's?

Along with what we eat and how we exercise, our sleep habits didn't form overnight. How we sleep developed over long periods and took time to improve. Prioritizing sleep is well worth the effort. Sleep is another keystone habit that has a terrific impact on daily living. Changes in how one sleeps trigger a domino effect, making other habits easier to modify. Sleeping well means you'll be more successful at exercising, eating a healthy diet, and reducing stress.

Sleep deprivation is a crisis in today's America. About 20 percent of people sleep fewer than five hours a night, compared to only 3 percent in 1942, according to a Gallup poll. There are many reasons for this crisis, including a "strong work culture" that prioritizes productivity over rest; technology and screen time before bed that suppresses melatonin and delays sleep onset; chronic stress and mood disorders that keep people up or prevent them from falling back asleep once they've awakened; unhealthy diets and consumption of alcohol and caffeine; sleep disorders like obstructive sleep apnea, insomnia, and restless leg syndrome; family and caregiver responsibilities where personal slumber is sacrificed for that of a loved one; and lack of sleep education and the understanding of the importance of sleep. One or more of these reasons likely applies to everyone. Restless sleep happens to all of us, but when it occurs chronically, the toll can be dramatic.

Although all the ways in which sleep benefits us have yet to be fully understood, we know it is essential. From the brain's perspective, sleep is vital for learning and memory consolidation (transferring recent memories into long-term storage). Experiences deemed unimportant are also pruned from existence. During sleep our brain also processes emotional events and feelings, helping us to stay regulated and balanced the next day. Research using functional MRIs has shown that brain regions responsible for creativity and problem-solving show heightened activity during REM (rapid eye movement) sleep, which is when dreams occur. While our bodies appear to be "resting," our brains remain highly active.

At a biochemical level, sleep also helps clear waste matter from the brain, including neurotoxic proteins like amyloid and tau, the same hallmark proteins used to define Alzheimer's disease. In fact, research is still investigating why these proteins accumulate in the brains of affected individuals. The lack of sleep is believed to be a potential factor.

The WRAP (Wisconsin Registry for Alzheimer's Prevention) study investigated the impact of sleep in 619 healthy participants. This study failed to find a relationship between poor sleep and the development of amyloid proteins; not surprisingly, it did show that erratic sleep was associated with worse cognitive performance on testing, including in areas such as learning, memory, and executive function. Those who reported poor sleep also tended to have higher body mass indexes, higher waist-to-hip ratios, and greater insulin resistance.

Quality slumber has health benefits, too. It reduces stress, lowers blood pressure, and supports heart health by reducing the risk of cardiovascular disease. It also aids in weight management and enhances immune function by reducing inflammation. Deep sleep supports tissue repair and growth hormone release, which are critical for recovery after exercise. Better yet, some studies have shown that consistently good sleep is associated with lower risk of developing diabetes and some forms of cancer, and with having a longer lifespan.

But people don't love sleep just because it prevents unhealthy conditions from developing. Sleep also helps people feel good. Quality sleep boosts creativity, feelings of sharpness and focus, and emotional resilience. Sleep reduces cortisol levels and promotes relaxation and the feeling of well-being. It obviously has a restorative role, and we feel that when we wake after a good night of rest.

The impact of sleep in those with cognitive impairment is even more profound. Think of the brain with cognitive impairment as being more vulnerable to perturbances. When someone with MCI or dementia sleeps poorly, they may exhibit more cognitive or behavioral symptoms the next day. In dementia, as the underlying disease progresses, people tend to sleep more, sometimes up to eighteen hours each day. Prior to this point, however, improving sleep—its duration and quality—may slow the disease's progression or at least symptoms of cognitive impairment. This may be related to the direct cognitive benefits of sleep or to the habit stacking, such as exercising, eating healthy, and engaging in mentally stimulating activities, that sleep affords.

Super Sleep Suggestions

Everyone's goal should be seven to nine hours of nightly sack time. Less than six hours and more than ten have been shown to have negative effects. A 2021 study found that even being deprived of sleep for one night can frustrate the brain's ability to rid itself of waste matter. The quality of slumber matters, too. You don't want to wake frequently in the middle of the night, even if you're lying in bed for the target number of hours.

If you wake frequently, get up feeling tired, or nod off at inappropriate times, you may have sleep apnea. There is no firm proof that this sleep disorder heightens Alzheimer's risk, but some researchers suspect that if the brain can't get its natural rest every night, a causal link may exist.

Improving sleep habits, though challenging, is essential. Here are seven tips for improving your sleep hygiene:

1. Exercise. Being physically active and ideally working out every day will make your body and mind more eager for sleep.
2. Avoid alcohol after dinner and drinking caffeine after lunch. Alcohol has a dreadful effect on sleep. It shaves time off REM sleep, reducing dreaming, and though alcohol may make it easier to slip off to slumber, it will make you wake up. Even worse, its ill effects make it more difficult to go back to sleep. Finally, alcohol makes sleep apnea worse because it unnaturally relaxes the muscles that keep your airway open.
3. Limit fluids before bedtime. In fact, avoid eating and drinking anything after dinner to prevent the need to urinate in the

wee hours of the morning. If you go from 6 PM to 7 AM, that's an easy-to-accomplish mini fast, and you'll wake up eager for a high-protein breakfast.

4. Keep your bedroom cool, dark, and free of pets. (Even before you go to your bedroom, turn off bright overhead lights in other rooms.) If necessary, install blackout curtains, buy a white noise machine, or use earplugs. A bath or sauna an hour before bedtime is relaxing and lowers your core temperature, which signals your body it's time to rest. Studies have also shown that keeping your bedroom between sixty and sixty-seven degrees at night encourages your body to rest.
5. Create a sleep schedule by going to bed and waking at the same time each day.
6. Have a relaxing pre-sleep routine. Turn off your mind an hour before turning off the lights. If you watch the TV news before going to bed or doomscroll on your phone in bed, you're getting a major dose of stress. Keep your phone out of your bedroom, turn off the TV at least an hour before bedtime, and while you're at it, get the TV out of your bedroom. No mousing, scrolling, or typing on your laptop before bed either! Besides getting you worked up over the day's news, screens emit blue light, which interferes with the sleep hormone melatonin.

   Millions of Americans use melatonin supplements because it creates a sense of quiet wakefulness prior to shutting their eyes. Melatonin is available over the counter. But before trying it as a sleep aid, talk to your healthcare provider. Melatonin can interfere with blood pressure medications, affect blood sugar levels, and have a bad effect on other health conditions. If you're currently taking other over-the-counter sleep medicines on a regular basis, tell your doctor, as their effects could be harmful.
7. Use your bedroom only for sleeping and sex. You want your mind to associate that cozy place with only those activities, not with paying bills—though you might consider making an exception for reading an old-school, paper-and-ink book like this one.

Playing Video Games as Therapy

One of my patients loved video games. She did this between 11 PM and 3 AM every night. Waking up at 11 AM didn't bother her, but because she did, her whole day was shifted. She missed out on many activities, including seeing her family and friends. Because her daytime period had less sunlight, she found herself less active and mentally stimulated. Often, she would skip meals and even her medications (i.e., following AM and PM dosing was difficult).

Her husband and I convinced her to play games from 7 PM to 9 PM so she could go to bed around 10 PM. Melatonin at night and light box therapy (exposure to a bright, artificial light source for a set time) in the morning helped her make this transition.

For a year, she was in the best shape of her life. Adjusting her sleep schedule led to habit stacking. She was more physically, socially, and mentally engaged. She ate three meals each day and never missed her medications. Her well-being, cognition, and daily function improved.

At one point, in her jubilation, she told me, "Dr. Chin, you reversed me. I no longer have mild-stage dementia." I smiled and calmly replied, "No, you still have dementia, but you're thriving because we're improving every aspect we can in your health. While we can't stop the Alzheimer's from progressing, we can do our best to strengthen your brain and build your buffer to resist the changes that will come."

Enjoy your life, especially the present moment, because you don't know what tomorrow brings. I try to find the silver lining in any situation while still meeting my patients wherever they are with whatever goals they have. If you want to play video games, then let's find a way to incorporate that into your day. But I want you to have the best possible quality of life playing those video games and living every other aspect of your day.

Despite not having a cure for diseases like Alzheimer's, Parkinson's, and Lewy body, we can always find ways to improve someone's day. When we focus on that outcome—on the person and not their disease—we achieve success.

NURTURE RELATIONSHIPS

Loneliness doesn't just anguish the soul, it sours the brain, too. In addition to the increased risk of depression, research has found that having poor social connections has negative health impacts equal to smoking fifteen cigarettes a day because isolation worsens cardiovascular and cognitive health. Many studies have revealed that having few, if any, social connections is linked to higher risk of premature death from all causes, not just Alzheimer's.

It's common sense—we engage our brains when we are with other people. Now that I have children, I'm playing cards and board games more than ever before, and I certainly wouldn't be doing this if I were home alone.

Socializing gives many brain regions a workout. Even the simple act of talking to someone creates a symphony of harmonious activity in the mind. It stimulates language-focused cognitive regions such as Broca's area, Wernicke's area, and the primary auditory cortex. Meanwhile, your memory is retrieving relevant information and past experiences to maintain context. Your amygdala is interpreting and controlling your emotional tones. Your attention center and executive function are organizing thoughts and directing your focus to the person you're speaking to. Your executive function is also assembling the list of things you plan to say in response. As if that's not enough, your somatosensory cortex is processing feedback from facial and body language while your motor cortex is controlling muscles in your body and face. It's incredible what happens during a "simple" conversation.

Studies across the globe have demonstrated that people who are socially active tend to perform better on cognitive tests. Social engagement provides a sense of support and connection, which can be mentally stimulating and protect against cognitive decline. Furthermore, social support helps prevent people from feeling lonely or isolated, factors that can also impact well-being and lead to behaviors detrimental to health. Interacting with others through in-person gatherings, phone calls, or online forums depends on one's preferences. Volunteering or participating in group activities further enhances social and cognitive engagement.

People who are socially isolated tend to have more unhealthy habits than people who interact frequently with others. They are less physically active, more likely to smoke, and have worse diets, all of which put them at higher risk for physical and mental health conditions like cardiovascular disease and depression, which are independently associated with dementia risk.

Loneliness and the sense of isolation can make you feel like you're buried under an avalanche. Whether self-imposed or not, the feeling can be crushing, its weight making it harder to breathe. When such solitude is left unaddressed, digging out from it can be an ordeal.

Can volunteering reduce the risk of dementia? At least one study shows that serving others has protective cognitive value. It doesn't matter whether volunteer work involves helping schoolchildren read, visiting patients in a hospital program, working in a soup kitchen, or serving at your church or synagogue. Research at the University of California–Davis found that no matter what your race or income level, serving others benefits the brain's executive functioning and memory. The study found that those who volunteer several times a week had higher levels of cognitive skills. Truly, it is better to give than to receive.

While the solution is obvious—get out there and join some community programs, clubs, or activities—it's not always so easy to implement. For many older people it's hard to make friends. Here's a suggestion I share with my patients—it's easier to meet or talk to people doing an activity when the focus is directed elsewhere. Investigate offerings at your local senior center. One place I know of has a *sixty-page* catalog of activities that range from taking dance lessons, creating Valentine's Day cards, and making bracelets to learning photography, playing bridge, and taking knitting classes—everything but playing shuffleboard. Even if nothing immediately grabs your interest, pick something and give it a try. It might surprise you. Most of us can remember being told as kids to "just go outside and play," maybe for our own good, or maybe because we were driving someone a little crazy. Either way, the advice still holds: Go out, join in, have fun. Just go play.

Attending Memory Café meetings is a great option for people with mild cognitive impairment. What is a Memory Café? It's a meeting where people with memory loss and their caregivers, family, and friends can come together to share concerns, do activities, or simply socialize. Some cafés have speakers, educational events, arts and crafts lessons, and musical performances. The concept got its start in Europe in the 1990s and quickly spread to America. They first appeared in Santa Fe, and now there are hundreds across the United States. Unlike other social events, everyone in attendance at a Memory Café knows what it's like to journey through memory loss. If friends or other relatives have fallen by the wayside, cafés are a place to share concerns and find support. Support groups just for caregivers are commonplace and can be found through your local senior center or the Alzheimer's Association. If it doesn't sound like a natural fit for you, go anyway. Just once. You might be surprised by how much lighter the load feels when you're not carrying it all alone. I took my mom and dad to a few different cafés. She enjoyed talking with other caregivers. And my dad? He was mostly there for the cookies.

Being with others can bring hope to someone with dementia, put a spark back in their eyes, and give them renewed vigor. The family of one of my patients wanted to move their mother to a nursing home for her safety. Since she had belonged to many clubs, I sensed that assisted living might be preferable because it offered opportunities for socializing. When she got there and was surrounded by people, activities, and structure, she thrived. Her family's safety concerns vanished. All she needed was an environment where she could be a social butterfly.

If you can be social while volunteering, you're combining the best of both worlds. Every retired person needs a purpose in life after they stop working. Even if you hated your boss or didn't enjoy your job, it still gave you a reason to get up in the morning. It also gave you the structure most people need in their lives. Some studies indicate that having a purpose—

any purpose—helps keep older people, including Alzheimer's patients, alive. Like good food, exercise, and sound sleep, volunteering does wonders for the mind and body. Helping others is a protective factor—for those you help as well as for yourself. As an old saying goes, "Doing for others is the most selfish thing you can do, because it's so good for yourself."

Keep in mind that social activities must be personalized to who you are. We all hate being told what to do. Do what gives *you* the support and stimulation you need. You don't need to see friends five days a week or join every social club. Ideally, you should feel you are a part of *something*, a group or charity that does good deeds for others. If you go to church, synagogue, or religious service of another faith, that's wonderful. Attending services has social benefits, and faith in a higher power encourages gratitude, compassion, and hope in difficult times.

If you're the child of a parent with Alzheimer's, you might be asking yourself, *How can I help Mom? How can I help Dad?* Little gestures can make a big difference. Come for a visit, and do an activity together—paint together, sing together, and bring the grandchildren so your parents can enjoy them. Don't wait for a caregiver parent to ask you for help. Make offers yourself while respecting your parents' wishes regarding ways you can pitch in.

My dad loved to eat and be around other people. Alzheimer's didn't take that from him. I frequently brought him to small local cafés to get him out of the house so he could see other people and give my mom a break. Being a lover of all things sweet, he always wanted ice cream, and occasionally I would stop so we could get ice cream cones.

A dish and spoon became a problem since he immediately wanted to dig in. We sat down at a booth one afternoon and were enjoying our cones when I noticed he was eating the paper wrapper around the cone. These are the times you can either laugh or cry. I gently removed the holder without taking the cone out of his tightly clenched hand while he continued to eat, and then he looked at me with his wonderful smile I miss so much.

So don't let perceived embarrassment stop you from going out socially. As we left, an older couple who'd quietly been observing us patted me unobtrusively on the back to express their admiration for how I dealt with my dad's Alzheimer's. There was no need for words. Their simple and gentle act reminded me that we're all in this together. Some of my most profound learning moments haven't come in school but in the alleyways and ice cream shops of life.

UPLIFT YOUR INTELLECT

The first modern crossword puzzle ran in an American newspaper in 1913. A few years later, solving these across-and-down challenges became such a mania that a *New York Times* editorial called them "madness" and a "sinful waste in the utterly futile finding of words." How wrong that was.

We now know that routinely engaging in mentally stimulating activities like playing checkers and solving puzzles is associated with better performance on thinking tests. Challenging mental activities may lead to new or stronger neural networks, which enhance brain efficiency, create a buffer for age-related atrophy (brain cell death), improve blood flow, and enhance proteins that support brain cell survival and repair.

Cognitive activity should be an enjoyable daily practice, but one that challenges you and forces you to learn. How difficult should the activity be? Here I tend to apply what I would call the Goldilocks Principle. An easy game may be fun because you feel good succeeding; however, you're likely not learning and recruiting new brain cells into a neural network. You may continue to play that game, but you're not building resilience over time. A super-difficult game challenges you to learn and build neural networks, but it can also be so frustrating that you abandon it entirely. Instead, find the middle ground, an activity that is enjoyable and challenging *enough* that you still want to do it day after day. That game is going to be the best one for you, not one that I or your doctor recommends.

It turns out, my Goldilocks approach has a scientific cousin. Psychologists call it the zone of proximal development (ZPD)—a concept introduced by Russian psychologist Lev Vygotsky. The ZPD refers to the range between what a person can do independently and what they can do with some guidance or support—from a teacher, coach, or teammate, among others. It's often described as the "sweet spot" for learning: somewhere between "I've got this" and "What fresh hell is this puzzle?" This is where your brain is challenged just beyond your current ability, but the task is still achievable with the right kind of support. Educators use it to scaffold learning. Team-building professionals use it to design ropes courses. And you can use it to choose the right crossword, brain game, or new skill to learn. So if you feel like you're coasting in your chosen activity, ramp it up. If it makes you want to launch your iPad across the room, maybe dial it back a notch. Your brain thrives on the stretch—not the snap.

Even in aging the brain retains the capacity to change. New brain cells, synaptic connections, and neural networks form that allow the older adult brain to adapt to ever-changing environments. Many studies have found that complex mental activities reduce the risk for dementia. However, there is little consensus on what is the best type of complex mental activity. How long should one do it in a single session? Is a group activity better than one done alone?

Old-style puzzles may be better than electronic ones. A 2023 study examined individuals with MCI. One group played computer-based cognitive games while another did computer-based crossword puzzles. After a year, both groups showed improvement in cognitive tests and symptoms, but the crossword-solving group performed better. Results for men and women were identical. Those early in the disease process got equal benefits from computerized games and crossword puzzles, but those later in the disease excelled more at crosswords than games.

Why are thinking games good for the brain? No one knows exactly, but there are several plausible reasons. Crosswords employ the brain's language areas and require sharp reasoning, thus strengthening existing neural pathways while building new synaptic connections and neurons. If the maxim "Use it or lose it" is true, then word games give our mental muscles stimulation they otherwise wouldn't get. As with other habits, ritually doing crosswords may cause the brain to rewire itself by carving new problem-solving pathways just as plowing a field helps germinate seeds.

How much time should one devote to mental games? Science doesn't offer a set number, but thirty minutes a day should suffice, as with exercise, and more is usually better. The same, in my opinion, may be true of curling up with an engrossing book. I've seen this kind of deep concentration benefit some of my patients, encouraging neuroplasticity in the brain in ways that shallow engagement by browsing the internet may not. An analogy can be made to how bread is prepared for baking. It takes intense kneading to produce a delicious loaf. Briefly brushing the outside of the dough, that is, the equivalent of web surfing, won't have the same effect. Still, doing something is better than doing nothing. Five minutes of crosswords is better than thirty minutes of watching TV, especially if you're willing to gradually increase the duration over time.

If the numbers game sudoku or finding words with Wordle works for you, go for it. If you enjoy learning a language through a fun smartphone app like Duolingo, swipe away. Routinely involving yourself in any complex mental activity does the trick. If you're going to read, take the next step and talk to someone about it. Challenge a different region of your brain by hearing what they say in response. A stimulating conversation with a friend or loved one can be one of the most enjoyable of all activities.

Does Playing a Musical Instrument Have Benefits?

My father understood that mental stimulation might slow the progression of his disease and took up the guitar. I suspect his doctor suggested it. He had never played one before. It's a tricky instrument. He thought learning a few songs would be cognitively productive. I thought so, too.

The problem was the disease impacted his ability to learn and to remember. When people complain about forgetting, they assume the information is in there and the difficulty is retrieving it. But as we learned in chapter 1, Alzheimer's disease diminishes your ability to encode recent events (i.e., to learn) as well as recall them. This is why giving an iPhone to someone with mild-stage dementia who's always used a flip phone may not work.

For my dad, all the guitar did was lead to frustration. It became yet another activity he couldn't do. It sat in the corner, a symbol of his inabilities. And for me, it was a symbol of what *not* to suggest to my patients.

Music can be helpful for some people. A patient with advanced Alzheimer's lived with her son, who had a guitar. If it was given to her, she enjoyed strumming it to make sounds. For her, at that point in the disease process, she probably found it soothing to merely hug it and get it to make noises.

At a much earlier stage of the disease, another patient, Sally, had been diagnosed with mild-stage dementia. She had been a professional pianist. Her mood was low. When her family asked me to prescribe something to boost it, I did, but I also asked her what she enjoyed doing. The answer was a common response: "I watch TV." I probed deeper to learn what she enjoyed in her twenties, thirties, forties, and fifties. Though her answer was that she loved raising her children, her daughter instantly blurted out that she once played the piano beautifully. Her daughter teared up with pride while Sally blushed and whispered, "Yes, that was a long time ago."

So my second prescription was playing the piano. I was hesitant to do this given my father's experience; however, Sally had a prior history, and I was relying on her established neural networks to still be in place so she wouldn't have to create new ones. It was a gamble, but her daughter bought her an electronic keyboard.

At first, trying to recapture her skills upset Sally, but her daughter encouraged her by saying, "No one expects you to be in top form. Playing will address boredom and improve your mood." She began practicing daily, got pretty good, and persisted in her mild stage for years longer than anyone thought she would. At our subsequent visits, she mostly wanted to talk about music.

One last word: Music hath charms to soothe not only the savage breast but any soul, especially those of people with Alzheimer's. The right music, especially when played routinely, can have a calming effect. Just be sure you're playing music *they* enjoy, not what *you* prefer. If your dad grew up loving the Beatles, the Fab Four might be just the ticket. After all, all he needs is love. But if he swings to Frank Sinatra, and you don't exactly dig the Chairman of the Board, well, daddy-o, that's life. Play him the music that'll fly him to the moon.

PROTECT YOUR SENSES AND TEETH

Step 1: Correct Hearing Loss

Impaired vision or hearing and poor oral hygiene dramatically increase a person's odds of developing dementia. Taking care of eyesight, hearing, and teeth should be a priority to boost quality of life. Corrective action in each of these areas is one of the easiest things anyone can do and will cut the risk of future cognitive decline.

Out of all the fourteen modifiable risk factors reported by the *Lancet* commission (see sidebar on page 165: "Fourteen Alzheimer's Risk Factors"), one that might come as the most astonishing is the danger of unaddressed hearing loss (8 percent of dementia cases). Compared to people with normal hearing, those who have mild hearing loss are twice as likely to be at risk of dementia. Those with moderate hearing loss are *three times* more likely, and those with severe hearing loss are *five times* more likely. Most people with severe hearing deficits have hearing aids. The greatest benefit is for people with mild to moderate hearing loss. They have adapted to hearing less and don't think it's a problem. It is, and it's one you can remedy today. All it takes is an appointment to be fitted with a hearing aid—in most cases no prescription is needed. Walk in and walk out hearing the world again.

I spoke with Dr. Frank Lin about his pivotal study that looked at how hearing aids can reduce cognitive decline in older adults with hearing loss. The study was called ACHIEVE (Aging and Cognitive Health Evaluation in Elders). It compared two groups of research participants, one healthier than the other. When Lin removed the more fit group from his analyses, he found that when the less healthy group used hearing aids, the result was a 50 percent reduction in cognitive decline. This was significant.

There are three interrelated ways in which hearing loss increases risk for cognitive decline and dementia, according to Lin. First, when you can't hear, your brain receives a garbled signal and must reallocate resources to help interpret the message. This action comes at a cost. Your cognitive reserve is being drained so you can hear. Second, when your brain is deprived of the appropriate auditory signal, it atrophies, withers in a way, because these mechanisms directly damage brain cells. Third, if you aren't hearing properly, you are unable to fully participate in conversations and engage in mentally stimulating activities. You will not be building brain resilience.

No one should be shy about getting a hearing aid. Nearly 25 percent of people over age sixty-five have a disabling hearing loss, a figure that rises to 75 percent at age seventy-five. There's no stigma about wearing glasses, and they dramatically change one's appearance. Today's hearing aids are almost unnoticeable.

For people with mild to moderate hearing loss, no prescription is needed. The newest generation of Apple AirPods even includes a simple built-in hearing test, and many users find them surprisingly effective. Not only are they far less expensive than most traditional hearing aids, but they also come without stigma—everyone walks around with those small white earbuds today. What once might have felt like a medical device now doubles as an everyday accessory, blending seamlessly into daily life while providing meaningful support for hearing. And of course, they also allow you to enjoy excellent music—just be careful not to crank up your favorite songs too loudly, or you'll undo the very help they're giving you.

Many of my patients see me with their adult children, who often bring up concerns about hearing loss. While some brush it off, their loved ones ask about screening and referrals for testing. I love it when children gently encourage parents to prioritize their health and be proactive. As with any relationship, patience, politeness, and persistence can go a long way in helping someone make a beneficial decision.

My clinic worked with Drs. Pamela Souza and Kimberly Mueller on the first clinical study that investigated over-the-counter hearing aids in a memory clinic population. I witnessed patients' apprehension about hearing aids diminish when they learned they are economically priced and can be bought without a prescription. Nearly everyone was willing to be screened for hearing loss, too.

Step 2: Address Vision Issues

As for eye care, poor vision can increase the risk of Alzheimer's. The reasons why would be similar to those regarding hearing loss—if you have to strain to see, you are overstressing your brain in one or more ways.

About 20 percent of people over sixty-five have cataracts, a clouding of the eye's transparent lens, a share that rises to 50 percent at age seventy-five. Having cataracts makes it harder to read at night, and driving becomes more difficult. They can literally make you feel like the light is going out of your life because insufficient light is getting to your brain. Studies have found that people across all demographic categories who had their cataract-clouded lenses removed and replaced with artificial ones had an almost 30 percent lower risk of developing dementia compared with people who decided against surgery. (Glaucoma surgery, which doesn't restore vision, has no meaningful association with dementia risk.)

Cataract surgery is a medical miracle. The incision to remove the original lens and insert the artificial one can be as small as one-tenth of an inch. The procedure's success rate is 98 percent. It uses local and brief general anesthesia and is done on an outpatient basis. The new lenses last a lifetime. Depending on the type a patient chooses, a person can see with 20/20 vision or vision that no longer requires glasses for driving. Patients often see the results of the surgery immediately on opening their eyes.

Step 3: Maintain Oral Health

If eyes are the windows to the soul, then a person's teeth and gums speak volumes about the body's overall health. After all, how well a person cares for their teeth over their life could reflect how well they've cared for themselves in general.

Regular toothbrushing and flossing prevents plaque buildup on teeth and lowers the likelihood of gum inflammation. A connection has been found between periodontal (gum) disease such as gingivitis and the likelihood of being diagnosed with Alzheimer's and heart disease. That's because bacteria associated with oral inflammation get in the bloodstream and release enzymes called *gingipains*, which destroy nerve cells in the brain. The old dentist's joke "You only need to brush the teeth you want to keep" might have a corollary—keep your teeth clean if you want to keep your brain, too.

Daily oral care is a must. Brush twice a day, in the morning after breakfast and before going to bed. If you don't, bacteria in the mouth take food particles, break them down, and create acid, which dissolves teeth. Floss daily and see your dentist twice a year to have your teeth checked and professionally cleaned.

The better your teeth look, the more you will want to smile. And smiling has been proven to have health benefits for your brain. Showing off your pearly whites lowers stress, boosts your immune system, and actually makes you feel better. Even if you don't feel like smiling, that happy expression releases neuropeptides and neurotransmitters that reduce anxiety. Plus, smiling is contagious. It makes other people want to smile, too. As Louis Armstrong sang, "When you're smilin', keep on smilin' / The whole world smiles with you."

THINK POSITIVE

Everyone wants to have control over their life. A diagnosis of a disease like Alzheimer's, which has no cure, can shatter that sense of control. We do, however, know that lifestyle interventions can have an uplifting impact on daily living. We are not solely our genes or the amyloid proteins building in our brain—one aspect we can control is the decisions we make. For better or worse, our actions, habits, and behaviors can make a difference. While there's no guarantee that creating good, healthy habits means you won't develop disease later in life, you may delay its progress and keep feeling better for longer.

Patients who commit to lifestyle changes often return for checkups feeling better. However, after a couple of years, they may still experience cognitive decline despite their best efforts and "doing everything possible." This can be understandably disappointing, but here is a different perspective—if they had not adopted those new habits, they would have done *much* worse on the testing, and they would not have had the last two years of better abilities and overall quality of life. While the next two years may be challenging, they will still be better than they would have been without the courageous decision to act years before. It's important to compare oneself not to an ideal but to a version who didn't make those changes—a version that would be further along in the disease because they were still eating poorly and remaining inactive.

One of my favorite books is the bestselling 1988 novel *The Alchemist*, by Brazilian author Paulo Coelho. It tells the tale of a young shepherd who believes he has a purpose but doesn't know what it is. During his mystical journey, he travels the world. He learns that all things are connected and no matter what obstacles one faces, a person's duty in life must be to achieve his unique reason for being.

In the book's introduction, Coelho writes, "The secret of life . . . is to fall seven times and to get up eight times. . . . Once we have overcome the defeats—and we always do—we are filled by a greater sense of euphoria and confidence. In the silence of our hearts, we know that we are proving ourselves worthy of the miracle of life. Each day, each hour, is part of the good fight."

Some people might call this Pollyanna thinking. But part of a doctor's job—something you won't find in a chemistry textbook—is to give patients hope and courage. That doesn't mean sugarcoating reality. It means recognizing that even when a disease like Alzheimer's enters the picture, there is still room for moments of happiness.

I'll never forget Joe, one of my patients. He owned a hardware store in a small town, and by the time he met me, he had handed the day-to-day management over to his son. That freed him to pursue his true love—fishing. He went after everything from trout in mountain streams and walleye through the ice to bottom-dwelling lake sturgeon. In truth, it wasn't the fish he loved but the peace of mind the experience gave him. As Henry David Thoreau supposedly said, "Many men fish all their lives without realizing that it is not fish they are after."

When Joe came to my office, his family shared that he had fallen into a deep funk after his diagnosis. He'd stopped caring, they said. He'd lost interest in nearly everything. Instead of diving into medications or staging, I asked him about his life. What had brought him the most happiness? What were his fondest memories?

His face lit up when he talked about fishing. He and his brothers had gone on annual trips for years, he told me, and he loved hiking to the streams and sitting in ice shacks, even when the fish weren't biting. I asked why he wasn't doing it anymore. He shrugged. He was afraid of what lay ahead in the disease. "What if I can't do it later?"

I understood that fear. But I reminded him—that's a tomorrow problem. Alzheimer's wasn't preventing him from fishing today. And, frankly, something else could take away that chance just as easily: a stroke, cancer, even a freak accident. I took a risk being that blunt with him. But the greater risk, I thought, was saying nothing and watching his world shrink.

That day wasn't really about fishing. It was about reclaiming agency, even in the face of a progressive illness.

If you have been diagnosed with mild cognitive impairment, dementia, or Alzheimer's, fight. Be strong. Make healthy decisions. If your loved one is walking that path, hold his hand, maybe put your arm around his shoulder, and go with him. Walk the good walk together.

6

"I See the Bright Future Ahead"

A NEW ERA OF ALZHEIMER'S TREATMENT IS DAWNING

Do Lecanemab and Donanemab Work? • Who Is Eligible to Take Them? • What Are Their Risks? • Why Have Research Results Been Slow in Coming? • Is Amyloid the Fire or the Fireman? • Why Alzheimer's Is Not a Type of Diabetes • Are Inflammation and Oxidation Possible Causes of Alzheimer's?

A diagnosis has been made and treatment options explored. Anxiety about symptoms and their meaning has now been replaced by a different concern—what's next for me or my loved one?

Prescription drugs can play a meaningful role in the answer to that question. You've likely heard about the groundbreaking Alzheimer's drugs lecanemab and donanemab. Both are FDA-approved medications that target and remove amyloid from the brain. You may also be aware of four other drugs—donepezil, rivastigmine, galantamine, and memantine—that have long been prescribed for Alzheimer's.*

* These drugs are marketed under the following brand names: lecanemab (Leqembi); donanemab (Kisunla); donepezil (Aricept); rivastigmine (Exelon); galantamine (Razadyne); and memantine (Namenda). While I have served as a consultant to pharmaceutical companies, this book received no funding or support from any such company, and no outside entity had any role in its content or conclusions.

The specific type of neurodegenerative disease a person is diagnosed with and its stage of progression will help a doctor determine treatment options, including what medications to recommend. Depending on the exact diagnosis and other health factors, a patient may choose to use one or more of the above drugs or none of them. These choices will influence the direction of care and the course of the disease.

The goal of this chapter is to explain what these drugs do and when and if someone should take them. Before getting into the nuts and bolts of that, it's important to share some background on how medical science arrived at its present state of knowledge. To be an informed patient, it helps to know some of this. So, for a history lesson on how Alzheimer's was discovered and the decades-long and sometimes rancorous twists and turns of Alzheimer's research, read on. (To jump to the section on the drugs your doctor may prescribe, turn to page 242.)

THE HISTORY OF ALZHEIMER'S RESEARCH—MEET MRS. DETER

Like Parkinson's and Crohn's disease, Alzheimer's is named after the doctor who identified it—in this case, the German psychiatrist and neuropathologist Alois Alzheimer. In 1906, he performed an autopsy on Auguste Deter, the wife of a Frankfurt railway clerk, who had spent the last years of her life suffering from memory loss. "Her behavior is characterized by total helplessness," he wrote after first examining her several years before her death.

Mrs. Deter puzzled Dr. Alzheimer. When he first met her, Mrs. Deter's mental woes were pronounced, yet she had no history of events such as a stroke or alcoholism that could cause neurological deterioration. What really caught Dr. Alzheimer's interest was her age. When he first saw her, she was in her early fifties, not elderly. She died at age fifty-six.

By today's definition, Mrs. Deter had younger-onset dementia since her diagnosis occurred prior to the age of sixty-five. Despite dementia being typically associated with older people, a study in *JAMA Neurology* estimates that 119 out of every 100,000 will be diagnosed with it before sixty-five, a number that is higher than most scientists initially thought. In Mrs. Deter's case, the cause was early-onset Alzheimer's, which was later found to be inherited through a single faulty gene, a pattern known as *autosomal dominant inheritance.* Her mutation was in a gene called *presenilin 1,* but scientists have since discovered two other gene culprits: *amyloid precursor protein (APP)* and *presenilin 2.* Mutations in any of these three genes can lead to early-onset Alzheimer's, a form of the disease that is distinct from the more common late-onset type. It is interesting that the first person diagnosed with Alzheimer's had a rare form of the disease that occurs in fewer than 2 percent of all cases.

Dr. Alzheimer's autopsy of Mrs. Deter's brain revealed that a mysterious "special substance" had infiltrated the dead neurons. The technology to identify what it was didn't yet exist. We now know it was amyloid, a protein that is normally present throughout the body but can cause health conditions when found in excess in the kidneys, bladder, heart, and brain.

More than a century later, I found myself pondering those same mysterious brain changes when my own father's brain was examined. During that process, the outward appearance and initial brain specimens did not shout amyloid, but that protein, among others, was found on closer inspection. Without the autopsy, our family wouldn't have had a definitive or complete understanding of the brain diseases that shaped his final years. That closer look linked our family's experience to the very protein that has defined the disease since its beginning.

Amyloid, the protein that clogs and apparently helps destroy the neurons of Alzheimer's patients, has been the defining characteristic of the disease since it was first discovered. Our bodies naturally produce amyloid proteins, but sometimes, for reasons yet to be discovered, these proteins start folding incorrectly. When this happens, their shape changes, and they begin to clump together. In the brain, these clumps form deposits called plaques, which then trigger other harmful processes. Researchers are still investigating what causes amyloid misfolding. Possible factors include inflammation, genetic mutations, and other underlying conditions. What we do know is that when this normal biological process goes awry, it leads to serious diseases like Alzheimer's. Unfortunately, we currently have no way to prevent it or stop it once it begins.

In autosomal dominant Alzheimer's disease like Mrs. Deter's, there is an overproduction of amyloid protein. In late-onset Alzheimer's disease (the most common form), overproduction of amyloid is not the problem. Instead, the plaques form due to a decrease in the natural removal of amyloid from the brain. (The brain filters out chemicals it produces just as the kidneys and intestines remove other waste matter from the body.) While early- and late-onset Alzheimer's share the same name and pathological hallmark of amyloid, they have different underlying mechanisms.

LOST OPPORTUNITIES, THEN BREAKTHROUGHS

For much of the twentieth century little was understood about senility, a more common term for the mental deterioration of some older people. Doctors generally believed it was inevitable, a normal progression of aging. It had existed throughout human history and could not be prevented. Today, we know better. According to the CDC, only 4 percent of people over sixty-five develop dementia, proving that cognitive decline is not a consequence of healthy aging.

World Wars I and II and the Great Depression all conspired to stifle research into Alzheimer's. Not until 1984 did American scientists George Glenner and Caine Wong identify the "special substance" as amyloid. A year later, researchers discovered that another protein, tau, was also a key constituent in the dead tangles of neurons.

Think about it—nearly *eighty years* had elapsed before researchers identified the key suspects in the Alzheimer's mystery. That is a tragedy, but not necessarily surprising. In the mid-twentieth century, not that much money was spent on Alzheimer's research since doctors (and the public alike) thought senility was as natural for some people as wrinkles and white hair. Without enough financial investment, research into Alzheimer's disease could only go so far.

Today, we've reached a point where it's entirely possible that Alzheimer's treatments will follow a path similar to those developed for HIV (human immunodeficiency virus). Decades ago, having HIV was considered a death sentence, as it almost always led to AIDS (acquired immunodeficiency syndrome). But medical science transformed HIV into a manageable, chronic condition. Now, a mother living with HIV can give birth without passing the virus to her child. That's the power of scientific progress, even without a cure.

HIV research accelerated in the 1980s, fueled by major financial investments and the creation of the Office of AIDS Research. The 1990 Ryan White CARE Act not only boosted funding but also raised public and political awareness, helping sustain support for science. That momentum led to annual federal funding surpassing $1 billion and paved the way for antiretroviral therapy, the backbone of present-day HIV care.

Although Alzheimer's and related dementias affected millions, research lagged throughout the 1980s and 1990s. The NIH only allocated $500 million annually to dementia research until 2013, a fraction of what was needed. Not until 2016 did the government start to spend more than $1 billion per year on Alzheimer's and dementia research. This increase was driven by growing recognition of the disease's impact, thanks to advocacy groups, congressional support, and the National Alzheimer's Project Act (NAPA).

While we are diagnosing Alzheimer's more often today, that's partly because clinicians now recognize its signs earlier and have better tools to confirm the disease. Yet there also appear to be more actual cases, driven by the aging baby boomer generation, longer lifespans, and decades of rising health risks such as obesity, diabetes, and hypertension. Encouragingly, some studies suggest that the rate of Alzheimer's within specific age groups may be declining due to improved public health, but the overall number of cases will continue to grow as the population ages.

A major step forward in public consciousness came in 1994, when former President Ronald Reagan announced that he had Alzheimer's. In his letter to the nation, he wrote that he "hope[d] this might promote greater awareness of this condition. Perhaps it will encourage a clearer understanding of the individuals and families who are affected by it." Until then, a heavy cloak of stigma hung over Alzheimer's and other forms of dementia. Perhaps by coincidence, World Alzheimer's Day first took place that year, on September 21.

In the early 1990s, researchers around the world began to focus on what has come to be known as the amyloid cascade hypothesis (or the amyloid-beta hypothesis). In the United States alone, billions have been spent to fund research to cure Alzheimer's based on unlocking how and why amyloid appears in the brain. The theory is simple—stop amyloid from forming, and then tau never forms. Tau appears after many years of amyloid development and is more closely associated with neuron death and a person's symptoms. It is the combination of amyloid and tau that is so damaging to the health of our brains. But without excess amyloid there's no tau and no Alzheimer's. At least that's the theory.

For years, up to one-half of Alzheimer's research funded by the National Institutes of Health has gone to amyloid-related investigations. At times this has amounted to over $1 billion. (Bill Gates alone recently donated $100 million to the cause.) That means a great many scientists and doctors at universities and medical research facilities have built their lives, careers, and scholarly reputations around this hypothesis. It's no secret that it's easier to get research funding if you plan to study amyloid instead of a less favored theory into the origins of Alzheimer's. Unfortunately, the field has also been discredited by well-supported allegations that a few prominent Alzheimer's researchers have knowingly published fraudulent papers that other scientists have referenced for years. Careers have been ruined, and a shadow has been cast over legitimate work by upstanding scientists.

Progress is slow because science is inherently slow and diseases of aging are complex—not because less than 1 percent of scientists commit fraud. Should more funding go to other non-Alzheimer's neurodegenerative diseases and nonamyloid targets? Yes. Is the amyloid cascade hypothesis still the most viable theory to date? Yes. Has this been a wasted investment? Ask the people taking lecanemab or donanemab who now have months to a year of more cognitive and daily function. I don't think they'd say so.

TO TEST OR NOT TO TEST FOR APOE

In 1993, Japanese scientists and researchers at Duke University discovered the gene *apolipoprotein E* (written as APOE or ApoE), where *E* denotes its specific subtype. They identified three versions—APOE2, APOE3, and APOE4. The particular type a person carries can influence the chance of developing Alzheimer's, either by increasing the risk, decreasing it, or having no effect at all.

One of the most common questions I get from my patients' children is whether *they* should get tested to find out whether APOE4 is part of their genetic makeup. It's a question that weighs heavily on them. They understand what the results could mean, but they're also aware of the emotional burden that kind of knowledge can carry. It's not an easy decision, and so they often turn to me, their parent's doctor, who they know has faced the same question, for guidance.

Here's a summary of the differences between the three types of APOE. A person obtains one copy of at least one of the three APOE genes from his mother and one copy from his father. Having APOE2 can reduce one's Alzheimer's risk by up to 40 percent. More people have the APOE3 version, which has no effect on risk. On the other hand, APOE4 is considered a "risk gene" because carrying one copy of it (i.e., from only one parent) increases a person's risk by 200 to 400 percent, and carrying two copies of it (one from each parent) increases risk by 1,200 to 1,500 percent.

Someone who has both APOE3 and APOE4 in their DNA has a 25 percent higher lifetime risk of developing Alzheimer's disease, while someone who inherited APOE4 from *both* parents has a 60 percent risk of developing Alzheimer's dementia by age eighty-five. (This happens in only about 2 percent of the population.) About 25 percent of people carry one copy of APOE4; not only does it increase one's Alzheimer's risk, but it also lowers the age at which people start developing amyloid in their brains.

A genetic test for APOE has existed for decades. Until the introduction of new Alzheimer's treatments like lecanemab and donanemab, it was rarely used in patient care. Today many healthcare providers order the test after diagnosing mild cognitive impairment (MCI) or dementia and confirming the presence of amyloid. Essentially, genetic testing is ordered only after cognitive impairment due to Alzheimer's has been established.

For Alzheimer's patients, APOE4 testing is primarily used to assess the risk of side effects from lecanemab and donanemab. Patients with two copies of APOE4 face the highest risk for amyloid-related imaging abnormalities (ARIA), including brain bleeding. This makes them more likely to be excluded from treatment. Those Alzheimer's patients with one copy of APOE4 and one copy of APOE3 have a higher risk of ARIA than those with two copies of APOE3, but they can still receive treatment.

Understanding this genetic risk can inform treatment decisions and monitoring strategies. Sadly, the irony is that individuals with APOE4—those most susceptible to developing Alzheimer's—are also at greatest risk for severe side effects from these two new drugs. The very people who stand to gain the most are also those most likely to be excluded from treatment.

APOE testing for patients differs from testing for family members of those affected. While patients undergo testing to determine postdiagnosis treatment options, family members are typically healthy and seek this information for personal planning.

Before the approval of these new Alzheimer's treatments, the prevailing medical belief was that APOE genetic testing lacked "clinical utility" and was therefore unnecessary. According to the NIH Cancer Institute, clinical utility refers to a test's ability to prompt an intervention that leads to improved health outcomes. Because no specific treatments for APOE4 carriers existed, many medical professionals dismissed the test as irrelevant to patient care.

That perspective, however, is narrowly focused and seems paternalistic to me. Just because a treatment does not exist does not mean a test lacks value. It fails to consider the concept of personal utility. This counterpoint to a treatment-only focus encompasses subjective benefits such as a person's increased self-knowledge. Taking the test might motivate a person to make lifestyle changes, take part in clinical research, and begin future health and lifestyle planning.

Because the medical establishment largely ignored the demand for genetic testing, private companies stepped in. Direct-to-consumer genetic testing services now offer APOE results for a fee, allowing individuals to access this information outside the healthcare system. However, using these services comes with privacy concerns because individuals must consent to their genetic data being used for business and research purposes.

For cognitively healthy individuals considering APOE testing, the main argument in favor of getting tested is personal utility. While no APOE4-specific treatments exist, learning one's genetic status could encourage proactive health decisions. Being tested might also inspire participation in research studies that contribute to scientific advancements and possibly offer personal benefits. However, it's important to think carefully about why you would want this information and what you plan to do with it—once learned, it cannot be unlearned.

Before deciding whether APOE testing is right for you, consider the following:

1. **Understand Your Current Risk:** APOE4 is a risk gene, not a determinant. Carrying it does not mean you will develop Alzheimer's, but it is the strongest known genetic risk factor. If you already suspect you are at high risk due to your family history, confirming your genetic status might validate your concerns and inspire you to take steps to lower your risk through lifestyle changes.

   If you have never seriously considered your risk, receiving a positive result could be an emotional shock. It is essential to prepare for how you might react to this information. For those with a family history of dementia, do you know for certain the dementia was caused by Alzheimer's? Other cognitive disorders such as cerebrovascular disease have less of a genetic component, and in those circumstances, taking the test might have far less value.

2. **Assess Your Cognitive Symptoms:** If you are already experiencing memory issues or cognitive changes, it's important to seek medical evaluation before pursuing genetic testing. Many reversible conditions can cause cognitive symptoms, and an APOE4 result is not the same thing as being diagnosed with Alzheimer's. Moreover, learning you carry APOE4 could lead to a self-fulfilling prophecy—a psychological phenomenon in which an expectation influences behavior and perception. In this case, knowing you have APOE4 might make you more anxious about your memory, cause you to overanalyze normal forgetfulness, and detrimentally impact your quality of life.
3. **Evaluate Your Health Behaviors:** Many people considering genetic testing already engage in brain-healthy activities such as exercise, eating a nutritious diet, and being socially engaged. Would knowing your APOE4 status push you to do more? Would it motivate you to adopt additional protective behaviors, such as adhering strictly to a Mediterranean diet, prioritizing sleep, or reducing stress? If you already lead a health-conscious lifestyle, ask yourself whether this information would inspire meaningful changes or simply add stress to your life. On the other hand, not knowing your status may cause its own kind of anxiety for some people, especially those with a strong family history or lingering uncertainty. For these individuals, peace of mind comes from having clarity.
4. **Prepare for the Future:** Learning you have a higher genetic risk for Alzheimer's may influence how you plan for the future. It can impact decisions about finances, legal arrangements, and long-term care. It is crucial to understand the effect it could have on your insurance coverage. While the Genetic Information Nondiscrimination Act (GINA) protects against health insurance and employment discrimination, it does not cover life insurance, disability insurance, or long-term care insurance. Some people opt to

secure such policies before undergoing genetic testing. I encourage this approach, as it allows individuals to acquire coverage in advance and avoid the risk of being excluded based on genetic information discovered later.

Be aware that GINA protections only benefit some people. Those in the military, employees of small businesses, and individuals seeking certain types of housing (such as senior living communities) may not be protected. GINA also ceases to apply when a person is diagnosed with cognitive impairment—once Alzheimer's is confirmed, genetic test results could be used in ways that affect access to care and resources.

If you share your direct-to-consumer genetic results with your healthcare provider, it may become part of your medical record and would be regarded as part of a legal document. Such information could be accessed by insurance companies and other agencies that request your records.

5. **Decide Who to Share This Information With:** Genetic information does not exist in isolation—it has implications for family members as well. If you test positive for APOE4, will you share this information with your siblings? Even though siblings do not have identical genetics, they may feel anxious knowing they could also carry the risk gene. If you have children, will you tell them? If you are APOE4 homozygous (carrying APOE4 genes from each parent), you have certainly passed one copy to each of your children, increasing their risk. Having the test done under these circumstances is a deeply personal decision that requires careful consideration.
6. **Consider the Potential for Stigma:** Stigma surrounding Alzheimer's can affect your self-perception and how others treat you. If you learn that you carry APOE4, you may become hyperaware of memory lapses, and this could lead to unnecessary stress or anxiety. Other people, either consciously or unconsciously, may begin to scrutinize your behavior, attributing normal forgetfulness to impending cognitive decline. While you cannot control how others react, you can decide how much you wish to disclose and to whom you disclose it.

With great access comes great responsibility. Before seeking APOE testing, take the time to reflect. Consider whether having this knowledge will enhance your life or cause you unnecessary worry. The best decision is the one that leaves you feeling informed, prepared, and at peace with your choice.

My Family's APOE Decision

Shortly after my dad's diagnosis, my sister and I faced two life-altering decisions—whether to move home to be closer to our parents and whether to learn our APOE genotype. Despite no other evidence of Alzheimer's in our family history, my dad's young age suggested a high likelihood that he had the genetic mutation, specifically APOE, that caused his early-onset Alzheimer's. Did we want to learn if we had the gene as well? The choice wasn't simple. Whatever we decided would ripple through many aspects of our lives.

If you are the child of someone with Alzheimer's, you face the disease on two fronts. You are trying to focus on your parent, supporting them any way you can. At the same time, whether consciously or not, you face the reality that you are now at higher risk of sharing their fate. By simply having a first-degree family member with the condition, you have a 73 percent increased risk of having Alzheimer's disease. Your risk of being diagnosed with it is greater than if you had diabetes, hypertension, or obesity. Here is a double whammy—this doesn't even take into account the added genetic risk of APOE4, if you have that gene.

After much thought, I decided not to get genetic testing. My healthcare institution declined to offer it to me because it did not believe my father had the autosomal dominant form of Alzheimer's. Of course, I could have bought the test from an online company. Had I done so, I would have been giving my DNA to a private corporation that offered me no pre- or post-test counseling. More worrisome was its twenty-page small-print contract that outlined what it could and could not do with my "data." I read each line closely. The more I read, the more uncomfortable I became. As a researcher myself, I recognized the immense power and value of what they were collecting.

This company's lack of adequate data protection safeguards concerned me. So far as I could tell, the company could have shared the essence of who I was with others for financial gain. If it merged with another company, my data would have been considered an "asset" and sold with the business. My DNA would not have been mine anymore. I also wondered just how accurate this company's test was. There was no way I would ever know what its technological standards were.

In the end, I knew that the test results would not change my behavior. I was already modifying my lifestyle, habit by habit, and so I had little to gain from the test and much to lose in terms of my peace of mind.

This is a decision I'll revisit if and when prevention-focused clinical trials begin to show clear benefit—especially if enrollment requires knowing my genetic status.

THE AMYLOID MYSTERY

Not everything in Alzheimer's research is straightforward. For more than thirty years, Alzheimer's research has been focused on the amyloid cascade hypothesis. Some in healthcare reject this belief. Indeed, evidence suggests the amyloid story and its resulting pharmaceutical therapies will be a dead end, or at best a roundabout route to a cure. There's worry—even anger—among experts that this focus has delayed overall progress. Some respected researchers speculate that the cause of Alzheimer's lies elsewhere.

Many are asking, "Where are the results?" More than a dozen anti-amyloid drugs such as gantenerumab, crenezumab, bapineuzumab, solanezumab, and ponezumab have failed to pass human trials. (Just saying those names gives the brain and tongue a workout.) Lecanemab and donanemab are the first Alzheimer's-targeting drugs to be approved for use in decades.

Facing the Backlash

Current controversies in the field of dementia research and patient treatment have become intense. In August 2023, I coauthored the editorial "Ushering In a New Era of Alzheimer Disease Therapy" in JAMA, *the* Journal of the American Medical Association. *My colleagues and I wrote that lecanemab and donanemab had "an exceptional ability" to remove amyloid from the brain, though we also cautioned that patients taking them would only see "modest benefits." We emphasized that healthcare was not ready for their full implementation, and fundamental changes would be needed for them to succeed. Despite our balanced approach, I received feedback from colleagues on both sides questioning my position. Some said I was too eager to utilize an untested long-term pharmaceutical strategy, and others suggested I lacked the expertise to properly interpret the science within the clinical trials. It felt like I couldn't win.*

That fall, I joined a conversation as part of a podcast with two other leaders in the field—Dr. Sharon Brangman, a geriatrician who teaches at SUNY Upstate in New York, and Dr. Jason Karlawish, a geriatrician who teaches at the University of Pennsylvania. (He's also the author of the excellent book The Problem of Alzheimer's: How Science, Culture, and Politics Turned a Rare Disease into a Crisis and What We Can Do About It.*) The hosts asked us, "Are you going to prescribe these new medications—lecanemab* *and donanemab?" There was an awkward silence, and then we all said, "Yes, for certain patients and for certain reasons."*

After the podcast hit the internet, to say I got negative social media feedback would be an understatement. Commenters had harsh words. "How can geriatricians favor such drugs?" one person asked. "They've lost their way," said another. Insults like "They've lost their principles" and "Shame on them" hit hard. I was taken aback. I had never received criticism like that before.

Instead of turning away, I leaned in. I asked Drs. Karlawish, Brangman, and Eric Widera to write an article with me for the Journal of the American Geriatrics Society *that would address the role of geriatricians with these new therapies. It was published a few months after the podcast episode aired with the hope of bringing the field together. Whether geriatricians liked these drugs or not, the therapies were available, and I wanted our specialty to become stewards of their use.*

After the article's publication, the backlash was even worse. I read somewhere that I had been bought by pharma and was an antigeriatrician, a zinger that hurt. The experience caused me to ask the question, "What is the role of a geriatrician in this new era of Alzheimer's disease?"

My mission is to prevent people from dying of a disease that robs them of their memories and autonomy. We are all going to die, but a reasonable expectation would be to experience death knowing who you are and who the family is surrounding you.

There's no question that the amyloid cascade hypothesis has taken away investment, energy, and creativity from other areas of Alzheimer's disease research. Alzheimer's alone has diverted research energy from the other diseases of dementia, such as Lewy body, Parkinson's, Huntington's, vascular dementia, frontotemporal, and the most recently identified condition limbic-predominant age-related TDP-43 encephalopathy (LATE).

The issue of how research money is spent is made more complex by the fact that mixed dementia is more common than most people recognize. As many as 60–65 percent of patients with Alzheimer's, including my father, also have another type of neurodegenerative process such as Lewy body or frontotemporal or cerebrovascular disease. Excess amyloid is a key piece to the Alzheimer's puzzle, but it may have little to do with other brain diseases. So, while Alzheimer's research raises awareness, it doesn't always translate into help for those with other types of dementia—or those with more than one type. My father was one of them.

Early in his disease, my dad began acting out his dreams—talking in nonsensical conversations and gesturing dramatically in his sleep. It was so striking that my mother recorded it one evening for me and his medical team. Watching it, I understood why partners of people with REM sleep behavior disorder often sleep in separate rooms. At the time, we assumed his behavior was a medication side effect and adjusted his prescriptions. The dream reenactments improved but never fully resolved.

He also had other atypical symptoms: staring spells where he'd gaze into the distance for minutes, and difficulty judging spatial relationships. Sitting down required him to feel the chair first, as he often misjudged where it was. Because of his Alzheimer's diagnosis, we lumped these symptoms together without question. Only after his pathology report confirmed Lewy body disease did we fully understand his experience. That knowledge mattered—it explained his younger onset, rapid progression, and distinct symptoms. Yet, I've rarely identified myself as the son of someone with Lewy body disease, despite his mixed dementia. That is the power—and the problem—of Alzheimer's. It always takes center stage, even when it isn't the full story.

The cold, hard reality is that research dollars will continue to flow first into Alzheimer's, just as they do with cancer or heart disease, because of how many lives it touches—and how profoundly. Money in medical research, as in other fields, goes where the need is greatest. But that focus often leaves families like mine, living with more than one diagnosis, searching for answers that remain out of reach.

THE ALZHEIMER'S "DEFINITION" CONTROVERSY

Nothing captures the unsettled nature of the Alzheimer's community more than the fact that the field still can't agree on how to define the disease. That's right—even its very definition is still up for debate. The first widely accepted clinical criteria for dementia were established in 1984. In 1999, Dr. Ronald Petersen and colleagues at Mayo Clinic introduced mild cognitive impairment (MCI) to describe a stage between normal cognition and dementia. Twelve years later, the National Institute on Aging–Alzheimer's Association (NIA-AA) refined both stages, and in doing so also incorporated biomarker research into the definitions to link symptoms with underlying biology.

The Alzheimer's definition debate intensified in 2018. The NIA-AA introduced a research framework that defined Alzheimer's as a biological process rather than one that had to have symptoms. In other words, a diagnosis could now be made simply based on the result of imaging, blood, or spinal fluid biomarker tests that would reveal the excess presence of amyloid *and* tau, with or without the presence of accelerated brain cell loss. Now a person would not need to have any symptoms of Alzheimer's to be diagnosed with the disease—only positive test results.

This shift away from clinical symptoms rattled the research and clinical communities. Critics raised concerns about Alzheimer's biomarker tests. Would they be too expensive? Would they be available to everyone? Would they really live up to expectations? Would people without symptoms who were diagnosed face discrimination or social stigma? Would these tests somehow restrict future research? Would doctors misuse or misunderstand the tests? The questions went on and on. Over time, these concerns were addressed. Biomarkers have proven to be accurate, interpretable, and predictive. Once costly and inaccessible, such simple blood tests are now economical and widely available.

But that's not the end of the story. In 2024, the Alzheimer's Association redefined the disease once again. Now it declared that a diagnosis could be made solely by one thing alone—the presence of elevated amyloid on a biomarker test. This challenged the entire field, as many experts were still pondering whether Alzheimer's could exist without clinical (i.e., observable) symptoms. Unlike the prior framework, the new definition applied to clinical care and not just research. If the medical community accepted this new definition, an Alzheimer's diagnosis would not require symptoms or the confirmed presence of the second hallmark protein tau.

In the past, to tell someone he had Alzheimer's, you would expect him to have memory loss, changes in cognitive tests, and a biomarker—a combination of hard scientific biological factors and subjectively observed symptoms. However, doctors have long agreed that symptoms are unnecessary for a diagnosis in every other known disease—anything from the common cold to hypertension, diabetes, or cancer. There's always an asymptomatic stage where biological changes happen before a person or doctor notices them. Why should Alzheimer's or any brain disease be treated differently?

This debate over a definition affects me personally. First, as the medical director, I oversee the Wisconsin Registry for Alzheimer's Prevention (WRAP) study at UW-Madison. This visionary project has observed more than six hundred people for decades using amyloid and tau PET scans. The ability to do this is a triumph for Alzheimer's research. Amyloid and tau PET scans can only be done at a handful of major academic centers, making WRAP's ability to study so many people for so many years a substantial accomplishment. WRAP found that, on average, it took 6.2 years after development of amyloid for tau to begin appearing in a part of the brain called the *entorhinal cortex*. The likelihood of having tau increased significantly with each decade of amyloid presence, and after twenty years, only two participants in the study showed no evidence of tau. This illustrates a key concept in the amyloid cascade hypothesis—anyone with elevated amyloid who lives long enough will develop tau. All the participants who developed elevated amyloid eventually developed Alzheimer's as it is strictly defined. They may not have symptoms, but they have the two characteristic proteins in their brains.

The second way this evolving definition affects me is because I meet with these study participants, and explaining these linguistic somersaults to them can be upsetting. For years I've told research participants, "If you have elevated amyloid, you are *at higher risk* for developing Alzheimer's disease and the symptoms of dementia because you are now at higher risk for developing that second Alzheimer's protein called *tau*. The scientific community is not convinced that everyone with elevated amyloid develops elevated tau. If that's true, this means some people with elevated amyloid won't develop Alzheimer's." When you are healthy, being told you are at higher risk for Alzheimer's disease is different than being told you have it.

Now participants are calling me and saying, "Dr. Chin, you told me I was only at risk. Now the definition has changed. Do I have it or not?"

Many of these people never had symptoms. Now by definition they have Alzheimer's, a disease that carries a stigma. It is unfortunate that people have received this news in such a confusing way. This is yet another consequence of the ever-evolving and often uncertain state of the Alzheimer's community.

IS AMYLOID THE ARSONIST OR THE FIREMAN?

What causes Alzheimer's? Let's think deeply for a moment about Alzheimer's disease as a biological process happening in the brain. It has a sequence of events, and the first identifiable part of that process is the buildup of elevated amyloid. After amyloid appears, tau follows, and eventually brain cells begin to die. We can confirm this through PET scans or an analysis of spinal fluid or blood.

Here's the wrinkle—amyloid, tau, and the death of neurons are only one biological process happening in the brain. Other changes are likely occurring *before* the buildup of amyloid and *between* the buildup of amyloid and tau.

What if the amyloid isn't the disease itself but rather evidence of the damage it left behind? One prominent critic of the amyloid cascade hypothesis is George Perry, a professor of neuroscience and developmental and regenerative biology at the University of Texas–San Antonio. I've gotten to know him because we are both members of the Medical, Scientific & Memory Screening Advisory Board of the Alzheimer's Foundation of America.

Here is the ingenious way in which Perry turns the amyloid theory on its head. He believes that amyloid, instead of being destructive, is actually produced in overabundance by the brain's valiant, yet unsuccessful, efforts to defend itself. "It'll always be there like a fireman," he says in a video on his website. "In a well-managed city, when there's a fire, firemen are there. If you didn't understand the context of how fires start and stop, you would think firemen were destroying things. . . . They pour water on things. They poke things. They cause massive destruction. When you arrive, the fireman's there, but the arsonist is long gone. So, therefore, you're missing what's causing the problem."

Others, according to Perry, have used the analogy that airbags cause deaths. "If you look at [wrecked] cars that have airbags deployed, people very often have died," he says. "That doesn't [consider] the fact that the airbags reduced how many people would have died had they not deployed."

Researchers argue that amyloid is not inherently harmful and in fact serves a beneficial purpose. One such purpose involves how synapses function and how plastic or malleable they are. The brain may need amyloid at low levels for learning and memory. Some studies show that amyloid strengthens synapses that lead to long-term memory storage. Other studies reveal that amyloid reduces excessive neuronal activity that can be toxic. So perhaps amyloid protects neurons from being hyperactive the way coolant or motor oil keeps a car engine functioning within normal limits.

Other scientists say amyloid may have a role in creating new neurons and promoting healing at sites of brain injury and inflammation. Some suggest that amyloid acts as an antimicrobial agent, trapping and neutralizing bacteria, viruses, or fungi. The way they see it, plaques, instead of being dangerous, are how the brain stops microbes from spreading. In this way, amyloid is actually part of the brain's immune response. Indeed, examinations of the brains of Alzheimer's patients have found herpes viruses, bacteria from oral gum disease, and *Chlamydia pneumoniae*. Their presence supports the theory that amyloid has caught them like bugs on fly paper.

Meanwhile, other research shows amyloid may act as a protective antioxidant. It shields neurons from minuscule amounts of harmful copper, iron, and zinc molecules and thus prevents oxidative stress. When amyloid forms plaques, it loses this ability, which leads to oxidative damage. If amyloid binds to metal and renders it less harmful, it's plausible that plaque formation indicates excessive levels of iron, zinc, or copper. High iron levels, for instance, are known to promote oxidative stress, which can contribute to neurodegeneration. Here again, instead of being the primary driver of Alzheimer's disease, amyloid serves as the defense mechanism against a different root problem.

If amyloid isn't the driving force behind Alzheimer's, then what is? Over the years, scientists have proposed a range of alternatives to the amyloid cascade hypothesis, many of which downplay or dismiss amyloid's role entirely. Some point to chronic inflammation while others point to dormant viral encephalitis (brain infection). These theories rise and fall, each claiming to reveal the true cause. Researchers surf these scientific waves, because everyone wants the cause of Alzheimer's to be reversible. We all want to rush toward this hope. After all, no one wants this disease to be incurable.

IF NOT AMYLOID, WHAT THEN IS THE CAUSE?

Diabetes, inflammation, oxidative stress, and glycosylation (an attachment of carbohydrates to proteins in the blood) have all been suggested as causes. The most likely possibility is that the driving force behind Alzheimer's is multifactorial—in other words, it has its roots in an array of factors that include a person's genes and lifestyle. This is true of many other chronic diseases, including some types of cancer, which is why lassoing their causes and wrestling them to defeat proves so challenging.

Some earlier theories about what causes Alzheimer's have been abandoned. A few years ago, researchers suggested the culprit was insulin resistance in the brain. That is another way of saying Alzheimer's was a type of diabetes—type 3 diabetes. (In type 1, your pancreas lacks the ability to make insulin; in type 2, your body doesn't make enough.) So diabetes, they argued, made brain cells die. Further research put that theory to rest. Instead, studies showed insulin resistance was an important factor in the development of Alzheimer's but not a singular driving force.

Inflammation has been suggested as a root cause of Alzheimer's. Without a doubt, inflammation is a chronic driver of diseases of blood vessels, and it causes the hyperactivity of other processes that could lead to changes like amyloid buildup. When we talk about diseases of aging, inflammation tends to be an ever-present factor.

In fact, inflammation is so common in older people that there's a word for it—*inflammaging*. Dr. Claudio Franceschi, an Italian professor of immunology, coined the term in 2000. According to Franceschi, "Inflammation is an intrinsic component of all chronic disease." This ongoing, low-grade inflammation in older people is simply how their immune systems tend to behave. Inflammaging increases as people age, often depending on how well they're taking care of themselves with exercise, diet, and other behaviors. Inflammation drives a lot of aging processes and, likely, Alzheimer's, too. That's why it's important to brush your teeth and floss—gum disease (chronic periodontitis) sparks inflammation in the mouth that spreads through the body.

A Not-So-Sweet Habit

Many researchers believe that inflammation plays a key role in the development of Alzheimer's disease. There has long been agreement that inflammation is linked to up to 20 percent of cancer cases and that it's a culprit behind many heart and circulatory conditions.

Inflammation in the body is typically triggered by infections, injuries, or irritants such as allergies. These factors activate the body's immune response, leading to blood vessel dilation and the familiar signs of inflammation—redness, swelling, warmth, and pain. While this process is a natural part of healing, other factors, like smoking, alcohol consumption, stress, and poor diet can cause a more subtle, chronic invisible inflammation. Unlike acute inflammation, this "silent" form negatively impacts the digestive system, joints, and organs without obvious external symptoms.

My family has always wondered what triggered my father's Alzheimer's. He had no known family history of Alzheimer's or dementia. He didn't smoke or drink, but he did have one vice—he loved sugary sweets. For years when he was practicing medicine, one way he managed his stress was by reaching for a piece of candy, not a cigarette. (In his defense, my father did exercise regularly.) Candy, pies, ice cream, pastries—he loved them all. Even so, he was thin, had none of the typical Alzheimer's risk factors.

Could his sweet tooth have had something to do with his getting Alzheimer's? Maybe. A person's diet, especially an unhealthy one, might lead to chronic inflammation not only in the gut but in the whole body. A diet high in sugar has been linked to many metabolic disorders, which are risk factors for dementia, too. Sugar itself damages blood vessels, including the brain's tiny arteries and veins. What's more, studies have found a relationship between sustained inflammation in the brain and the presence of amyloid and tau proteins.

Toward the end of his career, everyone in the hospital knew Moe Chin liked his sweets. He went from nurse station to nurse station eating candy and cake. It was endearing, but I'll always remember my mom saying to me, "That is an unhealthy man." Eating sugary foods is a bad habit—perhaps not as bad as some vices, like smoking. But in my father's case, I believe sweets may have been just as damaging.

Then there's oxidation or oxidative stress, as it's also called. This results from an imbalance of two types of molecules in the body—antioxidants and free radicals, both of which are associated with the body's mishandling of oxygen. Oxygen is the life-giving gas our body needs to breathe, but it can be deadly. A pure oxygen environment killed *Apollo 1* astronauts Gus Grissom, Ed White, and Roger Chafee in a command module fire during training in 1967. One spark created an inferno in seconds. Too many oxygen free radicals (molecules containing oxygen that are highly reactive and unstable) in the blood have a damaging impact on tissues. Oxygen is what causes iron to rust, and it silently does similarly destructive work in the body. This oxidative stress can cause a buildup of cholesterol in blood vessels in Alzheimer's patients' brains. Neurons don't get enough nourishing blood. Inflammation increases, and Alzheimer's may be more likely to develop as a result.

Glycosylation is another potential contributing cause of Alzheimer's. This biochemical process is typically associated with diabetes. When you have too much sugar in your body, as diabetics do, it attaches to proteins. (*Glycan* is another term for carbohydrate.) Normally sugar is supposed to speed to your muscles or be stored in fat cells, but if it gloms onto proteins or other molecules in your blood, it will modify them and their function. This change in the proteins can impact how cells communicate, how they maintain their shape and function, and even how the body's immune system functions.

Hemoglobin is the protein in red blood cells that carries oxygen throughout the body. (It's also what gives blood its distinctive color.) Sugar in carbohydrate form attaches to hemoglobin, permanently changing it and giving it a different function, usually a bad one. When a protein is glycosylated, its new monstrous effect causes blood vessels to become inflamed, leading to high blood pressure and vascular disease. It can also cause inflammation in the brain, which can also lead to oxidative stress. So, not surprisingly, inflammation is associated with glycosylation and oxidation as well as with a person's genes and lifestyle.

There's been growing excitement about whether weight-loss drugs such as semaglutide and liraglutide might play a role in the push to end Alzheimer's. A flurry of studies suggests they not only reduce obesity but also lower inflammation, factors that improve outcomes in diabetes, heart disease, and kidney disease. Whether these benefits extend to the brain's memory regions, however, remains to be seen. Some observational studies have shown a modest reduction in Alzheimer's risk among people taking one form of the drug, but it's still unclear how significant that effect is, or how the medication might be working. Is it just about improving insulin and weight, or is something happening in the brain, too? It's worth remembering that these drugs are still relatively new in the brain health space, and beyond their approved uses, long-term data simply doesn't exist yet. One thing is certain: Given these drugs' popularity, many millions will be spent evaluating their usefulness fighting Alzheimer's.

The interrelatedness of all bodily systems and ways in which they malfunction reminds us how essential it is for each of us to practice preventive medicine in our lives. Take to heart the fourteen modifiable Alzheimer's risk factors listed by *The Lancet.* (See page 165 in chapter 5.) Build them into your life, and your body and brain will function better together like a proverbial well-oiled machine. That way you'll keep at bay the underlying forces that instigate Alzheimer's.

I don't know if amyloid is the fire, the ash, the firefighter, or some combination of these things. As with many issues in medicine and science, we are searching for a simple unifying answer, but as we do, we only reveal more complexity and nuance. For example, inflammation serves a beneficial purpose to the human body, but only at low, temporary levels. Even stress has a useful purpose in short spurts. Isn't it reasonable to think amyloid could also be both beneficial and harmful? Although a full understanding of amyloid eludes us now, I do know amyloid is important, and other doctors and researchers agree. As we become more sophisticated in our knowledge of brain diseases and cures, we're learning that there's rarely a single culprit or cure—most conditions arise from a complex interplay of complementary factors working together (or against each other) over time. For now, it's okay that there's disagreement as to amyloid's role, because whatever the truth is, lecanemab and donanemab remove it, and in doing so, patients are helped.

MANY PATHWAYS TO SUCCESS

My belief is there's not *one* Alzheimer's disease but rather multiple versions or pathways leading to toxic amyloid protein buildup, malfunctioning synapses, and death of neurons. Like other maladies of aging, such as cardiovascular disease, cancer, arthritis, and falls, these conditions are heterogenous, which means they result from the combination of multiple contributing factors.

Instead of reinventing the wheel and throwing out amyloid hypotheses, why not try to combine these competing theories? It's possible that chronic inflammation and/or viral infections lead to or are involved in the amyloid cascade process. Acknowledging amyloid and tau as two critical proteins in Alzheimer's disease benefits scientific exploration in the field. It helps frame future progress and serves as the foundation upon which other discoveries will be made.

Research from the Wisconsin Alzheimer's Disease Research Center (WADRC) and the Wisconsin Registry for Alzheimer's Prevention (WRAP) has illustrated that having amyloid above a certain threshold in the brain can't be ignored. It is problematic. Elevated amyloid sets the stage for cognitive decline and the development of other abnormal proteins, including tau. Other studies have demonstrated that amyloid proteins, even before they become plaques, injure neurons and synapses. Amyloid is a part of the Alzheimer's story, but it does not need to be mutually exclusive or diametrically opposed to other theories.

Ultimately, I believe Alzheimer's will be treated with an array of drugs and lifestyle interventions that attack multiple mechanisms related to aging and the amyloid cascade. To recognize the disease's complexity and then propose only simple solutions would be an error of grand proportions. In the interim, the FDA's approval of lecanemab and donanemab represents the most dynamic progress in the fight against Alzheimer's in a generation.

Sometimes I think doctors and researchers forget that all a patient wants is *some* certainty, not debate. You hope that your doctor can do something to delay disease progression until a cure is found. I firmly believe that in the next ten years we will reach a point where the degenerative effects of Alzheimer's can be blocked or slowed for longer and longer periods of time. Just as cardiologists manage cardiovascular disease from progressing to a life-threatening stage, Alzheimer's will be thwarted in similar ways.

Although some of my peers disagree, lecanemab and donanemab are the first steps to making Alzheimer's a chronic condition. These drugs successfully attack amyloid, and even if you do not believe amyloid is *causing* Alzheimer's, removing it from the brain has been conclusively shown in clinical trials to slow cognitive and functional decline. The issue facing doctors and their patients is whether patients who take these drugs will notice enough improvement to make doing so worthwhile.

SCIENTIFIC ADVANCES: LECANEMAB AND DONANEMAB

Lecanemab and donanemab are scientific marvels. From a clinical trial perspective, their effectiveness has been proven through research that culminated in two international Phase III studies. For example, testing on donanemab took place at 274 medical centers (or hospitals) in eight nations. It involved 1,736 patients between the ages of sixty and eighty-five who had either mild cognitive impairment or mild-stage dementia. This research adhered to the most rigorous standards—namely double-blind, placebo-controlled, parallel-group trials.

We live in a post-Covid age where many people are suspicious, perhaps justly so, of medical research and treatments. Sunlight disinfects, and an informed public benefits science and healthcare. The bottom line is that these drugs went through the wringer and succeeded where others failed.

The experimental hypothesis behind the clinical trial phases of testing was that amyloid is important, and by removing it, a meaningful slowing of decline in cognition and function would result. For this to be scientifically valid, the trial had to have clearly defined goals, a sound strategy for conducting the study, and proven tools to collect data from patients and their families, and the results would have to be accurate, statistically significant, and reproducible. Both clinical trials met these high standards, and the results were not faked. That's the scientific proof.

Now comes the rub—lecanemab and donanemab removed amyloid

and slowed cognitive decline in statistically significant ways, but does statistical significance translate in the real world to results patients would find helpful? Put another way, does that statistically significant result create a slowing of cognitive decline a patient would notice? Numbers on paper are one kind of evidence, but what a human being senses about his mental state is the bottom line when it comes to treatment.

For example, during follow-up visits in the memory clinic, my dad underwent brief cognitive tests lasting about ten minutes. He would be told his score was "stable" or that he had "only lost one point compared to six months ago." But those numbers didn't reflect how he actually felt. Instead, he experienced forgetting conversations moments after they happened, realizing he was repeating himself, searching for misplaced items, or coming to terms with the loss of his ability to drive. Those changes weren't "stable" or losses that felt like "one point." To him, they were dramatic. The truth is this: What looks good on paper may not feel good to the person actually living it.

This is where another Alzheimer's controversy arises. Some doctors choose not to prescribe these drugs. My response? This is exactly where shared decision-making comes in. I believe in educating my patients about the risks and benefits of all available medications and empowering them to make their own informed choices.

Beyond that, I question the ethics of any provider who withholds information about an FDA-approved medication simply because he or she doesn't personally support it. A healthcare provider's role is not to make decisions for patients—that's paternalism, and it should have ended long ago. Modern medicine requires informed consent. That means providers need to be knowledgeable about approved treatments in their field so they can guide patients toward the best decisions for them—not for the provider. Primary care providers are not experts on these medications, nor is it reasonable to expect them to be. However, they know their patients best, and at times it may be reasonable for them to offer opinions based more on individual circumstances than on scientific evidence.

The best evidence suggests that for some patients, lecanemab and donanemab slow cognitive decline for four to five months and at most for up to a year. These modest results plus the drugs' risks and cost ($27,000, which is covered by Medicare and Medicaid) are what deter other physicians from recommending them to their patients.

When these drugs are attacked because of their cost, I can feel my pulse quicken, my jaw tense, and a flush rise to my face. It makes me angry, and it's hard to hide. To me, this argument feels ageist, reflecting a society that places less value on its elders. I understand that cost is an essential factor in healthcare decision-making. It is not economically sustainable to always provide every possible medical intervention across all specialties for all patients everywhere. What frustrates me is that this scrutiny seems to apply disproportionately to geriatrics and eldercare. I rarely hear the same debates over the cost of third-line chemotherapy that extends life by mere months, expensive autoimmune medications that don't cure the condition, or neurological treatments that slow but don't stop disease progression—often for younger patients.

In geriatrics and dementia care, we are routinely asked to justify cost or prove a favorable cost-benefit ratio in order to have a proposal seriously considered. Other specialties don't seem to face the same hurdle. A study published in *JAMA Health Forum* illustrates this disparity. It found that widely used anti-obesity medications failed to be cost-effective when lifetime health gains were taken into consideration. Despite this, insurance companies had already approved these drugs and will likely continue covering them for years.

"We Don't Have Time to Wait": The Mike Zuendel Story

Mike Zuendel advocates for early diagnosis and intervention—and for good reason. He experienced remarkable results from his treatment with the first anti-amyloid drug, aducanumab (now replaced by other treatments). Amyloid in his PET scan became undetectable—as if it had never been there. "The therapy saved my life," he told me on my podcast, *Dementia Matters*. His memory loss stabilized. No new cognitive changes have developed, and he remains functionally independent.

Today Mike serves on the Alzheimer's Association's Early-Stage Advisors Group, but his success story may be the exception rather than the rule. Other patients and families report different experiences from these anti-amyloid therapies—no noticeable slowing of disease, only ongoing gradual declines in thinking and day-to-day abilities. Even so, his experience is inspirational. Here is what he told me.

The diagnosis hit me like a ton of bricks. I expected it, but it hit me in the gut. There were a lot of tears, but I picked up the pieces and asked myself, What am I going to do now? *I told my family not to worry because I was going to survive the disease and was going to go public to fight the stigma.*

I was fortunate to have caught this disease early because the current medications can only be prescribed to those in the beginning stages. I was determined to get aducanumab. One thing I've found on my journey is, you have to be your own advocate. I told my physician that was what I wanted. She told me the pros and cons and let me make my own decision.

I took monthly IV infusions of the drug for thirty-six months. The process was easy. You sit in a comfortable chair for an hour while the drug enters your body. I wasn't worried. I couldn't wait. I understood there was a slight possibility of side effects from aducanumab, but I also knew what Alzheimer's disease was definitely going to do if I didn't fight it. I wanted to stop it in its tracks.

Three years later my doctor told me I had a miraculous response because all or almost all the beta amyloid plaques had been removed from my brain. But I don't kid myself. I still have impairments from the damage that was done. I forget words. I misplace my phone. I forget why I've come into a room. That's an easy life compared to a disease that debilitates you.

I hope the damage won't get worse, but we're in uncharted territory, like the early days of chemotherapy. We do not have a cure for AIDS, the common cold, or cancer, but we have wonderful, incredible treatments for them. We now have good treatments for Alzheimer's, and they're going to get better and better.

My advice is, find a specialist who is up to date on the latest treatments. Don't worry. Do not let this disease define you or push you into a corner. There is hope, real hope, great hope, but it won't happen unless you get diagnosed.

WHO CAN TAKE LECANEMAB AND DONANEMAB

Lecanemab and donanemab cannot be prescribed to all Alzheimer's patients. FDA regulations forbid either from being prescribed to those who have progressed beyond the mild stage of dementia. (Dementia is divided into several stages—mild, moderate, and severe.) In mild-stage dementia, a person has an impairment in some or all of the instrumental activities of daily living (IADLs)—shopping, cooking, housework, managing finances, keeping appointments, driving, taking medicines as prescribed, and using technology. The moderate and severe stages share six activities of daily living (ADL)—dressing, bathing, toileting, standing, walking, and continence. Once you become impaired in even one ADL, you have progressed to the moderate stage and are no longer eligible for lecanemab or donanemab. This restriction exists because people in the later stages of dementia were excluded in the clinical trials. Researchers believed the drugs would have little to no significant impact at these advanced stages. Supporting this, one of the clinical trials found that participants with MCI responded better to donanemab than did those with mild-stage dementia.

This is yet another reason why an early diagnosis is important—it can make you a candidate for these treatments and may improve your response to them. If your doctor can remove the amyloid protein when symptoms first appear, he may be able to deflect and slow the trajectory of the disease so you remain in your best health longer. This gives you more time so that newer yet-to-be-approved drugs, perhaps ones that remove tau or address inflammation, can be used. Stability is indeed a victory after all, especially for those living with MCI. An important study published in 2025 showed that lecanemab and donanemab extended independence in daily activities by ten to thirteen months when used earlier in the course of the disease. Everyone wants that benefit to be longer in the future. An additional year of independent, fully functioning life is not trivial. It's a big deal and progress worth cheering.

This is the logic oncologists have long used when treating cancer patients. Chemotherapy drugs slow the growth of tumors or force the cancer into remission. This gives patients a window of three months, six months, a year, five to ten years, or even a lifetime of better health. Yes, sometimes oncologists only buy their patients a few months or a year. (And some who have been on chemo those last few months and lived in agony from the side effects might share a different story.) Patients understand this, and most welcome the possibility of even limited benefits.

For the time being, this is how Alzheimer's doctors like me want to help our patients. Until now we haven't even had that ability, something that oncologists, cancer patients, and the general public accept without batting an eye when it comes to cancer. Unlike second- or third-line chemotherapy, which is often used closer to death when quality of life has already declined, these medications for Alzheimer's are different. They extend the earliest stages of the disease, when individuals are still capable, independent, and experiencing the fewest symptoms. Instead of prolonging a lower state of ability, these treatments help maintain the highest quality of life for as long as possible, ideally carrying those benefits into the later stages.

These drugs are far from perfect. They have modest benefits, carry notable risks, require great resources to manage, and are a burden on patients and their families. They are, however, the beginning of a new era in disease-modifying treatments for Alzheimer's. One day these agents might be compared to nitrogen mustard, the first chemotherapy to treat cancer (specifically lymphoma) and zidovudine (AZT), the first treatment for HIV. Anti-amyloid monoclonal treatments such as lecanemab and donanemab are not the solution, but they are a part of it and mark the beginning of much better treatments to come.

For now, if we're going to slow the trajectory, even a little, it should be when results would be most noticeable to the patient. I have a patient in the earliest stages of mild cognitive impairment taking donanemab. She knows she's still going to decline, but she's so early in the process that her attitude is, "I want as much of that amyloid protein gone as possible. My hope is I can be stable in my current completely independent, functional state. If a tau-fighting drug is approved, I want you to prescribe it as well to remove even more of those proteins. Meanwhile, I'm going to exercise. I'm going to go on an anti-inflammatory diet, and I'm going to change other parts of my life that might slow the progression of my cognitive decline." For her, the risk of taking the drug is worth it. This is her informed decision. I'm going to be there with her each step of the way.

REASONS *NOT* TO TAKE LECANEMAB AND DONANEMAB

There are plenty of reasons *not* to take lecanemab and donanemab. First and foremost, they come with possible side effects, some that might be life-threatening. Approximately 20–40 percent of clinical trial participants who took them developed ARIA (amyloid-related imaging abnormalities). ARIA can manifest as swelling or microhemorrhages (small bleeding) in the brain. The great majority of the time these side effects have no symptoms and pose no harm. Of those taking lecanemab in the Phase III trial, 0.7 percent had noticeable symptoms of intracranial bleeding.

During the two Phase III clinical trials, 59 of the 3,531 participants died. Slightly more than half were taking the medication while the others received a placebo. Of those on the treatment, some were taking blood thinners and died from bleeding in their brains. Today most clinicians and healthcare institutions consider it unsafe or inadvisable to prescribe anticoagulants like warfarin (sold under the brand name Coumadin) or apixaban (marketed as Eliquis) to patients receiving the new Alzheimer's therapies. If a person is on a blood thinner for a short-term condition, such as deep vein thrombosis, treatment would be delayed until they have completed therapy and discontinued the anticoagulant. However, if long-term use is necessary for conditions like atrial fibrillation or a clotting disorder, these two Alzheimer's medications cannot be administered.

For some patients, another deterrent is the burden associated with obtaining the medication. These therapies are given not once but many times over years. Lecanemab is delivered by IV every two weeks and donanemab every four weeks for twelve to eighteen months. To receive one of them, patients must visit an infusion center for up to three hours for each infusion. (Infusion centers are where cancer patients typically go for chemotherapy.) Each infusion takes about an hour, and afterward patients must be observed for an hour or two longer to make sure they experience no immediate side effects. In the future, it may be possible to deliver some of these drugs subcutaneously like insulin, and patients will probably self-administer them at home. Other medications may still require an IV infusion but will be given only once or twice a year. This reduction in the "hassle factor" changes the cost-benefit ratio and will likely lead more doctors to prescribe them.

There's a saying in stroke care that highlights the urgency of treatment: "Time is brain." After a stroke, restoring blood flow to the brain is critical because every passing minute can mean the loss of brain cells and brain function. A similar concept applies to neurodegenerative diseases, except time is measured in years and decades rather than seconds and minutes. Patients don't want to waste the precious time they could be spending with their families pursuing interventions that offer little to no benefit.

Although chemotherapy has a reputation for harsh side effects, the possible side effects of lecanemab and donanemab are milder. A patient may feel feverish, cold, or nauseated during the infusion, any of which are typically well tolerated. Besides the repeated infusions, patients who receive lecanemab and donanemab must also undergo four or five MRIs over the eighteen-month treatment process to monitor them for signs of ARIA.

What is the difference between lecanemab and donanemab? Lecanemab targets amyloid earlier in the process of plaque formation and is administered every two weeks indefinitely, whereas donanemab targets more advanced, established plaques, making it more effective at reducing plaque burden on amyloid PET scans. Donanemab is given once per month and was shown in clinical trials to be slightly more effective than lecanemab at slowing cognitive decline, particularly in patients with mild cognitive impairment (MCI) and those with low to medium tau levels. However, donanemab has a higher rate of ARIA-related side effects.

When I discuss lecanemab and donanemab with patients, I want them to think deeply about this decision. My posture toward the drugs is conservative. First, I make clear that the side effects could be significant, far more so than nausea or diarrhea, so they know what the adverse consequences might be. Second, I err on the side of explaining the modest benefit and what that could mean for them. Third, I highlight the commitment they would have to make to complete the treatment. I usually conclude by making a recommendation based on their specific circumstances. That's what patients and families want from me. I tailor my counseling to each patient's situation, values, rate of change, and goals for treatment. I don't form such judgments lightly, nor do I base them merely on their diagnosis of Alzheimer's, their age, or a simple cognitive test score. People are complex. My recommendations usually are, too.

OTHER DRUGS PRESCRIBED FOR ALZHEIMER'S AND MCI

Each patient's situation is different, and decisions about which medications to take rest with the patient and family. I always take time to explain how each drug works and what its potential benefits and risks are before making a recommendation.

Donepezil, galantamine, and rivastigmine have been prescribed for nearly thirty years to patients with MCI and dementia (though the FDA approved them only for dementia). Unlike lecanemab and donanemab, none of these drugs remove amyloid from the brain. Instead, these drugs, known as acetylcholinesterase inhibitors, manage symptoms by slowing the breakdown of acetylcholine in the brain. Acetylcholine helps neurons transmit signals. These drugs reinforce the presence of this naturally occurring chemical, thus helping maintain a person's cognitive state.

None of these drugs address amyloid, tau, inflammation, or oxidation. They help brain cells work but do not repair those that are dying. They're not harmless. Their possible side effects include nausea, upset stomach, diarrhea, vivid dreams, nightmares, bradycardia (slowed heart rate), dizziness, and even confusion. While these adverse effects occur less than 10 percent of the time, they can result in emergency room visits or, at a minimum, difficult days and nights at home. One advantage of rivastigmine is that it is available in patch form, which allows the medication to enter the body through the skin, bypassing the stomach, where it can cause irritation.

A fourth drug, memantine, is prescribed for moderate to severe stages of dementia and works differently than donepezil and the others. Instead of targeting acetylcholine, it blocks the effects of the brain chemical glutamate. Under normal conditions, glutamate helps neurons communicate, but nerve cells injured by Alzheimer's overproduce it, so memantine blocks the effects of excess glutamate. Memantine is better tolerated overall but can still have side effects such as high blood pressure, weight gain, abdominal pain, constipation or diarrhea, and dizziness. Families do commonly report a beneficial calming effect on the patient. While this is not the purpose of the medication, it has been seen as an added bonus for my patients with anxiety.

Memantine works with the acetylcholinesterase inhibitors, and they are commonly used together as the dementia progresses. While donepezil is approved for someone living with dementia, many healthcare providers will use it in the MCI stage. I will prescribe it when someone with MCI has changes in memory or attention, both areas of the brain where acetylcholine is essential for proper functioning. Other cognitive domains, such as executive function and visual-spatial processing, may benefit from acetylcholine, too, but they are also dependent on other neurotransmitters, and so patients may receive less benefit from an increase in acetylcholine alone.

Memantine is meant for the later stages of dementia, and clinical research has not found it to be helpful in MCI or mild-stage dementia. A doctor might prescribe it for a person with mild-stage dementia who is unable to tolerate the acetylcholinesterase inhibitors. It is possible that an individual will see a benefit from it even though studies showed no benefits when measured across a large group. I tend to keep patients on this medication as they progress into the severe stage of dementia and end its use when they transition into hospice.

Many providers remain skeptical about all these medications and, as a result, won't prescribe any of them. They cite studies that show only mild subjective improvements for six to twelve months before patients return to the same level as the placebo group. To me, this perspective feels nihilistic. A year of benefit is still a year of benefit.

Of course, many providers recognize this and continue prescribing these medications for patients who tolerate them well and experience no significant side effects. When viewed through a palliative lens, they bring relief by reducing symptoms of cognitive decline. That in and of itself is a meaningful goal. Furthermore, small but important long-term studies have shown that these therapies provide symptomatic improvements over several years in comparison with untreated groups (or predicted scores based on historically untreated groups). In the end, even as the disease progresses, experiencing fewer or less severe symptoms for a longer period is a worthwhile benefit.

Nonetheless, I tend to deprescribe (or stop) these medications in the moderate to severe stage of dementia because the side effects outweigh any benefits. The drugs rely on healthy brain cells to be effective, and by the advanced stages of the disease, I worry that too many brain cells have been lost, making the medication more harmful than helpful. I explain from the beginning that we may stop the medication if, over time, it no longer provides a meaningful benefit.

My father started taking donepezil after his diagnosis, though my mother objected. He eventually went on memantine, too. I supported both decisions, as I would today. If you were to ask my mom, she would say they didn't work and instead gave him false hope. Despite her feelings on the matter, she was willing to go along with his wishes until he stopped taking most of his medications. In the clinic, I recognize the delicate balance between the patient's and the family's wishes, knowing they are not always the same.

NEVER, NEVER QUIT

It is probably too much to hope for a cure for Alzheimer's in the near future, but scientific and medical advances sometimes happen in sudden and surprising ways. Thomas Edison tested six thousand materials in his search to find the right filament for a lightbulb that would glow for months, even years. He never gave up. His first big breakthrough came in 1879, when uncoated cotton thread glowed for fourteen and a half hours. Finally, he tried bamboo threads. They glowed and kept glowing for months. Edison had succeeded, and he changed the world. When a reporter asked him what it was like to fail one thousand times, he is said to have replied, "I didn't fail one thousand times. The lightbulb was an invention with one thousand steps."

Right now in a laboratory large or small, some researcher might be conducting that one-thousand-and-first experiment on a chemical that will better unravel Alzheimer's mysteries. While our current attention may be on amyloid-removing therapies, the world of clinical trials has already broadened its view. Of the 495 clinical trials supported by the National Institute on Aging in 2025, only 12 were directly related to amyloid. Studies have diversified their approach to this disease. The belief that one factor causes Alzheimer's is losing favor. Researchers are increasingly casting a wider net and studying such diverse possible causes as neuroinflammation, tau, synaptic plasticity, neuroprotection, mitochondria, bioenergetics, circadian rhythm, oxidative stress, and the roles of neurotransmitters like serotonin. Having a multipronged approach to Alzheimer's disease that includes amyloid among other pathways is more than smart, it's necessary.

Quit is not a word in the vocabulary of most leaders, regardless of whether they are in medicine, science, or politics. Speaking to British high school students in September 1941, Winston Churchill said, "Never give in, never give in, never, never, never, never—in nothing, great or small, large or petty—never give in except to convictions of honor and good sense."

Surrender to Alzheimer's? Never.

7

"You're Not Meant to Do This Alone"

Prepare Now for the Future • Why Memory Cafés Matter • Every Caregiving Community Is Different • What About Grandchildren? • How Strong Routines Help • Why Some Routine Answers Are Hurtful • The Home Healthcare Decision • Driving: When to Stop • Adult Day Centers: Pros and Cons • The Power of Pets

Support comes in many shapes and forms, but it typically takes nearly two years for caregivers to formally reach out for assistance. That's a long time to go it alone. The more traditional route for finding help includes for-profit, nonprofit, local, state, and national sources, including the guidance you will find at your healthcare clinic. Families indicate that help starts informally with relatives, friends, and neighbors, as well as a form of support many people overlook—a dog or cat who gives warmth and love unconditionally.

I understand why many caregivers think they can do it all and wait to raise their hand for help. Up until the formal diagnosis, they have been doing just that. Hearing a diagnosis of mild cognitive impairment (MCI) or Alzheimer's can be overwhelming. It can feel like stepping off a cliff. How do you prepare for the future when you're still in shock in the present?

When I see new patients and their families, they have typically been living with symptoms—and the accompanying anxiety—for as long as three years. Their exhaustion is palpable. There's been denial, covering up, and compensating, and when those outlets fail, they come to the office not knowing what to do next. The last thing they want is to plunge into another emotional process that forces them to confront "the future," one where they learn "horrible truths" about losing abilities, behavioral changes, and dying. Unfortunately, the longer the wait, the more the finite reservoir of energy has been depleted.

At first, the need for outside help may seem unwarranted. If I'm making an early diagnosis and patients are still living with minimal assistance, families balk when prompted to connect with the Alzheimer's Association. Why talk to an agency about help when they don't need it today, tomorrow, or even next month? It is hard for people to overcome the stigma of Alzheimer's and force themselves to contact helper agencies when they're still getting by on their own. This is the double-edged sword of an early diagnosis.

When families are in my office, I advise them to address legal matters first. (See chapter 4 for advice on healthcare and legal powers of attorney.) By and large, patients and their families do take care of those matters.

But the other piece of advice to which I give high priority—build a close-knit community to help you—often gets ignored. And that's not just unfortunate; it's a serious oversight. Beyond diagnostics and treatments, this is the top recommendation I wish every patient and family would take to heart. You have to assemble your support system now, because when the crisis hits—and it will—you need people already in place who know you and are ready to come to your rescue. You are not superhuman. Unpreparedness by patients and families grieves me because this is what will happen: A swarm of bees will chase you through your house and make you leap in the shower with all your clothes on. That was the Alzheimer's crisis that befell my mother that I wrote about in chapter 4. It took being harassed by a mob of stinging insects before she realized she needed more help, that she couldn't take care of my father and their farm alone. She discovered she didn't have superpowers. None of us do. If you fail to start building your caregiver community, you will have a crisis. I guarantee it, though it probably won't be caused by a gang of crazed bees. The unhappy event might be a fall. It might be a behavioral symptom you are unable to handle. For example, it could be your loved one's hallucination from straight out of left field that leaves you dumbfounded because in your isolation no one had told you what could happen. Or you find yourself bleary-eyed, driving the streets of your city each night in an attempt to appease your spouse who keeps insisting he wants to go home. Worse, sometimes the crisis is a hospitalization—and it could be you or your loved one.

When this inevitable calamity hits, a family will suddenly lose its collective composure and realize, "Oh, my doctor isn't as helpful as I thought he would be," or, "The clinic is understaffed and not giving me direction. I have to find someone in the community to help me. *Now.*" That's when physicians like me get a frantic phone call. I'm pleased to help, and I do help, but addressing a family in distress is far different from advising a family that is calm and able to proactively make decisions about a loved one.

When you urgently need outside help, it's not as simple as ordering a pizza. Let's say you want to hire a home health aide. That process is not so different from finding a doctor, lawyer, or plumber. It will take time. It will almost certainly take you at least a week, sometimes longer, to hire an agency that will send an aide. You can add more time to that waiting period if you want to meet with multiple companies or interview the aide they plan to send.

You will also be expected to complete paperwork that may raise legal or insurance issues you had not anticipated. Before most reputable companies agree to work with a family, they typically send a representative for a home visit. Most check your home for potential safety risks, and you may be required to install gates or safety handles in bathrooms. These are all good suggestions, but they come at a time when you are already swimming upstream. Adding another layer of frustration, the company you select might be short-staffed and have no employee available to help you when you most need it—right now. Even worse, some agencies may already have more business than they can handle and decline your application.

THE SOCIAL PRESCRIPTION

The husband of one of my patients once asked me to write a prescription for finding caregiving help. He was joking (I think), but it's actually something I used to do, sort of. The Alzheimer's Association had what it called the "Direct Referral." It was a big sheet of paper that was a fake prescription. I signed it. The family signed it. Then I faxed it to the Association so it could call the family and schedule all manner of things. The gimmick didn't work. Many people simply declined to answer the Association's phone call.

Imagine that this chapter on building community is a kind of social prescription—one we create together. After all, 6.2 billion drug prescriptions are written every year. But what I'm offering here may be even more powerful than a daily pill. Instead of pop and swallow, make a phone call. Send an email. Visit a place in your community that can support you. Just make a gentle reminder to reach out. The dose is simple: connection.

As the legendary baseball player and philosopher Yogi Berra once said, "When you come to a fork in the road, take it." In other words, do something—maybe it's only a small step, but do it now.

Caring for someone with changes in their thinking involves more than just evaluations and medications. Being part of a community will be therapeutic, helpful, and essential as cognition continues to decline. With that in mind, this chapter has four themes—(1) community building, (2) establishing routines, (3) planning for the next stages of Alzheimer's, and (4) taking care of yourself.

We can't always prevent a crisis, but we can prepare for one. This chapter will help you build the support you need to do both.

YOUR CORE SUPPORT—YOUR MEDICAL TEAM

Your doctor won't be your number-one, go-to, speed-dial contact. A physician acting alone simply can't achieve what a full medical team can together. This multidisciplinary approach of physician, nurse, social worker, and occupational, physical, and speech therapists is a tried-and-true strategy. Don't be disappointed if your geriatrician or neurologist doesn't seem as involved. It's not that he is uncaring. The other team members are simply better suited to respond to your immediate questions.

The most important person after a diagnosis is the social worker in your doctor's practice. She helps connect families to the community and broader resources. She's the one who works hand in glove with the caregiver. She's the one who helps families form important relationships and guides them through the medical plan, clarifying recommendations, offering practical options, and ensuring they feel empowered to take action.

Your doctor's nurse can answer basic medical questions that arise and is a phone call away. Her counseling and advice are free and can be true sources of comfort. Nurses are knowledgeable because they have medical training, and they have heard the same issues, concerns, fears, and requests from countless other patients. Sometimes, what feels like a sudden decline—a change in behavior, increased confusion, or agitation—might actually be caused by a common ailment like a urinary tract infection. With a simple phone call and timely treatment, symptoms that seem like the brain disease taking a bad turn can stabilize and return to baseline. Nurses play a crucial role in triaging these kinds of calls and helping rule out acute medical issues. If your question is one the nurse can't answer, she will forward your message to your physician.

The sooner you begin building relationships with social workers, nurses, local agencies, and other members of the care team, the sooner you'll begin to build trust. And that trust is much easier to sustain and strengthen in moments of calm than in times of crisis. Caregiving for someone with Alzheimer's is a long journey, and anticipatory care is essential. Anticipatory care means planning for a person's future health needs in ways that are thoughtful, intentional, and in line with what matters most to the patient.

It takes time to become acquainted and comfortable, even with the medical team, which is why it's so important to start early. When sensitive decisions must be made, having a solid foundation of trust and comfort can make all the difference.

Initially, you might only talk with a social worker or nurse once or twice a month. As your loved one declines and more assistance is needed, these relationships, which have gone through many iterations, have solidified and become a source of strength. Difficulty arises when new help comes onboard, particularly when the family is physically and emotionally exhausted. For example, one possible aspect of dementia is paranoia, so suddenly introducing a new face can cause distress. If possible, bring new team members on gradually, with preparation and care. It's best to build these relationships early, when the sailing is fairly smooth, so trust can grow gradually and naturally. But if new help needs to come later, know that it may take time, and that patience, consistency, and compassion can still nurture meaningful connection, even in the harder stages of the disease.

What about occupational, physical, and speech therapists? What do they do? The title *occupational therapist* (OT) might sound like someone who helps with workplace injuries, and while that's true, he can be incredibly helpful for Alzheimer's patients. An occupational therapist can make daily tasks easier and safer by evaluating the home and recommending changes like installing grab rails, decluttering, taping down slippery rugs, and installing better lighting. He may suggest adaptive equipment you hadn't considered, like easy-to-use tableware and visual aids such as signs on dressers to help a loved one find clothing. He can also teach strategies for daily activities like eating, bathing, and dressing and will share techniques to support cognitive function.

You will be learning new ways to stay physically active, which energizes the body, spirit, and brain—and that's exactly where a physical therapist can help. As Alzheimer's progresses, it affects a person's mobility, balance, and coordination. A physical therapist works with caregivers and loved ones to build routines that keep patients active and flexible at every stage of the disease. She teaches exercises to help maintain balance, strengthen grip, and improve muscle strength and endurance by using tools like hand weights and resistance bands. These exercises have an added benefit—they can become part of a daily routine that makes caregiving easier and more predictable.

As the disease advances into the moderate stage, new challenges arise, including urinary and stool incontinence. Here, too, a physical therapist can help, offering pelvic floor muscle training to improve control and support patients' dignity and independence.

Beyond physical and occupational therapy, speech therapy also plays a vital role in Alzheimer's care. Speech therapists offer a range of tools to support communication and cognitive function. These include creating a "memory book" with pictures and familiar words, training exercises that teach patients how to handle moments when the right word won't come, and cognitive exercises aimed at strengthening language skills overall.

Therapists also provide strategies the patient can deploy to manage frustration when cognitive challenges develop and techniques to enhance attention and memory. They also coach families on how to effectively communicate so they can help loved ones stay connected while reducing emotional misunderstandings.

As the disease advances, a speech therapist's role expands to include swallowing therapy. Speech therapists can help diagnose dysphagia—swallowing disorders that often accompany moderate- and late-stage Alzheimer's. They develop exercises to strengthen the muscles involved in swallowing and suggest practical strategies to avoid aspiration. Aspiration, the inhalation of food or liquid into the lungs, can lead to pneumonia, one of the most common causes of death in people with dementia. By preventing aspiration, the therapist not only protects health but also helps patients continue to enjoy meals comfortably and safely, preserving their quality of life.

Last but not least, caregivers and loved ones living with cognitive impairment must take care of their own psychological well-being. Psychologists and psychiatrists are highly trained experts who have years of education and clinical experience providing essential support and counseling. Sometimes what's needed most is a licensed professional counselor (LPC) or licensed clinical social worker (LCSW) or therapist: someone who can listen, guide, and offer practical help through conversation. It's like talking to a trusted mentor or a wise friend, someone who listens, challenges you, and offers honest, levelheaded advice.

While my dad was dying, I never spoke with a professional about how I was feeling. Like many others, I buried my emotions and threw myself into work and family obligations. But at what cost? Years later, as I write this book, I realize I've blocked out many memories from that time. I've called upon my mom and sister to help me remember the quieter, less dramatic—but no less meaningful—moments of caring for him. I can't help but wonder how that period of my life might have left a different imprint if I had faced those feelings as they came.

Caregivers and patients alike can use therapy in many ways—to blow off steam, to seek advice about caregiving challenges, to learn how to manage or resolve issues with relatives, or to resolve long-standing issues that are preventing them from living their best life. For patients specifically, a therapist trained in health psychology can offer a focused program such as acceptance and commitment therapy (ACT). ACT typically involves five or six structured sessions designed to help individuals accept the diagnosis and its progressive nature while taking action to live meaningfully with this new reality. Counseling can then provide a safe space for coping with the ongoing changes, addressing emotions as they arise, and finding resilience throughout the disease journey.

Remember—even though its members are the heart of your care community, your medical team can only do so much. Your community team of local nonmedical helpers is who you will rely on when day-to-day living gets more challenging. Like any good investment, building your support system starts early. So, take the first step today—start developing your community!

What About Pets?

Bliss is a cat coiled in your lap or a faithful dog at your side. Beyond the comfort they bring in quiet moments, pets help caregivers and patients avoid isolation by offering steady companionship and emotional support. If you talk to a pet, it listens. Well, maybe dogs listen better than cats, but nonetheless, as Freud supposedly said, "Time spent with cats is never wasted." Pets offer companionship that is both unconditional and uncomplicated—they are a presence that listens without judgment and provides solace without words. Whether it's the soft purring of a cat or the eager tail wag of a dog, these interactions can elevate mood, offer a sense of connection, and create space for calm. When petting your four-legged friend, you give yourself a true release of endorphins that soothe the soul.

Research supports the therapeutic benefits of such companionship. A systematic review published in *BMC Psychiatry* found that animal-assisted therapy, particularly involving dogs, can lead to improvements in mood, social interaction, and even cognitive function among individuals with dementia. Similarly, a study highlighted by the BrightFocus Foundation demonstrated that the presence of fish aquariums in dining areas led to increased nutritional intake among Alzheimer's patients, suggesting that even passive interaction with animals can have positive effects.

My Portuguese Water Dogs Lorax and Wendell have been pillars of support during challenging times. Lorax, who was typically independent, would sense my struggles during my father's illness and offer closeness, nudging me toward walks that cleared my mind. Wendell, ever affectionate with endless licks to the face, insisted on being a lap dog despite his size, his enthusiasm and warmth providing comfort on the toughest days.

I love cats, too. Before my father was diagnosed with Alzheimer's, he never had a cat, because he supposedly was allergic to them. But we soon got him a ginger tabby named Sylvie. Throughout his disease, she was his best friend. We have so many pictures of the two of them together. Sylvie loved my father in a way that no human being could have. They were each other's devoted companions.

Having a pet early in the disease can provide a person with a sense of purpose. Helping to feed it, changing its water, cleaning its litter box, and taking it for walks are all noble duties. Moreover, owning a dog gets you outside into nature, opens conversational possibilities with passersby, and provides exercise.

It's important, however, to be realistic about the challenges of having a pet in the same home while you are a caregiver. Adopting a young or untrained pet demands time, energy, and consistency—and can quickly become overwhelming. In general, I do not recommend getting a puppy or a dog if you've never owned one before or if you're unable to fully commit to its care. While cats tend to be more independent, they still need daily attention and caregiving, which may not be feasible depending on the needs of the person with Alzheimer's.

If neither a cat nor a dog is right for your home, birds like parakeets can offer companionship with less demand. Studies have shown that a colorful flying friend can lower stress levels and alleviate symptoms of depression. Watching it chirp and flutter brings joy to the eyes and ears. You don't even have to have a bird in your house. One adult child who cared for his mother set birdfeeders outside windows of his home, including ones designed to attract hummingbirds. Watching birds come and go became entertainment, and his mother grew mesmerized by them for long periods. Having an aquarium offers similar benefits. Feeding fish adds a sense of routine, and watching them parade back and forth is comforting and stimulating.

For those for whom having a pet at home isn't practical, visiting places where animals are present—such as a friend's house, a community event, or even a local animal shelter—can provide meaningful interaction. If feasible, volunteering at a humane society or farm can bring both the joy of connection and the added benefit of purpose.

COMMUNITY—BUILD IT FOR THE LONG RUN

Caregiving for someone with dementia is uniquely challenging because the disease can be invisible. One moment your loved one may appear perfectly fine, chatty, clearheaded, maybe even independent, and the next she's confused, agitated, or unable to complete a basic task. Unlike caregiving for someone recovering from surgery or undergoing cancer treatment, there are no bandages, no IV drips, no physical signs that something is wrong. The brain can't wear a cast. There's no visual cue that says, *Oh, this is why Dad's not remembering my name today.* That invisibility can be disorienting. It can make it easy to forget why you're caregiving in the first place, or it can make you feel guilty for how tired, frustrated, or resentful you might be. And when you do forget why you are giving care, you might also forget to be compassionate.

This unpredictability creates its own kind of wear and tear. Dementia symptoms can come and go and differ from the steady decline that is also taking place but is often less obvious. Caregivers are elated on a good day but feel defeated the next when a loved one's behavior goes in circles or he fails to recognize his own home. Like a heavy surf hitting the beach, the emotional pounding of those erratic rhythms erodes a caregiver's confidence and well-being. As a caregiver, you find yourself rising and falling with the tides of behavior. We are wired to crave patterns—even painful ones—because they give us a sense of control. When nothing feels consistent, everything feels chaotic.

This is why habits and small rituals matter. They're like an anchor you drop for stability against the unpredictability of shifting behaviors. For example, my dad sometimes refused to put on his seatbelt. There wasn't always a reason. He just didn't want to. Instead of getting upset, we created a routine. I'd say, "Dad, let's take three deep breaths." After we did that, he usually calmed down enough to try again. While this practice didn't work every time, it became a familiar part of life when so much else wasn't.

This habit came in handy—sort of—the day I drove Dad to the funeral of a friend and parked in the church lot. I told him, "Wait until I release your seat belt." But by the time I opened his door, he was already struggling to get out. Because he still had a lot of upper body strength, it was difficult to release the belt against his pulling. A gentleman from a nearby car gently stepped in to help me restrain Dad while I untangled him. Was it embarrassing? Yes. Did I feel super frustrated? Not really, because I knew this could happen. This is the type of moment I think about when I suggest building strategies and habits. You don't do it because everything will always go smoothly; you do it so that when nothing works, you're still able to emotionally handle the situation.

These daily challenges are part of why caregiving for someone with Alzheimer's is often measured not in weeks or months but in years and possibly decades. No one is meant to shoulder that kind of load alone. That's why having a community, people who understand and can step in, listen, and simply be present, is foundational.

When you think about your Alzheimer's caregiving community, think long-term. Alzheimer's is being diagnosed far earlier than in the past. Not so long ago, most patients were diagnosed in the moderate stage of dementia and might live only another three to five years. Today people can survive a decade or more after a diagnosis. Caregivers must now build lasting resilience, maintain durability, and discover ways to sustain both their spirit and physical health over the long journey ahead.

The progress in Alzheimer's biomarker testing is reshaping how we think about time. We can now detect the silent but unfolding brain changes decades before memories fade. A new language among doctors is emerging, not just of patients and caregivers but of *pre-patients* and *pre-caregivers*, people who carry the knowledge of what may come long before any symptoms show. Living with this awareness can be both a burden and a blessing. It invites us to build strength into our bodies and minds earlier, before it is needed, and to weave resilience into the fabric of our days. What we do now shapes not just our future but the future of those we love.

We have to start to be aware of aging—and how to slow it—beginning when we are in our forties, not at age sixty-four. My mom loved playing the Beatles for my dad in his last years. He knew their music well, and it had a calming influence on him. So, in my idle moments my mind turns to the Beatles' song "When I'm Sixty-Four." Years ago, I never thought about the question the song asks—"Will you still need me, will you still feed me / When I'm sixty-four?" Now for me those lyrics take on a richer meaning, one that couples in midlife might be wise to ponder. Time slips away far faster for all of us than we think it will. The best day to start to plan ahead is today. One day we all will need someone to mend our fuses, knit us a sweater by firelight, or even just send us "a valentine, / birthday greetings, bottle of wine." Love is what we all need.

WHAT TO EXPECT—AND WHEN

What is a realistic timeline for a person with cognitive impairment? Most importantly, how soon will someone need help to get through the day? When newly diagnosed with MCI due to a brain disease like Alzheimer's, you should anticipate up to seven years of gradual changes in thinking, during which it may become increasingly difficult to keep up with daily abilities, even with compensatory strategies in place. In my clinical experience, however, people often progress to dementia within two to five years—likely because symptoms have been present for years before a thorough evaluation is completed. As discussed in the previous chapter, these daily abilities fall under the category of instrumental activities of daily living (IADL), such as managing medications, finances, appointments, driving, and cooking. The next phase is moderate-stage dementia, in which activities of daily living (ADL) decline. These basic functions include dressing, bathing, and toileting. This middle stage can last anywhere from one to several years. The final stage can be three years, though this varies greatly depending on whether the focus of care is on extending life or on comfort and quality of life through palliative and hospice support.

Adding up the number of years in the above paragraph might come as a surprise. A person diagnosed early with mild cognitive impairment may well have another twenty years of life ahead of him. Many or all of those twenty years could be at home and with gradual declines in daily living abilities. That's different from some other diseases. Most of us know people who have battled cancer for years, even decades. Patients receiving cancer treatments such as surgery, radiation, chemotherapy, or immune therapies can and often do live incredibly active lives. They drive to the office, chop wood, dice carrots, thread needles, change car tires, vacuum the carpet, go skiing, plant daffodils, mow the lawn, buy and sell stocks, you name it.

With Alzheimer's, however, as years pass, so does the ability to do those activities independently. You and your loved one will need rising levels of assistance. Even though the pace of the disease can be deceptively slow, that is no reason to put off community-building efforts. The small steps you take now will pay off later.

REACH OUT—SUPPORT WILL BE THERE

In moments of caregiving or personal crisis, remember that you are not meant to carry the weight alone. Support exists in many forms, and one helpful way to understand it is to visualize yourself at the center of a series of concentric circles. Each one represents a layer of trust and influence, beginning with those closest to you and expanding outward into your broader community. These are your circles of trust, whose orbits around you are as steady and dependable as those of the planets.

The innermost circle starts with your family: spouses, children, siblings, those most likely to know your daily rhythms and respond quickly when help is needed. Find out who is in your sphere and willing to help and then ask them to do specific tasks. For example, when someone dies or a baby is born, families sometimes create meal trains where people take turns providing meals on set days of the week. Consider drawing up a to-do list when family members take turns doing different chores.

The next ring is your neighborhood group—the friends, coworkers, and neighbors who live nearby. I have patients whose neighbors become quiet helpers—mowing lawns, bringing in the mail, reminding them of appointments, offering rides, or simply sitting together for company. Some even call faraway adult children to share updates on how a parent is doing. These everyday gestures weave a safety net that holds people together when it matters most.

The third circle from the center includes local government programs, nonprofit organizations, and for-hire services. Beyond that lies a fourth circle: state associations, such as regional offices of the Alzheimer's Association. Larger states will have chapters for big cities or geographic regions, making them almost akin to county services. For example, although Wisconsin has only one chapter, New York has ten and Texas has six. Each will have educational programs, support groups, volunteer opportunities, helplines, and updates on the latest in the field. Your state and county will also have online resources, as will local adult day centers and senior centers. A simple internet search will reveal local helpers who range from Meals on Wheels, massage therapists, and mental health counselors to home healthcare companies and building contractors who do eldercare home remodeling.

There's also a little-known but extraordinary network called the Area Agencies on Aging, made up of more than six hundred nonprofit organizations around the United States. Established under the Older Americans Act, these agencies have become a cornerstone of community support for older adults and their families. Like the Alzheimer's Association and Alzheimer's Foundation of America, Area Agencies on Aging offer a wide range of services—everything from nutrition assistance, home-delivered meals, caregiver support, in-home care assessment, and care plan development to providing information about long-term care facilities, insurance counseling services, and help coordinating nonmedical transportation.

What makes these agencies truly special, however, is the people who staff them. They are deeply knowledgeable, passionately committed, and often have a personal connection to the work they do. In my home state of Wisconsin, we are fortunate to have Aging and Disability Resource Centers (ADRCs) connected to this network. Many ADRCs employ a specially trained "dementia specialist" who helps patients and families develop care plans after a diagnosis, navigate the challenges of caregiving, and find the resources at each stage of the journey.

I rely on these specialists to help my patients after they leave the clinic. When patients are willing to share financial information, dementia specialists can guide them through eligibility rules for state-supported services, including programs that offer respite care possibly free of charge or at reduced cost. For many families, these connections provide not just practical help but emotional reassurance that they are not facing this disease alone.

Finally, the outermost ring of trust would be the national circle that includes the Alzheimer's Foundation of America, the Alzheimer's Association, and UsAgainstAlzheimer's. These organizations are pillars in the fight against Alzheimer's disease, offering a wealth of resources and support to patients, caregivers, healthcare professionals, and researchers. They are deeply committed to advocacy, raising public awareness, and advancing research to find better treatments and, ultimately, a cure.

Their websites serve as trusted hubs for information, offering educational materials, care planning tools, and disease management resources. They host virtual and in-person support groups, Memory Cafés, caregiver workshops, educational conferences, and seven-day-a-week helplines staffed by professionals. Many services are accessible by phone, video call, or online chat, making help available whenever families need it the most.

I've had the pleasure of working closely with these organizations, and I'm continually struck by the dedication of their leaders, staff, and volunteers. Many have been personally affected by Alzheimer's disease, allowing them to channel that experience into a deep, sustaining passion for helping others. Whether answering phone lines, attending evening events, or leading weekend conferences and lectures, they show up with sincerity, generosity, and purpose. Their work doesn't go unnoticed—families feel it. I always recommend these organizations to my patients, and I'm proud to collaborate with them.

The sidebar "Where to Go for Help," which lists support organizations, is the proverbial tip of the iceberg. Perhaps the simplest way to start is to visit websites of national nonprofit groups like the Alzheimer's Association, the Alzheimer's Foundation of America, UsAgainstAlzheimer's, the Centers for Disease Control and Prevention, Alzheimers.gov, and the National Institute on Aging.

Where to Go for Help

Administration for Community Living: acl.gov
AgingCare: agingcare.com
Alzheimer's Association: (800) 272-3900; alz.org
Alzheimer's Foundation of America: (866) 232-8484; alzfdn.org
ALZConnected: (800) 272-3900; alzconnected.org
Caregiver Action Network: (855) 227-3640; caregiveraction.org
UsAgainstAlzheimer's: usagainstalzheimers.org
Churches, synagogues, and other places of worship
Community Resource Finder: communityresourcefinder.org
County agencies
Eldercare Locator: eldercare.acl.gov/home and usaging.org/eldercareloc
Home Care Locator: agingcare.com/local
National Institute on Aging (NIA): nia.nih.gov

Once you dive into the world of support possibilities, you will find there is so much out there it can be overwhelming. For example, the Eldercare Locator website invites visitors to type in their zip code to get a list of community resources. When I put in mine, the search brought up more than ten state and county agencies where I live. The Alzheimer's Association also has a zip code locator that leads visitors to support groups, education programs, and events. The avenues for aid are seemingly endless.

If building a community feels overwhelming, take heart. It doesn't have to be. Start by making a simple list of the types of support you need. That way, instead of facing one large, daunting task, you're breaking it into five or ten manageable steps. Take your time. Every connection you make increases the chance of finding the right helpers. It really does take a village, and bit by bit, your circle will grow, and with it your strength.

Talk openly with your loved one about areas where you believe more support is needed. See if they agree, and if not, ask what they think is going well. If they do agree, then discuss options for how best to get that support. If you're living nearby—or in the same household—use this discussion to also be honest about your own needs. Let them know you cannot provide all the support alone. From there, connect with resources such as your local Area Agency on Aging, the Alzheimer's Association, the Alzheimer's Foundation of America, your memory care provider, or your primary care clinic, as many healthcare systems offer helpful programs. Even if you live far away, these conversations can still be valuable. You can reach out to the same organizations remotely, coordinate with local community services, and, if necessary, consider hiring a private care manager to help fill in the gaps.

Building your Alzheimer's support circle can make you lucky—and yes, there's science to back that up. In his 2003 book *The Luck Factor*, Dr. Richard Wiseman studied people who considered themselves lucky or unlucky. The lucky ones weren't born that way—they made their luck by meeting more people, trying new things, and saying yes to opportunities. By getting out and creating more connections, they boosted their odds of success. They bounced around like Tigger from *Winnie-the-Pooh*, always open to what the next moment might offer. Compare that to Eeyore, forever staring at the same patch of ground and wondering why nothing changes. Honey is out there waiting for you.

DRINK DEEP AT THE MEMORY CAFÉ

I'm a believer in local Alzheimer's support groups and especially in Memory Cafés. These are safe, welcoming spaces where caregivers and those experiencing cognitive changes can gather, connect, and, best of all, exhale. Memory Cafés are physical places—though some virtual ones now exist, too—hosted in a wide variety of locations. Some meet in restaurants, while others are held in community centers, libraries, museums, churches, or even office buildings that donate their space. Whatever the setting, these social lifelines remind you that you're not the only one navigating this unpredictable, exhausting, and deeply emotional road.

Memory Cafés often start as simple social activities—coffee, cookies, light conversation—but gradually become something much deeper. Like a neighborhood book club or a pickup basketball team, when you attend regularly you begin to recognize familiar faces. You develop a shared language of acceptance while telling stories about the good and the bad in your lives. Attendees who have attended longer offer advice. Someone cracks a joke that hits a little too close to home, but you laugh because it's real, and everyone else gets it. What begins as casual meetings becomes a union of allies. These gatherings grow into communities where caregivers bring questions, find support, and go home feeling stronger than they did when they woke up.

Such cafés are places where friendships are born out of shared challenges. They are where caregivers share practical tips like how to handle repetitive questions without losing one's cool or how to convince a parent to eat dinner when he insists he already did. You can cry, vent, and listen all in the same conversation. Perhaps most important, you don't have to explain yourself. These people understand because they are living what you are living.

Online forums and national resources are incredibly valuable, especially for getting general information or finding local services. But there's no substitute for being in a room with living, breathing people like yourself who see *you*—not just your role. That kind of understanding can change everything.

Of course, sometimes support also shows up in places you didn't expect. Asking a librarian a question could begin a friendship. A chance meeting with a neighbor could lead you to a home health aide. Going for a spin in your Saturday biking group might bring insights into dealing with stress. Certainly your hairstylist or barber will lend an ear to your concerns and worries. People often want to help. They just need to know how.

When I first went to a Memory Café, I accompanied my parents. My father's Alzheimer's disease was in the moderate stage. He sat quietly eating cookies, often smiling, and was usually content. There were moments, though, that caught me off guard, when someone would talk about a recent hallucination or a partner who could no longer bathe himself or who had stopped dressing in the morning. I would watch my father's face and see those comments hit him. He'd pause what he was doing. His face would change. It was clear he recognized what they were describing. That hurt. I had pushed for us to come to this group, but in those moments, I questioned whether I'd done the right thing. I didn't want these gatherings to be thorny reminders for him about what was slipping away.

The tricky part about support groups is the balance between grieving and gratitude. The time together is not meant to be a complaint session. The café is not supposed to be about what's broken. More often than not, there is laughter and lots of it. People share wonderful stories, old memories, and small wins. There is appreciation for food, for music, for connection. My group reminded me that life wasn't about what is lost, but about what remains.

My mom thrived there. She wasn't one to dwell on the hard things, but she wasn't afraid to speak up either. She'd offer advice when someone asked and would suggest practical ideas and lend kind words of wisdom. I was proud of her and proud to watch her become not just a caregiver to my father but a caregiver to other caregivers. I saw firsthand how much benefit there is in learning from others by picking up new techniques and fresh ways of looking at old problems. Café attendees weren't strangers anymore.

As for me, I was the only child in the group. That made me different, but never out of place. I wasn't the primary caregiver, and I respected that. I spoke when it felt right, offered a son's perspective, and sometimes answered questions about medication or research. It's funny how easily we fall back into our old roles—me, the science kid, always ready with the data.

But I had a new role, too. I was a support to the caregiver. I helped my mom, and I helped my dad. Being able to run errands, keep the room calm, and tell them stories when they were tired had value. The group made me realize we all have a place at the table. That's what Memory Cafés offer: a space where no one has to go it alone, where listening can help, where experience is shared with generosity, and emotional support is as vital as logistical advice.

Joining a Memory Café might feel like a small step. But small steps lead to new people, fresh ideas, and emotional grounding. Sure, you might try one and feel out of place. But try again. Like the motto says: "Ready. Fire. Aim." You'll miss a few times—but eventually, you'll hit something good. Something that sticks. And maybe, just maybe, you'll feel lucky again.

Top Ten Tips for Caregivers

The Caregiver Action Network is a remarkable nonprofit. It offers resources not only to Alzheimer's caregivers but also to those who care for people with cancer, addiction, multiple sclerosis, PTSD, and other medical conditions.

Here are its top ten pieces of advice for all family caregivers, no matter what medical situation they face.

1. Seek support from other caregivers. You are not alone!
2. Take care of your own health so you can be strong enough to take care of your loved one.
3. Accept offers of help and suggest specific things people can do to help you.
4. Learn how to communicate effectively with doctors.
5. Caregiving is hard, so take respite breaks often.
6. Watch for signs of depression, and don't delay getting professional help when you need it.
7. Be open to new technologies that help you care for your loved one.

8. Organize medical information so it's up to date and easy to find.
9. Make sure legal documents are in order.
10. Give yourself credit for doing the best you can in one of the toughest jobs there is.

THE MANY FACES OF THE CAREGIVING COMMUNITY

How one defines community varies. It can include immediate family or extend to friends, neighbors, and support groups. One of my patients had eight children who rotated caregiving duties, even sleeping at their parents' home to support both the parent with dementia and the caregiving spouse. When one child burned out, another stepped in. It helped that one child was clearly the ringleader, issuing all the orders—in a diplomatic way, of course.

Not all families are that large or cooperative. I know of another case where both parents had dementia and their only child moved back into his childhood home with his wife to care for them. With unwavering dedication, he left his job and provided daily care, quickly realizing the immense physical and emotional toll dementia takes. Instead of being overwhelmed, he sought knowledge and leaned into support. With the help of Alzheimer's organizations, he made the home safer—removing clutter, clearing trip hazards, remodeling a bathroom so his parents could sleep downstairs—and arranged home services for cleaning, meals, and medications. Only in the final stages did he transition them to a skilled facility. His journey was a lesson in humility, resourcefulness, and the power of asking for help.

In my practice, I see patients from many cultural backgrounds. Some families find the English word *caregiver* puzzling or even offensive, because in their culture it is assumed that family members care for one another. It is a responsibility assigned at birth. The idea of *caregiving* is already embedded in the meaning of the words *son*, *daughter*, *wife*, *husband*, and *relative*.

Yet even when caregiving is expected or unquestioned, it can still be emotionally and physically difficult. The role often involves tasks that are stressful or uncomfortable, like cleaning up after a broken dish or bathroom accident, managing medications, juggling finances, or navigating family tensions. I have noticed that these traditional caregiving bonds often weaken in second- and third-generation Americans, especially when families live far apart. I sometimes think back to a time before jet planes and interstate highways, when Americans tended to live in close-knit communities, both rural and urban. Family ties felt stronger then, too.

The word *care*, as in *caregiver*, is derived from the Latin noun *cura*, a word that implied great cost and was often associated with grief, sorrow, and emotional burdens. From its origin, caregiving has been a fraught and demanding role. Yet behind its weight and history, caregiving remains an intensely personal experience, shaped by the evolving needs of both the person receiving care and the one providing it. It is flexible, often evolving with changing circumstances. Some people step into the role naturally while others may not realize they are caregivers at all. Many spouses, for example, do not initially see themselves as caregivers, even though they are helping every day. Social workers often need to explain what caregiving means—and that it includes much more than medical tasks. Sometimes it is invisible, unspoken, or shared across multiple people.

At its core, a caregiver is anyone who helps another person maintain independence, improve quality of life, or manage daily activities. This may mean driving to appointments, picking up groceries, assisting with housework, or coordinating schedules. Sometimes caregiving is as simple as making sure a friend has a prepared meal waiting in the refrigerator. Every family has its strengths and limits. They must find what works—what they can manage, what they can delegate, or when they should ask for help. Even small gestures matter—a text or daily call can go a long way. From little acorns, mighty oaks grow.

BELONGING IN THE EVERYDAY

Be honest with family and friends about what you need. Perhaps you don't want certain types of help but would welcome other kinds. That's okay. Many people want to support you in whatever way they can. But it's important to be up-front and direct. Let people know what's truly helpful and what isn't. Some offers, though well-meaning, may actually add stress rather than relieve it. It's better not to waste time and energy, and instead focus on the support that genuinely makes a difference. If someone only wants to help on their own terms, it's okay to decline their offer. Over time, you'll find that new friends often appear, sometimes as if by magic, while others gradually fall away. It's all part of the natural rhythm of caregiving and life.

Even running errands can create community. My parents went to the farmers market every Saturday, where the atmosphere was cheerful and lively, full of friendly faces, free samples, and down-home music. It was more than just a trip for vegetables; it was a ritual. As my dad's Alzheimer's progressed, my parents adapted—he began wearing Depends, then they visited only familiar vendors, and eventually they navigated with a wheelchair. But they never stopped going.

When I asked my mom why, she said, "People in the community know your dad, and they need to see what Alzheimer's looks like. They need to see your dad is still a person and he's living with this disease. He and I are still *living*. We are a part of this community, and we feel a sense of belonging when we're there. It's good for him, and it's good for me." Events like farmers markets, local sports games, and neighborhood arts or music festivals offer more than fresh air; they open the door to connection, identity, and moments of shared life.

I was initially skeptical of my parents' daily errands until one day when I joined them. I could see my father liven up and truly enjoy their routine. Despite the physical effort of lifting him in and out of the car, my mom relished it, too. Getting outside, even to return free movies at the local library, brought them into a different yet supportive space. Those trips stuck with me and continue to influence the way I practice medicine.

Now when my patients reach the moderate stage of dementia, I offer them a disability parking pass. I know firsthand the value of simply "getting out of the house" and how something as small as a parking spot can become a barrier. I want my patients to have what my parents had—small freedoms that made life feel fuller, even in the face of loss.

Driving: When to Stop

Families are often surprised to hear that a diagnosis of Alzheimer's doesn't automatically mean a person must stop driving. In fact, in the mild stages, many individuals with Alzheimer's can continue to drive safely, particularly with compensatory strategies and some personalized precautions.

Research has shown that people with Alzheimer's tend to be safer drivers than those with other forms of dementia. That's because Alzheimer's usually affects short-term memory and language first—cognitive areas that, in the context of driving, can often be supported or worked around. By contrast, other dementias have a direct impact on skills essential to driving fitness and safety. For example, Lewy body dementia affects visual-spatial abilities, attention, and executive function. Vascular dementia can similarly impact attention and executive function, while frontotemporal dementia is often accompanied by disinhibition and risky behaviors that make unsafe driving more likely. Individuals with these non-Alzheimer's dementias tend to fail on-the-road driving tests at higher rates.

Many patients who come to see me in the memory clinic have already placed reasonable limits on themselves. For those who haven't, I suggest commonsense restrictions: Drive only during daylight, only on familiar routes, and only within a certain radius of home; avoid freeways; and use GPS guidance or have a family member in the car. Some states, like Wisconsin, have laws that govern these matters. Check with your local DMV to understand the laws in your jurisdiction.

If concerns arise—whether from the patient or family—the best next step is to talk with the doctor. I often ask families a simple question: *Would you let your child or grandchild ride with this person behind the wheel?* Their answer can be very revealing. No one wants to cause harm, but the fear of losing a driver's license and the independence it represents is real. To avoid confrontation or a formal DMV review, the doctor can refer the patient to an occupational therapist for a clinical driving evaluation. These tests are conducted in office and focus on the cognitive domains critical to driving. There are also on-the-road assessments available outside the DMV system, though these are often not covered by Medicare or other insurance. Both can be extremely helpful in clarifying fitness to drive and building a shared understanding among family members.

Doctors and families should start this conversation early, well before driving becomes unsafe, so there's time to prepare, not just react. No one wants to feel blindsided or suddenly cut off. With enough lead time, families can plan ahead, discuss meaningful destinations with the person living with dementia, and problem-solve how to get there. There are more transportation options today than ever before, and you'd be surprised how many friends are happy to offer a ride. Many of my patients ultimately come to enjoy being passengers.

Taking away the keys against someone's will or involving the DMV should be a last resort. But sometimes it's necessary—for the safety of the person and the public. International consensus recommends that individuals with moderate-stage dementia stop driving altogether. I share this with my patients early, not to scare them but to normalize the process and provide a timeline that removes the feeling of being singled out. It's not about punishment. It's about planning, protection, and peace of mind for everyone on the road.

For my parents, their local library also became part of their daily routine. It was "dementia friendly" and became a second home. They went there to see films, look at art, and meet friends. My mother felt comfortable knowing my father could wander the stacks unescorted. Librarians chatted with him. The staff got to know my parents well and supported them with kindness and by sharing their time. It was my parents' safe place, and it also had therapeutic effects because it was an intellectually stimulating environment.

Even your local grocery store can be part of your community. My neighborhood co-op is dementia friendly because its staff have been trained to work with all kinds of customers. My parents would stop by each time they visited me. Over time, the manager, cashiers, and clerks got to know them well. They learned my dad had Alzheimer's and always treated him with kindness and respect.

One day when I went shopping with my parents, we bought lunch at the in-store café. As we sat down, my father said he needed to wash his hands, probably because, as a doctor, he always needed to have clean hands. We had been there so often my mom casually pointed and said, "There's the bathroom." After he walked away, she and I fell into conversation. Minutes passed. My mom suddenly asked me, "Where's your dad?" We turned and saw a cashier walking him back to our table. One hand rested gently on my dad's shoulder, and the other lay on his forearm, just as he had been trained to do when assisting someone in need.

My father had wandered into the utility closet, likely because he saw a sink and assumed it was the restroom. Presumably, he washed his hands amid the mops. The cashier chatted kindly with him as they returned. My mom wasn't embarrassed. My dad sat, and we ate lunch as though nothing unusual had happened. Later, when my father was elsewhere, my mom and I laughed about it. We enjoyed the moment so much because my dad didn't care. Neither did we, and, best of all, neither did the store or anyone around us. What had happened was normal for us, and the store treated it that way. We were so grateful we had done our shopping at a dementia-friendly grocery store. It could have been a horrible experience, but it wasn't, and for that, we were relieved.

I know dementia-friendly grocery stores are not on every street corner. But in your town, you will find libraries, farmers markets, shops, restaurants, hardware stores, and ice cream parlors that are dementia friendly or run by people who treat everyone with compassion and dignity. Think about what you and your loved one enjoy doing, and don't let the stigma of the disease stop you. Maybe you already visit a favorite state park, attend concerts or sporting events, or buy your bread and butter at a kindly store. Whatever those places are, continue to frequent them. They are part of your community, and your presence matters there.

VISITS WITH YOUNG CHILDREN

Grandchildren bring wonder and purpose to the lives of many older people, especially if they live nearby. Caring for grandchildren can give any older person a renewed sense of purpose. I recommend physical, mental, and social activity for brain health—and caring for children fills those requirements for many patients. Many of my patients find such meaning and pleasure in the little ones' playfulness that they look forward to their grands' visits. Delight in grandchildren may be one of the few joys they have left. So "babysitting" is what they do, and they love it.

I've seen some grandkids become a significant underlying motivation for patients' well-being. One such patient is Cathy, a sturdy farmer's wife. She grew up in rural Wisconsin, married a man who also had Scandinavian heritage, and raised five children. Most moved away, but two stayed close to their small hometown, where they started their own families. Many days after school Cathy found herself looking after little ones while their parents worked. Preparing after-school snacks, reading to them, playing games, kissing boo-boos, helping them with homework, and cleaning up messes helped give Cathy a regular schedule, allowed her to avoid being isolated, and kept her mind focused on appreciating the gifts in her life.

There is a caveat—while this may be fine in the early stages of mild cognitive impairment and mild-stage dementia, actual babysitting becomes dangerous as the disease progresses. My role is to educate families and tell them when this becomes unsafe.

I've seen situations where the patient's adult child badly wants his parent and the grandchild to connect. The adult child recognizes their parent is going to pass away and wants him or her to spend quality time with the grandchild. Plus, they want the grandchild to have memories of the grandparent.

Unfortunately, young children can be too noisy or cause more stimulation than the elder parent can tolerate. As a person progresses in Alzheimer's disease, she becomes increasingly self-centered, though not in a negative, selfish way. The patient simply starts to focus more on herself and her basic needs. She grows less aware of her surroundings and has less interest or ability to play with or be attentive to the grandchild. The disease makes the person unable to care about the feelings of the grandchild. The child's loudness is irritating, and the child becomes an annoyance instead of a source of pleasure.

Many people with hearing problems, for example, experience separation in a less dramatic way. When you can't grasp the essence of the conversation because you've missed parts of it, it's harder to stay interested, and so you tune out instead of participating. When adult children come to me about tension over the lack of a close relationship between a parent with Alzheimer's and a grandchild, I explain that their father or mother has passed the point where he or she wants to spend more time with the grandchild. This lack of interest is not intentional. It is a biochemical consequence of what Alzheimer's does to the brain. This typically does not happen until much later in the disease.

When a Loved One No Longer Recognizes You

One of the most painful changes families face is when a loved one with dementia no longer recognizes them. This usually occurs in the later stages of the disease, but it can happen earlier with acquaintances, distant relatives, or people who are less involved in the person's daily life. Much like how short-term memories fade while long-term memories often remain, recently formed relationships tend to be forgotten before those that span years. This is why spouses, children, and parents are usually the last to be forgotten, if ever.

My dad may not have remembered my name when he died, but I knew he recognized me at his bedside. One moment I'll never forget is when I knelt beside him for a hug, and he looked at me and with quiet confidence said, "I know your face." I saw the recognition and love in his eyes as he reached for my hand.

Even so, there often comes a time when familiar faces become unfamiliar. For grandchildren, this can be especially confusing and heartbreaking. They may not understand why their grandparent suddenly doesn't know them, and that disconnect can feel like rejection.

In these moments, how we respond matters. It's natural to feel hurt or to want to correct the confusion, but trying to reorient a loved one rarely works and can sometimes escalate stress. Instead, the best approach is one of calm acceptance. Introduce yourself gently, change the subject, or ask a question to redirect the conversation. It is an act of compassion to carry the emotional weight yourself so your loved one doesn't have to.

My own mother falls in the camp of "I've raised my children, and your children are yours." She loves my boys, but she's never been one to volunteer for babysitting. If one day she develops Alzheimer's, her attitude will likely only be accentuated. Dementia doesn't erase the relationship that existed before the condition; it tends to magnify what was already there.

My maternal grandmother was deeply thoughtful, a voracious reader, and loved spirited conversations in which she debated on a wide range of topics. She never hesitated to wade into controversial territory and was always comfortable discussing death, even in the final days of her life. As my sister and I grew older, we came to truly admire her. That relationship deepened into one of my most cherished friendships. But as far as I know, she never baked a cookie or hosted a child's birthday party.

My wife's mother, on the other hand, watches our children once a week. Her patience and desire to help is saintly. My wife and I are deeply grateful, and our family has benefited in countless ways. Even strong routines can't override a person's underlying philosophy on life. The key is to embrace the best of each family member and allow those gifts to flow through.

As for family relationships in general, as I've written in earlier chapters, every family has its own strengths, weaknesses—and conflicts. For more detailed guidance on how siblings can either support or unintentionally hinder the efforts of a primary caregiver, turn to chapter 4, page 146. To recap, adult children must learn to respect how the primary caregiver—whether a spouse or another family member—is managing daily life. This doesn't mean the caregiver is always right or beyond question, but they are the one living the reality hour by hour. Their perspective deserves attention, their decisions deserve space, and their well-being deserves support. Caregiving works best when families lead with trust, flexibility, and a shared desire to honor the person they all love.

MAKE THE ROUNDS—DO THE ROUTINES THING

For more than a century, doctors have made rounds in hospitals. Typically, interns and residents trail beside the senior physician, and together they gather around the bedside of one patient after another. The purpose? To assess patients' progress, discuss care plans, and improve communication among team members. For a young doctor this is a terrific learning experience.

Rounding in the intensive care unit is always sobering. These patients are critically ill, and the weight of that reality is present in every room. One morning, as our team entered a patient's room and began reviewing her medical issues, she suddenly became unresponsive. Her pulse vanished. Her blood pressure plummeted. Her heart rate spiked into the

130s—she was entering septic shock. My resident, steady and composed, quickly directed me to place a central line, a thin tube inserted into a vein in her neck, to rapidly deliver fluids and medications. There was no time to second-guess, no room for hesitation.

Under pressure like that, your mind turns to muscle memory. That's why we practice procedures whenever we can. The routine prepares us for the unpredictable. Preparation doesn't prevent crisis, but it gives you the ability to respond with calm and competence when crisis comes. That's how doctors benefit from following a regular routine in the hospital.

Of course, routines aren't just for doctors, they're built into the fabric of everyday life. From bus schedules and school bells to government economic reports, the world runs on rhythm and repetition. We all have our own routines—that grande iced half-caf triple-mocha latte macchiato made the way you like it, the 9 AM Monday meeting at work, going for a walk every day after dinner, or reading that book in bed before you turn out the lights. These patterns bring structure. They have a calming influence. Even when work or life gets chaotic, we find comfort in knowing we can escape to the gym at noon or settle into a familiar routine at day's end.

The same principle applies in caregiving, especially for someone with Alzheimer's disease. Like the rest of us, someone with cognitive impairment benefits from consistent routines: regular times for medication, meals, visits to adult day centers, and eventually toileting. Performing the same action at the same time each day reduces stress for both the patient and the caregiver.

When the brain follows a routine, it doesn't have to work as hard. A consistent schedule allows someone with Alzheimer's to rely less on memory and problem-solving and more on pattern and repetition. Not only does this make daily life more manageable, but it can help preserve function longer. And for caregivers, structure brings its own rewards: It makes it easier to plan for outside help and creates room to tend to one's own needs.

Routines are grounding. They offer the security of knowing what comes next for everyone involved. That may sound ordinary, but in caregiving, it's anything but. It's a quality-of-life anchor. And it may be the most meaningful form of stability we can offer.

ROUTINE ANSWERS THAT MAKE THINGS WORSE

How we respond to our loved one matters. We cannot control their disease, but we can control our behavior toward others. Falling into the habit of automatically replying to an Alzheimer's patient in a dismissive, unthinking way is unhealthy. We've all had the experience of scratching our heads and staring in puzzlement when a repairman, mechanic, or doctor uses technical terms to describe what the problem is with the refrigerator, car, or elbow. At best we feel dumb. At worst we feel demeaned, as though someone is speaking down to us and doesn't care enough to explain something in terms we can understand.

The same thing happens all too often with some Alzheimer's caregivers when they give hasty automatic responses to their loved one. It is entirely normal for an Alzheimer's patient to repeat the same question not twice but four, five, six, or seven times. His hippocampus deep in his brain has lost the ability to store your reply.

Confronting patients with brusque retorts, which chastise their short-term memory, is cruel and doesn't work. I will always remember the time I was seeing patients in my clinic while accompanied by a medical student. We entered the exam room where a wife and her husband were waiting, and straightaway the wife said, "He's upset about the testing. Tell him, tell him, tell the doctor what you just told me." The husband looked blankly at her. He had forgotten what he had said to her seconds earlier. Before I could say, "I'm sorry to hear that. I know the tests are hard," she again verbally prodded her husband, saying, "Well, you said the test was bad. Tell him. Tell him." When the student and I left the exam room, he turned to me, his eyes wide, and gasped, "Oh, my God, she was berating that man with Alzheimer's disease."

You can't control your loved one's memory loss. All you can do is control your reaction and give a loving reply. Think of it this way: If your loved one were blind, you would never think of speaking thoughtlessly or harshly because she couldn't see a color or the chair that blocks her path.

With an Alzheimer's patient, do not try to win an argument or even get into one. Overcorrecting does not work. Worse, it's counterproductive.

Don't be confrontational, and don't take anything your loved one says personally. Instead, adopt one of these strategies:

Agree with your loved one.
Give a brief answer.
Distract him.
Accept the blame for what's gone wrong, even if it's imaginary.
Respond to the person's feelings, not his words.
Be patient, cheerful, and reassuring.
And most of all, be forgiving.

I have counseled many Alzheimer's caregivers who overcorrect their loved ones out of a misguided sense of duty, an obligation they feel to keep their loved one "in this world." You cannot "fix" the statements of an Alzheimer's patient. Instead, what I find myself doing is helping the family member understand how her efforts at correctness are like chasing a rainbow. In such a situation, it is the family member whose behavior needs to be mended, not the patient's. You must meet the Alzheimer's patient where he is at, and you must do this routinely as a part of your daily conversations.

Communication Misstep to Correct Early On

As dementia progresses, families must adjust how they communicate. Unfortunately, many of us fall into unhelpful patterns—often out of habit or frustration—that unintentionally undermine our loved one's confidence and strain the relationship. These moments don't stem from bad intentions but from communication styles that no longer fit the person's changing needs. With awareness and effort, they can be improved.

One particularly common and unproductive pattern is how families give instructions. A familiar example I hear in my memory clinic: Someone in the house, often in another room, calls out a list of tasks for their loved one to complete. The television is on. There's no eye contact. No effort to confirm whether the person is paying attention or has even heard the request. The instructions include multiple steps, spoken quickly and without repetition. Nothing is written down.

Later, when the tasks go unfinished, the family member feels frustrated and the person with dementia is blamed. Yes, memory loss may play a role, but the environment wasn't set up for success either.

When I counsel patients and families, I recommend minimizing distractions, making eye contact, giving one-step instructions, writing down lists, and asking the person to repeat what they've heard. Just as important is giving time—pausing after you've spoken and waiting for a reaction or recognition before moving on. People with dementia want to contribute. With the right accommodations and new communication routines, they often can.

This can involve doing a certain amount of improvisation or "therapeutic fibbing," as it's also known. Let's say a loved one believes his late brother Bob is sitting with you in the den. Instead of telling an Alzheimer's patient he is imagining things—or worse, that his brother is dead, a response that could be upsetting—it's far better to do some innocent playacting. There are times when you have to live in the world of the Alzheimer's patient and respond on that basis. A kind response might be, "Oh, what is Bob wearing?," "What's he doing in the chair? Is he reading a book?," or even something vague like "That's nice." The moment will pass. Challenging the loved one or being confrontational may instigate a scene, one that leads to unnecessary embarrassment or shame for the patient.

In my dad's last year, he often said his mother had visited him during the night. She had been dead for decades. I took that opportunity to ask him what she said when they were together. He told me that she missed seeing him. Because my dad was afraid of death and had talked about it openly after his diagnosis, this gave me the opportunity to express my joy that his mother was waiting for him to come home. It always seemed to comfort him, and me, too.

Fibbing like this may seem unethical or wrong, but sometimes it is the kindest policy to practice. The Uncle Bob scenario happened with the family of one of my patients. They insisted they had to tell their loved one Bob had died. I told them that telling the truth would be traumatic for their loved one. Indeed, that is what happened. They later came back to me and confessed they wished they had taken my advice and given diplomatic or reassuring answers instead. The trauma passed because this Alzheimer's patient ultimately forgot that he had been told Uncle Bob was dead.

For ingenious ideas on how to have conversations with an Alzheimer's patient, see the sidebar "The Power of Imagination" below. The strategy described there relies on engaging with the loved one's creativity, not their memory.

The Power of Imagination

What Alzheimer's does to the brain naturally leads doctors and caregivers to focus on memory. But people can get bogged down reacting to their loved one's memory deficits—and that can interfere with good care.

So what would happen if wonder, not memory, inspired Alzheimer's caregiving strategies? That's the question Dr. Anne Basting, the founder and president of the nonprofit TimeSlips, asked. Her book *Creative Care: A Revolutionary Approach to Dementia and Elder Care* advises caregivers to use storytelling and what she calls "beautiful questions." Dr. Basting was my guest on my podcast, *Dementia Matters,* and had this to say:

Everyone has a story inside them, and you want to bring those stories out. I encourage caregivers to connect with people living with dementia by asking "beautiful questions." If you ask somebody a question that relies on memory for an answer, there's a good chance that that answer—because it's a fact—involves a pathway in the brain that is most likely broken.

If you ask a beautiful *question, there are a thousand possible pathways and answers. That means there's much more opportunity for a person to express themselves positively based on a strength rather than feeling ashamed at not knowing that one answer. A beautiful question is confidence building. It invites the person to express himself out of his strength rather than loss.*

What do I mean by a beautiful question? One of my favorites is, "If you could lift up right now and fly anywhere you wanted, where would you go?" Another is, "What do you treasure in your home?" Those kinds of questions have no right or wrong answer. Imagine you're walking by a window with a person who has dementia. You invite her to look outside and ask, "What sounds do you imagine outside? What smells? Can we trace that tree with our hands? What would that be like?" Questions like these open up a moment to wonder.

Ask open-ended questions that have no right or wrong answers. They invite the person to say whatever they want in that moment. That's empowering because people with dementia can get conditioned to think they're going to say the wrong thing and might as a result say nothing. An open-ended question invites the person to express himself using whatever strengths he has, and that response might be a sound, gesture, word, or phrase. You're inviting that light and that spark inside that person to come out and create a sense of shared wonder.

You're not giving up on memory by shifting to imagination. You're creating a new way for memory to come out.

THE HOME HEALTHCARE DECISION

Hiring home healthcare is ideal, and while it may not be necessary early on, as time goes by, most Alzheimer's caregivers begin to give serious thought to implementing this. The goal is to keep a loved one with Alzheimer's at home as safely as possible for as long as possible—because in the end, everybody wants to be in their safe, familiar place.

Home healthcare can be what you want it to be. A place to start is with an eldercare consultant who can visit your home, identify potential hazards, and suggest practical solutions. On the other end of the spectrum, home health might mean having someone live in your home or hiring an agency to provide one or more caregivers on a regular basis. How often they come and what they do is entirely up to you. You want someone trained in dementia—not just in general home care—because those nuances will matter when times are hard.

One of the tricky aspects of home care is that while it's preferable to moving into a facility, it also introduces someone into your private space. It can feel awkward. Ideally, you want to establish a relationship with a home caregiver early on—before things become overwhelming—but that also means bringing someone into your home when you may not truly need the help yet. So what do you have them do? It often starts with companion care, which means helping with social engagement or light activities. This can include walks to the local parks, shopping, or reading the newspaper together. Often, your loved one won't like it at first. You may need to get creative to help them feel comfortable with this new presence. Over time, that role gradually expands: more household support, then personal care, and eventually skilled nursing.

Besides bringing relief to the caregiver, such visits help keep the caregiver and the person with Alzheimer's socialized, because there can be a tendency for caregivers and patients to become isolated. Being alone and trying to do everything yourself for your loved one is dangerous. For the person with the impairment, isolation and loneliness lead to the development of behavioral and psychological symptoms of dementia (BPSD). These symptoms often arise during the moderate to severe stage of the disease and include depression, anxiety, agitation, restlessness, aggression, hallucinations, paranoia, disrupted sleep, and sundowning. Sundowning is a neurological phenomenon in which symptoms become more severe later in the day, often triggered by fatigue, mood shifts, or overstimulation. These behaviors can be exhausting, disheartening, and overwhelming. No one wants to see a loved one struggle in this way. Any thoughtful caregiver would naturally want to minimize these symptoms, but without help, even the most devoted person can burn out. That's why building a support system is more than helpful—it's a lifeline.

For many families, that support begins with in-home healthcare. This often becomes essential during the moderate stage of the disease, when your loved one will need help with dressing, bathing, and personal hygiene. She may wander, become disoriented, or exhibit behavioral changes such as agitation or restlessness. Communication becomes more difficult as well, which can add frustration for both the person with dementia and those trying to help. Having a trained professional involved at this stage can ease the strain on families and improve safety and quality of life for everyone involved.

The level of skill among home health aides can vary widely, especially when it comes to caring for people with dementia. Some may be better at providing companion care—offering conversation, activities, and supervision—while others are adept at more personal tasks such as bathing, dressing, or eating. Support may be scheduled for just a few hours a day, one or two days a week, or expanded to full-time daily coverage, with some agencies even offering overnight coverage. Costs depend on both the type of services provided and the aide's level of experience, making it important to carefully match the support to your loved one's needs. Health insurance, including Medicare, typically does not cover these services, though long-term care insurance often does.

Compared to life in a long-term care facility, home care is typically less expensive, helps preserve your loved one's independence, and can ease the eventual transition to residential care if it becomes necessary. It's also more adaptable to the unique needs and preferences of someone living with Alzheimer's, something that can be challenging in institutional settings.

If you've done the work of building a support network—whether through local groups, online chats, or books like this—these changes won't feel like surprises. Your community can also help you find leads for good home care providers. Good help in the home can often be hard to find, so don't wait for an emergency to make these decisions—line up the help you need before you think you'll need it.

Trying Adult Day Centers

Having a loved one spend time at a local adult day center can be a solace for everyone. For caregivers, it provides valuable time to run errands, rest, or manage other responsibilities. For someone with dementia, attending once or twice a week—even for just a few hours—can offer mental stimulation, social connection, and light physical activity.

My dad attended a church-run center that worked well—for a while. He went twice a week from 8 AM to noon and stayed for lunch. Before he started, we visited the center with my dad to meet its staff and chatted with other participants. It felt like a solid fit.

At first, he seemed to enjoy going. By the third month, however, he began to protest. He said he didn't want to attend and started resisting getting into the car. This went on for a few weeks. We kept taking him, though my mom checked in with the staff to see if anything unusual was happening. They reassured us that everything was fine. He was safe, engaged, and seemed to be doing well. We remained uneasy but believed the routine was still helping him. And I knew my mom needed respite.

Then one morning, a staff member called. My father was shaking and visibly upset. They thought he needed help in the bathroom, but he refused to let them in. When they finally got inside, nothing seemed obviously wrong, and to this day, we don't know what happened. That incident changed everything, however. We decided not to send him back. The experience was upsetting for all of us—my father, my mother, my sister, and me. My mom carried guilt for a long time about those final visits. My father never spoke about it. Fortunately, I don't think he remembered. My mom believes he did, and I think that's why she still wonders whether we should have stopped sooner.

In fairness, we could have done more to work with the center to prevent another incident. The staff was willing to collaborate and open to finding solutions. Alternatively, we could have explored a different facility with more advanced care—somewhere that offered on-site nursing or specialized support for behavioral changes in dementia. Our family didn't pursue those options at the time, but they were fortunately available to us.

Ending his visits was hard. Still, I don't regret trying it. He enjoyed it in the beginning. It gave him a new environment and gave my mom time to herself. But when his distress outweighed the benefit, we had to stop.

That's the reality of this process: Nothing is permanent. A strategy or activity can work for a time, and then it won't. Families need to stay flexible—willing to try, willing to stop, and ready to move on. It helps to be grateful when something does work, even if only for a little while.

As a caregiver, you must keep looking forward. Educate yourself about what lies ahead and be mindful of how the disease progresses. This is another reason why being part of a support group can be invaluable. You'll meet people caring for loved ones at every stage of Alzheimer's. Their stories—about what went well and what didn't—can provide tested and practical strategies. Learn from their mistakes instead of waiting to make your own.

I encourage you to read the sidebars in this chapter that offer life lessons from Dr. Arthur Kleinman and former Wisconsin Governor Martin

Schreiber. Both men cared for their wives for many years, and both made the decision to bring paid helpers into their homes. During the final stage of Alzheimer's, each husband decided to place his wife in assisted living. Whether that decision would be best for you and your loved one demands much consideration, and I encourage you—and your loved one—to visit such facilities so you can learn more about future options, get your name on waiting lists so those options are available to you when you need them, and perhaps make better decisions now about the future.

A Doctor's Wife Has Alzheimer's—What He Learned

Dr. Arthur Kleinman was his wife Joan's primary caregiver for eleven years. In his book *The Soul of Care: The Moral Education of a Husband and a Doctor*, he chronicled his emotional and physical journey. Kleinman is a professor of medical anthropology and cross-cultural psychiatry at Harvard. I spoke with Dr. Kleinman in 2020.

Lots of my friends read my book and were astonished when they learned what my caregiving involved. They knew I was doing certain things but didn't realize how basic many of those activities were.

You do the care because it is there to do. You're sort of thrown into it, and it's got to be done. The person has to have a bath. Someone's got to do it. You're there, and you end up doing it. Over time, you begin to figure out ways that you can be assisted.

My wife Joan was four or five years into her dementia before it became absolutely clear to me I had to have someone in the house to help. So I was late in understanding how crucial it was to have a home health aide. I benefited enormously from that assistance.

When it comes to caregiving, we get caught up in a rose-colored Hollywood vision of resilience. We think we can automatically expand our capacity, get stretched like a rubber band, and come back to who we were before. That idea is erroneous. None of us is like a rubber band that can be stretched. Everyone is wounded, even broken, by what they must do as a family carer.

Nonetheless, positive things come out of it—the sense of purpose and meaning in life. There are joys along the way. The fact that you are doing care doesn't obliterate the happiness in the rest of life. It channels joys in different directions.

As time passed, Joan wasn't present enough to say, "You can do this, Arthur," or "Keep going, Arthur." Because I loved her and because her presence brought out my devoted presence, I kept going. That's what helped me endure. Other times I endured thanks to the home health aide, my family, and the sensitivity of my work colleagues who realized the pressure I was under.

You can give care mechanically. You can give it in an institutional bureaucratic way without being fully present, but when you are fully present, you put the care *in caregiving. That care—worrying about people and then caring for them—is a universal feeling, an elaboration of the love we have for others.*

Care is a crucial part of who we are in relation to others. It's as universal as anything you'll find.

CAREGIVERS NEED CARE, TOO

When you are taking care of someone over a long period of time with any sort of chronic illness, it can easily lead to burnout, depression, and high blood pressure, to name just a few mental and physical woes. Caregivers often face an impossible task: balancing their loved one's needs with their own. That's why they must have their own team—doctors, therapists, and support groups—like the person with dementia.

During my geriatric training, I learned about the concept of the "invisible patient"—the caregiver. Using only two words, it captured the plight of many family members, especially those looking after someone with Alzheimer's. As clinicians, we're taught—rightly—to focus on the patient.

But in doing so, especially under time pressure, we often overlook the caregiver's voice and health. Their experience becomes secondary, even though their well-being is directly impacted by the progression of the disease. It's a flaw in the system that needs to be addressed.

I'll be direct: Caregivers must prioritize their health, because their loved one's decline will inevitably take a toll. I recognize how hard this is, and it's easier said than done. In many cases, it feels nearly impossible. But it's worth acknowledging and striving for. Small steps are still steps, and they matter. Research and clinical experience make clear that the health of the person giving care directly impacts the health of the patient, too. Burned-out care partners simply provide worse care. Those with stronger self-efficacy and emotional well-being provide better care and feel more satisfied in their role. They're more adaptable in crisis, and they recover faster. They endure longer.

Tending to someone with dementia is unlike supporting any other chronic condition. Dementia progresses steadily, and physical needs often increase at the moments when caregivers are the most depleted. That's why support is not merely helpful; it's necessary. Carers need a network of family, friends, hired in-home help (when possible), adult day centers, Memory Cafés, and support groups. They also need medical care for themselves and the time to devote to it. Therapists, psychiatrists, and primary care doctors can keep them strong, grounded, and resilient. Everything in chapter 5 about brain health applies to family members, too. In fact, they should adopt those strategies alongside their loved one.

The Triumph of Letting Go

Former Wisconsin Governor Martin Schreiber wrote his book *My Two Elaines: Learning, Coping and Surviving as an Alzheimer's Caregiver* to honor his wife's memory and share lessons from his journey with her. Governor Schreiber spoke with me in 2018 on *Dementia Matters* to reflect on his caregiving experience.

Being a true caregiver to me meant joining the world of the person who is ill. When I joined Elaine's world, every time she didn't know who I was did not become another body blow. You must get to the point where you can let go of the person who once was and embrace the person who now is to better share with their heart and soul moments of joy that ordinarily wouldn't be there. Joining the world of the person who is ill will make such a big difference, reducing your anxiety, pain, hurt, depression, and some of the sadness.

One of the biggest challenges to caregivers of those with this disease is that it is progressive. You give every ounce of love, strength, and energy and wake up the next morning to find you're five paces backward. You ask, What am I doing wrong? What should I be doing better? *Suddenly guilt grabs you. So, when we talk about changes as the disease progresses, we're also talking about direct changes in the caregiver's life.*

The diagnosis is not the end of the world. It is the beginning of an opportunity to enhance our relationship, prepare our bucket list, and do things. To take the diagnosis and crawl under the covers to hide is a huge mistake.

Early on, Elaine and I had many wonderful experiences and opportunities. We talked things through and shared and understood that no matter what the end might be that our life together was worth it all. Sometimes you will cry together. Sometimes you will pray together, and sometimes you will share hurt and pain. But as you travel your journey together, you both gain strength from it. That strength builds up in a reservoir. As the disease progresses, you draw from it because you better understand the courage of the person who is ill.

Caregivers need to sleep, exercise, eat well, reduce stress, socialize, stay mentally active, and keep their vision, hearing, and oral health monitored not only for general wellness but because they are at higher risk for cognitive decline themselves. The constant stress accelerates aging.

I learned this firsthand by watching my mother. She was never an invisible patient. Anyone who has met her knows she's a force of nature. She advocated fiercely for my dad, directed his care, and made decisions alongside him and the medical team. My father was in good hands. Even so, her well-being went largely unnoticed. Only the social worker thought to pull her aside to ask how she was doing.

When my dad was diagnosed with mild-stage dementia in his early sixties, it was devastating and felt deeply unfair. No one should start to lose their memory so young, though many sadly do. One small silver lining was that my mom was young, too. She was physically and mentally healthy, which made it possible for her to care for him longer than many could. With minimal help from me and a few friends, she kept my dad at home until the day he died. Her selflessness and devotion were remarkable, but caregiving took its toll. It aged her, as it does so many in that situation. While we may not be able to prevent all these changes, we can try. We should try, because the cost is real, and it accrues quietly, day by day.

If you are caring for someone, your brain is being tested constantly, and your body is under stress. Building resilience through healthy habits is not optional—it's survival. For the care partner and the person with dementia, aloneness and isolation are dangerous. Caregivers need connection, rest, and support. They need to live a full life, not a life of disease.

Carve out time to enjoy life as a person, not just as a caregiver. See friends. Go for walks. Watch a movie. Get lunch and share freely. Laugh, cry, and connect. Don't wait for the "right time" to care for yourself. Use respite care when possible, and accept offers of help so you can truly step away, even for a little while.

I spend time on this point because the statistics are sobering. Caregivers for people with Alzheimer's report higher rates of depression than those caring for any other chronic illness; 30 to 40 percent experience depressive symptoms. Many report anxiety, poor sleep, and emotional exhaustion. In one national survey, 59 percent described their stress level as high or very high. Burnout doesn't just make you feel worse—it puts your health at risk, increasing chances of heart disease and even early death.

Earlier in the book, I used the airplane oxygen mask analogy. Put on your mask first, then help those around you. If you neglect your own needs, you'll be less able to care for your loved one. It is anything but selfish to care about your well-being. Prioritize your own health—address your medical conditions, move your body, eat nourishing food, stay connected to others, and find time to take a deep breath. This isn't indulgence. It's the foundation that allows you to keep showing up with strength, grace, and love. Most of all, this is what your loved one wants you to do. My patients tell me this all the time: More than anything—other than a cure—what they want is for the people they love to stay healthy.

8

“I’m Looking at the Future”

MY LIFE IN CLINICAL RESEARCH AND DAY-TO-DAY PATIENT CARE

Creating a New Purpose in Life • Surprising (and Easy) Ways to Volunteer • How to Find Close-to-Home Dementia Research Opportunities • What Is a Study Partner? • “We Need More Participation” • The Many Research Roles for Caregivers • Why Brain Autopsies Are Vital • Questions to Ask Before Participating in Research

I lead two professional lives. In one, I sit with patients and families, helping them navigate the uncharted terrain of memory loss. In the other, I help lead pioneering research at the Wisconsin Alzheimer’s Disease Research Center (ADRC). By advancing clinical trials and research into blood biomarkers and brain imaging, our program, alongside others, is moving us toward real treatments and possibly, one day, prevention.

These two roles don’t compete; they reinforce each other. Clinic visits shape the questions we ask in research, and discoveries from research inform how I care for patients. The connection is personal, too. I’ve watched my own parents move between the memory clinic and research programs—my father as a patient and participant, my mother as a caregiver and study partner.

If you’ve been diagnosed with mild cognitive impairment or Alzheimer's, you should strongly consider becoming a research volunteer. Taking part in clinical research has the power to change the trajectory of your health and belongs in your care plan. Many people do volunteer for research after a diagnosis, and, increasingly, individuals are enrolling while still cognitively healthy. Doing so opens the door to interventions and resources not yet available to the public.

I encourage everyone to get involved with Alzheimer's research: caregivers, individuals experiencing MCI or dementia, those worried about their memory, and those simply curious about how their brain works. The opportunities are nearly endless, and studies are easy to find online.

One of my tennis heroes, the great Arthur Ashe, said, "To achieve greatness, start where you are, use what you have, do what you can." That advice has guided me in my own life, and if you are considering becoming involved in Alzheimer's research, the most meaningful progress often begins with the small steps you're willing to take.

* * *

None of the progress we've made would have been possible without community participation. Participation means far more than only helping yourself. It benefits future generations. It advances our understanding of disease onset and progression, risk factors, and approaches to care. And it's not just about testing new drugs. Some studies focus on lifestyle, mood, family history, or long-term health. Some involve a simple blood draw or an online survey. Others require more time and commitment, but there truly is a study for everyone.

There's also something wonderful happening. I'm increasingly seeing the line blur between clinical trials and clinical care. Many participants first come through our research program as healthy volunteers. Over time, as subtle memory changes emerge, cognitive testing declines, or biomarker results shift, it's easy to pivot and schedule a clinic consultation. This two-way street between research and care was rare years ago. Now, it's becoming the norm—and a powerful tool in how we deliver personalized medicine.

This chapter is about why you—regardless of your age, background, diagnosis, or current level of concern—should consider participating in Alzheimer's or dementia-related research. It will help you understand who can take part, how to determine which studies make sense for you, what's involved, and what questions to ask before signing up. It's an invitation to be part of the solution. Research isn't just something scientists do. It's something we can all do together.

CASE STUDY: THE DANCING DATA SCIENTIST

One of my goals as a leader at the Wisconsin ADRC is to raise awareness about Alzheimer's. I travel around the state giving talks to audiences at women's clubs, Rotary meetings, senior centers, and other community gatherings. I tell listeners about our NIH-funded studies and share what we're learning from research. I offer tips on brain health and explain how everyday habits might stave off Alzheimer's and other types of dementia.

My outreach is part of the Wisconsin Idea, the university's philosophy that research should strive to solve problems for everyone in the Badger State. (We are tenacious here about everything from football to medicine!) This ethos was the brainchild of president of UW-Madison Charles Van Hise, who in 1904 said, "I shall never be content until the beneficent influence of the university reaches every family in the state."

The poignant story of Arlo and Beverly symbolizes how research, volunteerism, and philanthropy can unite to change lives. In 2021, I gave a talk in Milwaukee, and they were in the audience. Arlo had just retired at sixty-five after a career as a data scientist. Beverly was the same age and had taught in local public schools. They had been married for forty-one years and were inseparable. Their shared passion was ballroom dancing. The cha-cha, foxtrot, and waltz composed the rhythm of their social life. They tripped the light fantastic with such grace that they scored high in ballroom dance competitions.

My speech struck a chord, especially with Arlo. Since retiring, he had started to notice occasional memory slips, enough so that he had shared his concerns with Beverly. They were honest and open with each other, a hallmark of their long marriage. Arlo wondered if the changes, including missteps on the dance floor, were simply part of adjusting to life without work or something more concerning. His mother had died of Alzheimer's, and he understood his increased risk.

Their mutual anxiety had brought them to the community event where I spoke. I didn't meet them that evening, but what I said caught their attention. They began reading about Alzheimer's and listening to back episodes of my podcast, *Dementia Matters*, in which I interview leading experts from around the world. (Past episodes are archived with transcripts on UW's website.)

Six months later, Arlo's mental fogginess had not abated. "I felt like I was slipping a little bit on my intellectual dance floor," he told me. Beverly shared his worries, supporting him every step of the way. They knew they had to act and took the initiative to call my clinic. They requested the next available consultation with me. (This happens from time to time when listeners of the podcast reach out. It's always an interesting moment to meet someone who feels like they already know me from what I've said online.)

When they came in, Arlo completed our standard three-hour cognitive evaluation (as described in chapter 3). He and Beverly were good sports about the detailed interviews, cognitive testing, and waiting for our team to deliberate. Based on his cognitive scores and the team's clinical assessment, I diagnosed Arlo with mild cognitive impairment. At that time, in 2022, we didn't yet have easy access to Alzheimer's biomarker testing. I told Arlo I suspected Alzheimer's, though I acknowledged I couldn't be certain. Back then, the only ways to confirm the diagnosis were through a lumbar puncture, which was only done on rare occasions involving an atypical case, or a brain autopsy after death.

That was the reality of Alzheimer's care only a few years ago. I often felt envious of my colleagues in cardiology, oncology, and other specialties. They had concrete diagnostic tools such as X-rays, blood tests, CT scans, and even the humble stethoscope to guide their decisions. Meanwhile, neurologists and geriatricians like me still relied on observation, conversation, and basic cognitive testing—not so different from what doctors did a century ago. We listened, we watched, and we evaluated using our five senses, interpreting memory complaints, mood changes, and behavioral shifts with pen-and-paper tools and clinical judgment. Many of us yearned for a technological breakthrough, a tool that could help confirm what our instincts and training already suspected. Only recently have we begun to use diagnostic tools that put us on more equal footing with colleagues in other fields.

This is where my story about Arlo dovetails with Alzheimer's research. Because I work in clinical care and research, I explained to him that even though the amyloid biomarker test wasn't available in my clinic, it would be available through his participation in an ADRC research study. If Arlo volunteered, he could have an amyloid PET scan that would reveal with high certainty whether he had Alzheimer's.

Arlo had already been poring over the latest Alzheimer's news. He had begun to consider the research path after hearing my first presentation and was motivated to participate to find answers for himself and help others. Within days, Arlo signed up as a volunteer, changed his diet, and reformed bad sleep habits. In addition to my clinical judgment, he wanted proof he had amyloid in his brain. Moreover, he wanted the support and resources that he would get from being in a research program, particularly one focused on brain health.

Arlo soon went to the UW hospital for two days of testing. This consisted of giving an exhaustive medical history; submitting to lengthy cognitive testing, an MRI, and a PET scan; and having a lumbar puncture. (For a detailed description of what this latter test entails, see page 319.) Given his background in data science, he found the process intellectually engaging, even if it was tiring and mildly uncomfortable.

Six months later, I sat down with Arlo to share the results of his testing. (A cautionary word—not every research center discloses information to participants. This relatively new practice, called "returning results," is a trend in which medical researchers share test data with volunteers out of a sense of ethical duty to them. It is rooted in the idea that participants deserve to know what has been learned from their data.) It was now a year since he heard me speak in Milwaukee. Unfortunately, I had to tell Arlo the biomarker test revealed he did indeed have Alzheimer's.

It was hard news for Arlo, but the blow was cushioned because he had long suspected this outcome. I also shared information that heartened him. Because he had a clinical diagnosis and biomarker confirmation of Alzheimer's (technically the presence of the amyloid protein), he would likely qualify to receive the disease-modifying drug lecanemab as soon as it was approved by the FDA. A few months later, it was, and Arlo was among the first patients eligible for treatment.

Since then, Arlo has continued to return to Madison every year to repeat the two-day testing. He remains my clinic patient and an active research participant, receiving the most current, evidence-based care. He is fully integrated into both settings. That connection benefits him, supports my clinical decision-making, and contributes to the larger research effort. This is an ideal model of care—science and medicine inform one another in real time.

The only way we will stop this disease and continue to alleviate its effects is with the participation of concerned individuals like Arlo—people who seek answers early, ask questions, and choose to volunteer for the research process. Not only does their willingness drive discovery, it often gives them earlier insight into their own health and care options.

One last note about Arlo and Beverly: Their lifelong love of dancing may be helping them more than they realize. In a 2022 study of people at risk of dementia, one group walked on treadmills twice a week for ninety minutes, while another group attended ballroom dance classes for the same amount of time. Those in the dancing group performed better on memory and executive function tests and showed less hippocampal shrinkage. This is likely because dancing activates multiple brain systems at once, including spatial navigation (the ability to sense where your body is in space), balance, memory, coordination, and emotional expression. It also raises your heart rate, fosters social connection, and brings joy. It is a splendid activity for people with MCI and one of the best ways to support brain health and overall well-being.

Arlo and Beverly still dance. Their story continues—step by step.

MANY WAYS TO HELP: EXPLORING RESEARCH OPTIONS

A volunteer can take an array of paths in the world of Alzheimer's research. In the field of drug studies alone, as of 2025, 182 ongoing clinical trials assessed 138 Alzheimer's drugs that targeted 15 different mechanisms. More than 50,000 volunteers are needed to participate in the United States and around the world. Those numbers only include people enrolling in trials to test new medications—not the vast spectrum of studies on other aspects of dementia-related research.

Alzheimer's research is sometimes criticized for overemphasizing the amyloid theory. That might have once been the case, but it's not true now. As of 2025, only 23 percent of trials target amyloid directly. In contrast, 35 percent of Phase III studies (the final stage before FDA approval) home in on neurotransmitters like serotonin, choline, and dopamine. Another 10 percent explore inflammation, while other studies investigate the roles of metabolism and bioenergetics, tau, synaptic plasticity and neuroprotection, other protein issues, circadian rhythms, neurogenesis, growth factors, and hormones.

It's impossible for anyone to keep up with all this exploration, except on a superficial level. I scan multiple scholarly journals online every day, attend four or five conferences a year, work in a research center, and rub shoulders with top experts on my podcast—and even I can't keep up with everything in my field. It would take a superhuman effort to keep track of research in other areas of medicine while still seeing patients regularly. It's not unusual for well-informed patients and caregivers to tell me about new studies in another medical discipline that they think might benefit Alzheimer's research or themselves. More than once I've had to admit I hadn't yet heard of the study one of them was curious about.

So if you're considering volunteering, it's understandable if the options feel overwhelming. Your decision depends on what kind of commitment you want to make, what you're comfortable doing, and how much time you're able to give. While some studies last for years, others only take months to complete. Some are not invasive: They can be done entirely from home by filling out a yearly survey or mailing in a sample of your saliva or stool to help researchers study the gut microbiome.

Learn About Brain Research near You

If you're interested in exploring research opportunities related to cognition or brain health, visit ClinicalTrials.gov or Alzheimers.gov to browse hundreds of studies. You can search by location, disease type, stage, and method, that is, whether the study is interventional or observational.

You can also contact the Alzheimer's Disease Research Center (ADRC) nearest you at usaging.org/adrcs or explore information from the National Institute on Aging at nia.nih.gov.

The Alzheimer's Association offers a clinical trial locator. Enter your zip code to see what trials near you are enrolling volunteers.

Here is a rundown on the types of research open to volunteers:

Observational Studies: Arlo participated in this type of research. These studies monitor changes in cognition and biomarkers over time, with no treatment given. They often include individuals at risk of Alzheimer's as well as those already diagnosed with cognitive impairment. Researchers in this type of study cast a wide net—they also want to learn more about volunteers' genetic background, lifestyles, and what are called "social determinants of health," such as where they live, their exposure to pollution, income, level of education, and even access to healthcare.

Biomarker Studies: This research aims to discover and develop biomarker tests for conditions such as Lewy body disease, Parkinson's, frontotemporal dementia, vascular disease, and limbic-predominant age-related TDP-43 encephalopathy (LATE, which was only officially discovered in 2019). None of these diseases currently have FDA-approved biomarker tests. Alzheimer's is presently the only cognitive disease to have such a test. One promising biomarker study, called CLARiTI (ADRC Consortium for Clarity in ADRD Research Through Imaging), launched in 2024 at the Wisconsin ADRC and is enrolling two thousand participants. (For more on this study, see page 327.) Twenty-five percent of these individuals will come from historically underrepresented communities, and 60 percent will have cognitive impairment.

Interventional Trials: These often test experimental drugs, though some explore new uses for older, existing medications—an approach known as drug repurposing clinical trials. For example, trials are investigating whether metformin or semaglutide (a medication developed for diabetes and now used for weight loss) might reduce Alzheimer's disease risk. Most interventional trials use a randomized, double-blind, placebo-controlled design—some participants receive the drug, others a placebo, and neither the volunteers nor researchers know who is receiving which. (*Placebo* is a Latin word that means "I will please.") This approach minimizes unconscious bias and provides a rigorous way to evaluate whether the drug is truly effective. The goal is to determine whether a specific drug produces the benefits that researchers predicted, mainly by slowing decline, improving memory or mood, or supporting quality of life.

Not all interventional trials involve medication. One example is the U.S. POINTER study, which was recently conducted with the support of the Alzheimer's Association. U.S. POINTER stands for Protect Brain Health Through Lifestyle Intervention to Reduce Risk. Starting in 2023, this two-year trial enrolled twenty-one hundred cognitively unimpaired adults from a range of racial, ethnic, and socioeconomic backgrounds who are at risk of dementia because of their lifestyles. Participants were in their sixties and seventies and led sedentary lifestyles, had less-than-ideal diets, and did not exercise regularly. They were divided into two groups—one followed a self-guided program while the other entered a structured program. Both regimens focused on making changes in exercise, social and intellectual stimulation, and diet.

This study found that both interventions appeared to improve cognition. Participants in the structured group showed more improvement compared to the self-guided group. The results on cognitive tests—for both groups—were similar to those of people who were one to two years younger. The bottom line is that if you improve your lifestyle, you can have some control over the possible trajectory of mental decline.

The scope of interventional trials currently enrolling participants is striking. Researchers are exploring dietary strategies like fasting and ketogenic diets, as well as brain-focused treatments involving electrical and magnetic stimulation, infrared light, and focused ultrasound. Others are testing the effects of supplements such as citicoline and mitocholine and evaluating how tai chi, dance, and music therapies might support people with mild cognitive impairment. Some trials are investigating the potential of psilocybin and CBD.

Others are delving into gene therapy. This approach repairs or replaces faulty genes and is already being used to treat cancer, hemophilia, and sickle cell disease. One active trial is examining whether introducing a gene that produces BDNF—a protein that fosters the growth of new neurons—into spinal fluid can slow neuronal loss and promote regeneration. If effective, this strategy could reshape brain architecture and help restore memory in people living with Alzheimer's.

Looking ahead, I'm particularly excited about the rise of multimodal interventional trials—those designed to address multiple biological pathways that contribute to disease, brain cell death, or cognitive decline. Rather than focusing on a single target, these studies combine medications with lifestyle-based strategies, such as exercise, diet, sleep, and stress reduction, while simultaneously testing drugs that act on amyloid, tau, inflammation, insulin signaling, and neuronal resilience. I would also like to see more research specifically focused on APOE4 carriers, who face the greatest genetic risk for Alzheimer's. These comprehensive approaches hold the most promise for truly changing the trajectory of the disease.

Exploratory Studies: This research asks novel, sometimes unconventional, questions. Such topics have yet to be studied in depth, and these trials are usually smaller in scale. One current study is investigating if the microbiome in a person's digestive tract can influence the development of

Alzheimer's. Another is pursuing a link between a person's consumption of ultra-processed foods and cognitive decline.

Digital Reserve: Rethinking Technology's Role in Brain Health

In an age where smartphones, apps, and AI assistants permeate daily life, questions abound: Is this digital overload impairing our minds? Are we forgetting how to remember?

Clinical neuropsychologist Dr. Jared Benge wants to debunk the doom-and-gloom narrative surrounding technology and brain health. His research has revealed a surprising trend.

Older adults who use technology tend to have better cognitive outcomes than those who don't, according to Benge, who teaches at Dell Medical School in Austin, Texas, and practices at UT Health Austin's Comprehensive Memory Center. While correlation doesn't equal causation, he believes there's more to the story than coincidence.

Benge explained his findings to me on my podcast, *Dementia Matters*. His "technological reserve" hypothesis builds on the well-established concept of *cognitive reserve*—the brain's ability to function despite age-related or disease-related changes. This new framework explores how engagement with digital tools may offer similar protective benefits. He breaks it down into three Cs: complexity, connection, and compensation.

- *Complexity* reflects the cognitive stimulation required to use modern devices. Navigating smartphone updates, pop-up ads, or evolving interfaces isn't always seamless, especially for older adults. Yet this mental effort—akin to doing a puzzle in an unpredictable environment—may keep the brain sharp.
- *Connection* speaks to the social dimension of tech. While digital interactions aren't perfect substitutes for in-person con-

tact, Benge contends they're far better than isolation. A simple text thread, social media update, or video call can counteract loneliness—a well-known risk factor for cognitive decline.

- *Compensation* refers to the way technology helps people manage memory challenges. From alarms and calendars to GPS and auto-pay, digital tools offload cognitive tasks. That helps people preserve their energy and independence. Benge likens it to a "trusted system" that enables users to focus on what truly matters.

Benge is quick to clarify that this isn't about over-relying on apps or replacing clinical care. Rather, it's about creating adaptive, digital environments that flex to users' needs and cognitive abilities. From biometric log-ins to AI-powered reminders, the goal is to make the digital world more accessible—and protective—for those facing cognitive challenges.

He sees technology not as a threat to cognition but as a tool—one that can be designed, studied, and personalized to support brain health. Importantly, Benge isn't claiming technology is a cure-all. In fact, he cautions against overuse or assuming tech use *causes* cognitive improvement. His findings reflect bidirectional relationships—just as walking supports brain health but also declines as cognition fades, technology may both influence and reflect our cognitive state.

In short, it's not about fearing the smartphone. It's about harnessing its power to help our minds thrive. "We built this digital world," Benge says. "Let's build it better."

Diagnostic Studies: These evaluate the effectiveness of tools that assess cognition and brain health. Current work in this field includes the development of new cognitive tests, particularly digital tests for smartphones to replace traditional pencil-and-paper tests. Other researchers are creating wearable technology that could precisely measure how well patients are sleeping or how physically active they are.

Cognitive Testing—There's an App for That

Remote cognitive assessments via smartphone apps are not only feasible, they're increasingly reliable. So says Dr. Lindsay Clark, a neuropsychologist and researcher at the University of Wisconsin. She and Dr. David Berron at the German Center for Neurodegenerative Diseases validated an app that delivers visual memory tests in real-world settings. Their findings showed strong alignment with gold-standard in-office clinical assessments.

Unlike traditional neuropsychological tests, which offer only a snapshot of performance, this approach captures cognition over time and in the user's natural environment. "It's about ecological validity," explains Clark. "We're not just testing what someone can do under observation—we're seeing how their brain works in daily life."

The bottom line? They concluded that digital tools used by unsupervised patients can meaningfully detect cognitive impairment. Their app not only correlates well with in-clinic testing but may also identify individuals experiencing early signs of decline—an important breakthrough for clinical trials and intervention research.

"People can take these tests at home over time and without the white-coat pressure of a clinic," says Clark. "They may provide more accurate and representative views of how someone's memory is functioning day to day."

In the future, subtle changes in how a person uses a phone or laptop—like slower typing or errors in online purchases—might serve as early warning signs of cognitive decline. Such digital inefficiencies, dubbed "digital dyspraxia," may complement formal testing in identifying memory changes before they become obvious. In much the same way that word clouds and internet search data can reveal where contagious diseases are spreading before official case counts rise, these everyday digital patterns could alert us to cognitive shifts well before symptoms become undeniable.

Of course, challenges remain. From digital access disparities to environmental distractions and potential "cheating," remote assessments require thoughtful design. But the benefits—accessibility, lower costs, and the ability to reach underserved populations—make the effort worthwhile.

"One of the greatest potentials is to expand who gets tested," Clark notes. "We can bring cognitive health tools into people's homes, particularly in communities that have historically lacked access to specialized care."

Berron agrees and envisions a future where cognitive health is managed like diabetes: regular self-monitoring via digital tools, coupled with periodic expert evaluation. "We're moving toward a model of continuous cognitive care, not just crisis intervention," he says.

---

* * *

Careful screening is part of every study to ensure researchers are enrolling the right participants. Arguably, many earlier Alzheimer's trials failed because researchers weren't studying people with Alzheimer's disease. It's possible, and likely, they were instead enrolling participants with memory loss due to other causes. After all, memory loss is a symptom of many brain diseases, not just Alzheimer's. Without a biomarker to prove the presence of amyloid, scientists had no way of knowing exactly what was happening in volunteers' brains. Today, that has changed. Volunteers can now be screened for amyloid and in some cases tau before joining a trial. Research can only go as far as the tools allow. You can't study what you can't see, and you can't solve what you haven't learned how to measure.

Regardless of the study, all volunteers go through a screening process to determine eligibility. Some trials require specific age groups, cognitive levels, medical histories, or genetic risk factors. You may be asked to complete cognitive tests, provide medical records, or share information about your medications and family health history.

There are also research opportunities for Alzheimer's caregivers. Such studies aim to deepen our understanding of the caregiver experience and identify ways to improve the quality of care for the person with impairment and the overall well-being of both individuals. (For more on caregiver research, see page 336.)

It's important to remember two aspects of taking part in a study. First, researchers do not provide medical care or treatment during studies, though they may refer you to appropriate clinical providers. Second, your research data is confidential. Outside of standard clinical tests and newly emerging acute findings, the information doesn't go into your medical record or to your insurance company. But it is your data. If you choose to share it with your doctor, you can.

OBSERVATIONAL RESEARCH—WHAT A VOLUNTEER DOES

In chapter 3, I wrote at length about the multihour visit a patient and their loved ones experience when a doctor like me makes an Alzheimer's diagnosis. Taking part in some types of Alzheimer's research can require an even more extensive visit—one that is exhaustive in its medical scope and can be draining for many people.

I want to walk you through what it's like to participate in an observational research study, one designed to collect medical information. (This is different from a drug trial, which administers treatment.) A perfect example is the Wisconsin Registry for Alzheimer's Prevention study, known as WRAP. I may be biased, as I'm one of its principal investigators, but WRAP is among the most important long-term studies of individuals at risk for Alzheimer's disease. Healthy volunteers visit once every few years for testing. No interventions are given, but their results are analyzed in the search for future Alzheimer's diagnostic tools and treatments.

Even when motivated by altruism, many volunteers, understandably, still find research visits stressful. Most Alzheimer's research takes place in hospitals, where the necessary equipment like MRI and PET scan machines is located. In addition, these studies often involve clinical procedures such as lumbar punctures, blood draws, and extensive neurological testing. At my hospital, a volunteer's visit is spread over two days, In other places, everything might happen in a day. In Madison, the first day lasts four to six hours and consists mostly of answering questions; the second day is devoted to imaging and the lumbar puncture.

In the memory clinic visit, a patient might be accompanied by multiple family members hoping to offer input leading to a diagnosis. For research visits, only the volunteer's study partner, typically a spouse or child, attends. (For more on the study partner's role, see page 332.)

On the first day, a research coordinator greets the volunteer and her partner and then chaperones them to the hospital's clinical research unit. A team of nurses checks her height, weight, waist circumference, and vital signs. Then comes the taking of blood samples—between ten and twenty vials. (This may sound like a lot, but it amounts to only three to five tablespoons.) More blood is drawn than at a typical annual checkup because it will be analyzed in far more ways.

One of the most important uses of a volunteer's blood is the development of blood biomarker tests for cognitive diseases. Currently there are still no blood tests for frontotemporal disease, Lewy body disease, Parkinson's disease, cerebral vascular disease, or TDP-43. The same was true for Alzheimer's disease until 2025, when the FDA approved the first blood-based biomarker test for amyloid confirmation. Remarkably, up to 40 percent of the data used in that landmark approval came from WRAP and the Wisconsin ADRC.

Since volunteers fast before their blood is drawn, they're treated to a well-deserved breakfast afterward. Then a study coordinator or clinician begins a long question-and-answer session in a setting similar to an exam room. The questions start with basic demographics—race, sex, gender, primary language, and education. They continue with topics such as marital status, number of children, zip code, type of housing, and military service. The coordinator also asks how the volunteers perceive their memory compared to years past, whether they own a car, how financially secure they feel, whether they feel supported or isolated, and how often they seek medical care. Additional sensitive questions explore experiences of discrimination and other societal stressors. Medical history is then reviewed in detail. This includes past and present health problems, current medications, history of substance use, cardiovascular and neurological diseases, thyroid issues, vitamin deficiencies, sleep apnea, mental health history, and (for women) menstrual history. After this comes a neurological exam to investigate for signs of Parkinson's disease and a clinician's assessment of mood, behavior, and daily functioning ability.

Then comes the cognitive testing. Unlike the version used in clinic settings, which may take forty-five minutes, this version can last up to three hours. These tests probe every domain of cognitive function—reasoning, memory, spatial and verbal abilities, pattern recognition, and visual processing. Many of these tests are the same as the ones administered in my clinic. The extended time, however, is necessary for two reasons. First, more tests are included. Second, each cognitive domain is examined more exhaustively. If you've ever had a hearing test, you know that the clinician administering the exam will send super-quiet sounds to your headphones beyond your hearing abilities simply to confirm the limit of your hearing range. Cognitive testing in research works the same way. Volunteers continue answering questions until they reach their point of failure, which doesn't happen in the clinic. This level of detail helps researchers distinguish between normal and abnormal aging and allows us to track changes over time. Interestingly, many volunteers tell me they prefer the lumbar puncture to the cognitive testing. The testing feels endless and demanding, and many research centers don't even provide feedback on how well a person performed (though some do).

At some point in the day, volunteers also complete questionnaires about their diet, exercise, sleep, and mental activity. Another form assesses apathy and stressful life events. These are unique to our program because of the interests of our scientists, although other programs may ask similar questions. Meanwhile, the study partner is asked about changes he's observed in the volunteer's memory, daily functioning, mood, and behavior compared to years ago.

The second day's visit can be shorter but may still last up to six hours. As with the cognitive tests and blood samples, the MRI and PET scan imaging takes longer than in clinical care. If an emergency department patient has an MRI to evaluate dizziness or a headache, the scan might take thirty to forty-five minutes. In research, the scanning lasts an hour or longer. A clinical PET scan may take the same amount of time, but in research we usually do two or more scans. That's because researchers are looking at and evaluating things like synapse density or specific proteins rather than a patient's current symptoms. While researchers have different goals than a doctor in a hospital or clinic, the volunteer/patient experience of the MRI or PET scan is similar. Their involvement is passive—they lie down and listen to music while the machine buzzes, clicks, and whirs. At UW, volunteers also have the option of listening to episodes of *Dementia Matters*. It's not Bach, but it is an option.

Last but not least comes the lumbar puncture. During this procedure, vials of spinal fluid are drawn, similar to how blood samples are taken. Because this is a sterile procedure, the setup takes ten to fifteen minutes, during which time the volunteer would be sitting on an exam table in a gown. For the brief procedure itself, the volunteer would lean forward—doing so makes the insertion site of the needle more accessible. An injection of lidocaine numbs the area, and the lumbar puncture begins. A thin spinal needle is then inserted, angled carefully so its tip slides between vertebrae and passes through the soft tissues into the subarachnoid space, where cerebrospinal fluid circulates. Once in place, the clear fluid—often described by clinicians as "champagne," a lighthearted tribute to a job well done—is slowly withdrawn or allowed to flow naturally into a collection tube.

The entire process typically takes just a few minutes. Despite the fears many have, it's not painful. The pain-numbing injection causes a sting, like a novocaine shot at a dentist's office, and that's the worst of it. Most people feel little or nothing after the initial pinch. In fact, the clinicians performing this procedure do this routinely. They are well trained and credentialed by the healthcare institution. Like a phlebotomist (a person who draws blood), their experience goes a long way to greatly minimize any discomfort.

A common misconception is that lumbar punctures can cause paralysis. This is not true. In fact, it's nearly impossible when following the standardized protocol. The "tap" or insertion of the needle happens near the base of the spinal column. The spinal cord, which transmits nerve impulses from the body to the brain, ends about five inches above where the needle is inserted. While the needle might briefly touch a descending nerve and cause a brief "electric" tingling sensation, there is almost no chance of paralysis or nerve damage. Afterward, volunteers lie down for thirty minutes to reduce the chance of a headache.

One woman I met, an African American office manager in her late sixties, had first come to our memory clinic because of concerns about forgetfulness. After her evaluation, she expressed a strong desire to contribute to research—not only to better understand her own symptoms but because she felt it was important for more African Americans to be represented in science. "There just aren't enough of us in these studies," she told me. "I want to change that." She enrolled in an observational study at the ADRC and completed a full research visit.

What surprised her most wasn't the scan or the blood tests—it was how much information she received about brain health. "I thought I knew a lot from coming to clinic," she said, "but the research staff gave me even more—conversations about blood pressure, stress, sleep, and the role of healthy eating. They explained things I didn't even know to ask about." When she returned to my memory clinic for a follow-up, she brought her PET scan results with her. The scan showed no signs of amyloid. She didn't have Alzheimer's disease—her symptoms were due to cerebral vascular disease. She hadn't come back looking for a new drug but rather for guidance on how to reduce her vascular risk factors. She left feeling more empowered and grateful to be part of a research movement working to improve lives.

Though the research visit demands time and the generous contribution of one's body, its impact reaches far beyond a single day, powering discoveries that will change how we understand and treat Alzheimer's. The extensive nature of the testing reminds me of the arduous tests NASA required of Mercury program astronaut candidates in the early 1960s. Alzheimer's volunteers aren't going into orbit, but I hope their generosity will take our understanding of the disease where no one has gone before.

WHAT IT'S LIKE TO BE IN A DRUG TRIAL

Clinical trials are not casual undertakings. They are serious, demanding, and highly structured. People interested in participating should do so only after thoughtful consideration. These trials are not like routine medical care or observational studies; they involve risks, close monitoring, frequent appointments, and a significant time commitment. Yet they also offer the possibility of meaningful improvement—slowing disease, halting progression, relieving symptoms, or enhancing quality of life. Because there is a possibility of real benefit, trials often carry a deeper sense of hope.

At the same time, trust must be earned. Doctors and researchers go to great lengths to protect trial participants. This hasn't always been the case. The Tuskegee study, which ran from 1932 to 1972, deliberately misled Black men with untreated syphilis, denying them information and withholding penicillin once it became available. The memory of that study—and others like it—still casts a long shadow. In response to the injustices, the U.S. government and medical institutions established strict safeguards, institutional review boards, and oversight mechanisms to protect every participant and prevent such abuses from ever happening again.

Clinical trials are also very specific. To be scientifically valid, they must control as many variables as possible. Not everyone is eligible, and, in fact, most people aren't. For example, someone who has already been treated with anti-amyloid monoclonal therapy might be excluded from studies focused on amyloid. They could, however, be eligible for trials targeting tau. Even lifestyle intervention studies have strict criteria. Researchers have to be particular. They must not unfairly exclude some people. At the same time, they need to ensure their results are accurate and meaningful, even if that limits the generalizability of the study's findings. The success of a clinical trial depends on its precision.

Dr. Cynthia Carlsson, who leads the clinical trials program at the University of Wisconsin, has spent much of her career making these studies safer, more inclusive, and more accessible. She served as the site principal investigator for the landmark A4 and AHEAD prevention trials, which studied whether Alzheimer's could be slowed—or even prevented—by starting treatment before symptoms appear. As she often says, "We have to be precise. The best results come from carefully designed studies that prioritize both scientific rigor and participant safety. That's how we move the field forward. That's how we get approved new treatments for our patients."

One man came to see me in clinic because his friend had participated in Alzheimer's research. Through that experience, he had learned what to look for when it came to cognitive changes—symptoms like word-finding difficulties and increasing trouble recalling the names of his neighbors. He noticed those signs in himself. Although he had no prior diagnosis and hadn't planned on seeking one, the education and exposure he received through his friend's involvement helped him recognize something wasn't right.

He scheduled an evaluation, and after a thorough assessment, I diagnosed him with mild cognitive impairment due to Alzheimer's disease. The news was hard to hear, but we had caught it incredibly early. Because he had already learned about research from the inside, he was ready. I immediately connected him with the clinical trials coordinator, and he was able to enroll in a trial shortly thereafter—having already completed much of the enrollment process during his clinic visit.

Drug trials resemble clinical research on steroids. Because the FDA is involved, the oversight is even more intense. There are more rules to follow and hoops to jump through. Every drug trial has a data-monitoring safety board as well as groups of overseers who check that everyone is following the rules in the most precise ways possible. Clinicians observe participants for adverse events and monitor every aspect of the trial. This level of oversight protects participants. It also explains why drug trials are expensive and time-consuming.

Your doctor, whether he is a geriatrician or neurologist, would rarely be the one running the trial. He might let you know about studies and offer basic information, but your enrollment and participation would be handled directly by the research team. If you meet the eligibility criteria and proceed, you would be thoroughly screened, required to give your informed consent, and then randomly assigned to receive either the active drug or a placebo. Usually no one, including the researchers, knows who gets what.

Participation involves more than taking a pill and attending frequent follow-ups afterward for side effects and progression of symptoms. It can mean regular cognitive assessments, blood draws, MRIs, PET scans, or lumbar punctures. Some drugs are taken by mouth or via a patch, but others are injected into the spinal fluid or infused into the bloodstream—procedures that require time, patience, and physical resilience.

Is it dangerous to take drugs that have yet to be approved by the FDA? That is the first question potential volunteers ask. Next on their minds is *What are the side effects?* The answer is that nearly all drugs go through animal testing first. If no dangerous side effects are observed, such drugs enter Phase I testing with a small group of healthy volunteers. If that phase goes well, Phase II trials follow with a few hundred volunteers to determine the correct dosage and gather early data on the drug's effectiveness. People may or may not see positive results at this point. Finally, Phase III testing involves thousands of people at many top medical centers around the world. It produces the evidence the FDA uses to determine drug approval for healthcare. I only wish the same level of rigor was applied to dietary supplements, which are not FDA approved yet remain widely available and commonly used by the public.

As with any treatment, there are risks. Common side effects may include nausea, stomach upset, and headaches. A rash, which happened to my father, can sometimes be a side effect. These same side effects often occur with prescription medications or over-the-counter supplements. Because dementia drugs target the brain, effects such as confusion, headaches, and changes in vision can occur.

In addition to the side effects of the medication, drug trials require the participant to make repeated trips to the hospital or clinic to have blood drawn and possibly be required to undergo a lumbar puncture or brain imaging. Some Alzheimer's drugs now being tested would be delivered by subcutaneous injection the same way diabetics self-administer insulin. Being in this type of trial would require injections, which could lead to pain, infection, and swelling at the injection site.

Before enrolling in a clinical trial, you and your supporters should get answers to all your questions. Participating in a drug trial is a serious commitment, and you deserve to feel confident and informed about your decision. The research team should explain the study's goals—what outcome they're hoping for and how the drug might help achieve it. They should walk you through the risks, the design of the study, how the drug works, how long the trial will last, and how often you'll be asked to return for follow-ups. You should know what procedures are involved and whether you'll learn the results of those tests. They should also tell you if you'll be compensated and whether you need a study partner. No one expects you to make this decision blindly or to rush into it. Good research teams will welcome your questions.

Questions to Ask Before Volunteering

Before joining a research study, ask questions so you can feel confident about your decision. Here are some to consider:

What are the goals of the study?
Have similar studies been done? What were their outcomes?
What steps will be taken to protect my health and safety?
How will my information be safeguarded?
What are possible side effects and risks?
How long will the study last? What will be required of me, and where will I need to go?
Will I learn more about my overall health and brain health?
Will you share my research results with me?
Will the study provide information about reducing my risk factors?
What happens if I leave the study early?
Will I (or my study partner) be compensated or reimbursed for my time and travel expenses?
Can I continue to take my regular medications during the study?

What happens if a new drug becomes FDA approved during the study?
Will I learn any of the study's findings?
If I'm assigned to the placebo group and the treatment proves beneficial, will I have a chance to take the drug later? (To phrase this in medical terms, ask if there is an open-label extension period.)

It's also important to know that not all clinical trials are the same. Some are brief, lasting just a few months, while others extend over several years. Some may involve complex drug infusions or invasive procedures, while others are far less demanding, such as taking a pill once a month and checking in periodically. The level of commitment varies, and it's worth finding a study that fits not only your medical profile but also your comfort level.

There's something else you should ask about—a promising development in trial design called an open-label extension. Traditionally, participants never found out whether they received the drug or a placebo. Now, in some trials, if the drug shows signs of benefit, all participants are offered the opportunity to receive it after the study ends—this time knowingly. To me, that feels ethically right. Volunteers contribute so much of themselves to the research process. If the results look promising, it's only fair that they get early access to a treatment they helped make possible.

Finally, there's also an intangible but powerful benefit: human connection. Research volunteers often spend more time with study staff and clinicians than they ever would with their regular doctors. They are monitored closely, given time to ask questions, and often feel they are part of a mission larger than themselves.

FOR PATIENTS—"A SENSE OF PURPOSE AND CONTROL"

I think of research participants as explorers, especially volunteers who are patients. They are the heroes who break ground where others have not yet gone. Volunteering gives a patient a revived sense of purpose in life. It allows them to play a more active role in their care at a time when so much can feel out of their control. Involvement in research often opens doors to people, conversations, and knowledge that can give a sense of what might lie ahead. Many patients describe feeling more engaged, hopeful, and connected.

That desire to give of oneself, especially when facing a diagnosis like Alzheimer's, can be a powerful motivator. It doesn't erase fear, but it can lessen anxiety. A patient might think to himself, *I'm not only enduring a disease, I'm contributing to its solution.*

When I think about Alzheimer's research, my father naturally comes to mind. He was, in his own quiet way, gung ho about joining research, committed and deliberate. Like many of my patients and their families, he gave of himself selflessly. Taking part enabled him to play a more active role in his own care and gave him hope that his involvement might slow the course of his disease. Volunteering felt meaningful because he knew that, thanks to his efforts, current and future patients might benefit.

He enrolled in two different types of research. One was the Alzheimer's Disease Neuroimaging Initiative (ADNI), a long-running study designed to improve how we understand and diagnose Alzheimer's. It didn't offer him a treatment, but it gave him a role to play in the scientific process—submitting to scans, blood draws, and tests over many months. This was his contribution to the movement that will one day lead to a cure or prevention, not for him but hopefully for his children and grandchildren. That gave him a sense of power and control, which disease so often takes away.

He also joined a pharmaceutical trial. As a retired physician, he understood the possibility of being, in medical lingo, "randomized to a placebo," an outcome no one wants but everyone accepts as necessary. Of course, my father hoped to be placed in the treatment group and, like anyone else, wanted the trial to succeed and bring real benefit. He focused on what could be gained. He took the risks in stride. What mattered most to him was taking action and being part of an intervention rather than a bystander to his own decline.

When I share a diagnosis with patients and loved ones, I always bring up the idea of research participation. It's not the first step in the care plan, but it is always on my agenda. Being an explorer isn't for everyone, and that's okay. Some people simply aren't ready; the weight of the diagnosis and maze of treatment decisions can be overwhelming. Others may not have the bandwidth, cognitive ability, resources, or capability of reaching the study site. But I believe everyone, no matter where they live, deserves the opportunity to participate. Offering research as an option is one way I show patients we're not giving up.

Introducing the idea of research in the same conversation as delivering a diagnosis is delicate. I never want to minimize the grief that comes with this news. But I also want patients to know we're in a different era—one of accelerating progress. What their parents or grandparents experienced with the disease is not necessarily what lies ahead for them. In my experience, talking about clinical trials brings relief. It gives people direction and offers a way to act and take control at a time when everything feels like it's being done to them.

Instead of patients leaving my clinic thinking, *Woe is me*, I have planted the seed of *Maybe I can help myself and someone else in this process.* They begin to understand they're part of the movement to overcome the disease. They're not helpless or powerless. They're needed. While I usually avoid military metaphors, in this case it feels right: They are the front line in the fight against Alzheimer's, and we're fighting with them.

BRINGING CLARITI—THE BIOMARKER REVOLUTION

One of the most exciting areas of dementia research is the development of new blood tests that detect the presence of Alzheimer's and other neurodegenerative diseases. Blood tests are, of course, nothing new. For decades, doctors have used them to monitor general health and diagnose conditions like dyslipidemia (high cholesterol) and hypothyroidism. But in neuroscience, we are only beginning to realize their full potential.

Thanks to advances in artificial intelligence, genetics, and molecular imaging, researchers and biotech companies are rolling out new generations of blood biomarker tests that promise to revolutionize how we detect and treat disease. For example, such a test is already available for colorectal cancer. Considering that 40 percent of adults shy away from colonoscopies, this simple, far less invasive test will diagnose far more cases before they reach a life-threatening point. Another new blood test can sniff out up to fifty different types of cancer, many of which had no previous early detection methods. Researchers are developing similar biomarker tools for autoimmune diseases such as lupus.

The same amazing developments are happening in Alzheimer's research. The first-ever blood test for amyloid, which the FDA approved in 2025, has an accuracy rate of about 92 percent. It is now recommended for people exhibiting signs of cognitive impairment and is used to confirm a suspected diagnosis based on a doctor's exam. Still, this is not a screening test for the general public—doctors like me generally advise against taking it without a clinical exam to put the results in proper context.

What is truly extraordinary is how far back this test can see. It can identify traces of amyloid in the blood *twenty years* before a person develops symptoms or shows cognitive impairment. One can easily imagine a future in which a forty-five-year-old receives a simple blood test during a routine checkup and learns they are at risk. If the amyloid is detected, the doctor might prescribe a drug—perhaps one not yet invented—to prevent further accumulation or even to dissolve what's already there. But even without medication, doctors and patients can begin early targeted risk-reducing interventions through lifestyle changes like exercise, diet, and restorative sleep. In a field of progressive, currently incurable diseases, lowering the risk or delaying the onset of Alzheimer's dementia is a meaningful win. This is the promise of personalized medicine, and it begins with biomarkers.

We also now know that Alzheimer's rarely acts alone. Most patients have "mixed dementia," meaning more than one type of brain pathology is present. That's why researchers are expanding biomarker development to include other neurodegenerative diseases such as Lewy body, frontotemporal, cerebrovascular, and LATE. Doctors want to know what brain diseases are active in a person and in what proportion to understand the root cause of symptoms and tailor treatment plans with precision. This requires identifying each disease's signature reliably, and biomarkers—

especially ones accessible through blood, spinal fluid, or imaging—make this possible.

One of the most important ongoing contributions to this effort is the WRAP study. Led by Dr. Sterling Johnson, it has shifted our understanding of when Alzheimer's begins—long before memory loss—and how we might detect and track it. The thousands of blood samples, imaging scans, cognitive test results, and lifestyle data collected through WRAP have helped make discoveries like the blood amyloid test possible. The study is expanding its focus to understand what factors in life might lead to elevated amyloid and tau, what interventions—lifestyle and medication—may meaningfully impact those proteins and eventual symptoms, and what other diseases may be contributing to the illness. Biomarkers open the door to disease understanding and intervention. While they are not treatments themselves, they are the step that leads to treatments.

Dr. Johnson is co-leading a new chapter in biomarker research through a major NIH-funded initiative called CLARiTI—short for ADRC Consortium for Clarity in ADRD Research Through Imaging. This project unites all thirty-six Alzheimer's Disease Research Centers (ADRCs) across the country in a collaborative effort to advance our understanding of Alzheimer's and related dementias. The goal is not simply to improve one test or measure, but to develop a comprehensive and reliable set of biomarkers that can detect multiple forms of dementia.

What makes CLARiTI especially significant is its scale and scientific scope. It will analyze PET scans, MRI scans, and blood samples and link them with comprehensive participant data from a subset of seventeen thousand diverse participants, many of whom have contributed to research for decades.

The CLARiTI study builds on the long-standing research infrastructure of the national ADRC network. It's a testament to what happens when researchers, clinicians, and participants come together with a shared mission. These NIH-funded centers are more than academic enclaves—they are engines of collaboration, designed to connect and amplify scientific discovery. Through CLARiTI, the strength of this network is being fully leveraged to refine tools that clinicians need to detect brain disease early, accurately, and affordably—ideally in your local healthcare setting.

This work will also help uncover the mechanisms—such as inflammation, insulin resistance in the brain, and oxidative stress—that drive Alzheimer's and related diseases. Future blood tests will likely tell us whether amyloid or tau is present and help determine why it is there. With research efforts like WRAP, CLARiTI, and the ADRC network, we are rapidly moving closer to a time when an Alzheimer's diagnosis may be no more daunting than managing high blood pressure—identified early, treated precisely, and kept under control.

TRY IT. YOU'LL LIKE IT.

Back in the day, people must have had a lot more indigestion. Brands like Alka-Seltzer ran TV ads night and day promoting their soothing stomach antacids. One commercial showed a businessman in a restaurant bemoaning his foolish decision to take a waiter's advice, a mistake that resulted in an undigested meal. As the ad ends, he sips bubbly Alka-Seltzer. It works, and he tells viewers, "Try it. You'll like it."

The ad was catchy because it captured a common occurrence: skepticism turning into surprise satisfaction. That's often how it goes with research volunteers. The overwhelming majority of volunteers at my Wisconsin research program are enrolled in multiple studies. Some participate in five, six, or even seven. Not every study is intense. Some involve little more than filling out a survey or mailing in a stool sample. But often what starts as simple participation evolves into a deeply meaningful experience. For many, research becomes its own personal journey.

Among the many remarkable volunteers I've met through research, Sara stands out not only for her dedication but also for the friendship that's grown between us. Her mother had Alzheimer's, and she was deeply motivated to do what she could to reduce her own risk. She started by participating in our ADRC observational long-term study. At first, it was straightforward. She came in every other year for two days of assessment. She was healthy, but not obsessively so. She only wanted to make smart choices for her future.

Then she signed up for an additional study, one that became a turning point for her. This twelve-week clinical trial, called BFIT (blood flow improvement trial), focused on metabolic health and lifestyle interventions. The study tested whether improvements in diet and exercise could enhance brain blood flow and boost cognitive performance.

The health-conscious Sara already taught yoga and dove into the program's low-carb diet and structured exercise routine. The study required multiple brain scans, blood tests, and regular educational support from clinicians and coordinators. She loved it.

Learning more about her body sparked her interest in how her brain responded to change, how the results of her blood tests shifted over time, and how different foods and habits made her feel. She felt healthier, lighter, and more energetic. She began sleeping better. She lowered her blood sugar and cholesterol and became mentally sharper and physically vibrant. She became, in her words, "obsessed in a good way" with food, movement, brain health, and aging well.

Sara became close with the study team and stayed connected long after the trial ended. Out of gratitude for what the BFIT study gave her, she made a modest donation to the lead researcher to fund a small pilot study to explore the gut microbiome and brain health. That sparked a series of events that led to a multimillion-dollar NIH study to investigate the connection between the gut microbiome and Alzheimer's. (Dr. Barbara Bendlin is the principal investigator behind BFIT. She is one of the leading figures in gut-brain research and is one of my colleagues at the Wisconsin ADRC.)

Sara gave more than money. She gave time, energy, and her heart. She joined the Initiative to End Alzheimer's philanthropy board to raise awareness and support for the program. Our relationship has outgrown the boundaries of a clinical trial. We're connected by a shared belief in the power of research and the idea that prevention doesn't have to be passive, it can be an enjoyable way of life.

Participating in research does more than help science, it can change lives. Sara's quest invigorated and empowered her, and her gratitude has brought new energy, new people, and new opportunities to our program.

You could be the next Sara. Your participation could launch a healthier path for yourself. You could inspire others to follow your lead. Try it. You'll like it.

THE STUDY PARTNER: A VITAL ROLE

Many Alzheimer's and related dementia studies involve individuals with some stage of cognitive impairment. As a result, they typically require the participant to have a study partner, someone who knows the participant well, such as a close friend or family member. They will go with the participant to appointments and are familiar with their memory, behavior, daily functioning, and history.

As a study partner in a clinical trial, you ride the emotional waves together. You worry about the risks of the drug being tested, of passing up the opportunity, and of choosing the wrong one. Your mind may constantly play *what-if* games. While your loved one faces the terrifying prospect of losing memory and experiencing drug side effects, you carry a different weight. Study partners hold their breath hoping their loved one will be selected for the "real treatment" group and pray that the treatment will make a meaningful difference in disease progression. They contend with doubt that their time, energy, and trust will be worth the investment. The hope is real, but so is the fear that their loved one's efforts might be for naught.

A study partner's role isn't passive. You are not simply along for the ride. You are an essential member of the research team. Participating in a similar way that you would in a memory clinic evaluation, you'll be interviewed at length and asked to report on your loved one's abilities. Your insights, particularly into the person's daily functional changes, could influence whether she qualifies for future interventions and how the medical team judges what stage of the disease she is in. Being a study partner can also offer an opportunity to share sensitive information that helps your loved one. You may be the first to gently raise concerns that the participant is not ready or able to discuss: changes in mood, judgment, or daily functioning with safety risks like driving, handling firearms, or operating heavy machinery. Your honesty with the research team can lead to conversations that protect your loved one and others.

In some cases, study partners confide things they've kept secret for years. They don't want to betray the person they're supporting, but they recognize that telling the truth may help their loved one and the research itself. That kind of contribution—emotional, practical, and deeply human—is vital to how research progresses.

One study partner, over years of participating in visits with her spouse, developed a close rapport with our research coordinator team. At one of the annual visits, she privately disclosed that her husband had been driving through a few stop signs, had a couple of minor fender benders, and had been pulled over a few times. He consistently dismissed her concerns.

During that research visit, our clinician brought up the topic of driving as part of the routine functional history review, something that happens every year. The participant felt safer during that review and acknowledged that he had noticed changes, but he feared that he would lose his license. Being outside the clinic made the conversation feel less intimidating. Together, we developed a plan for next steps, including speaking with his primary care doctor and eliminating distractions while driving.

Who's Right When It Comes to Alzheimer's Research?

When it comes to treatment decisions, a doctor's role should be that of a wise counselor—someone who educates, explains the pros and cons, and presents care options. For incurable, progressive diseases like Alzheimer's, referring a patient to research is a reasonable part of the care plan. Not all care comes in the form of a medicine, and not all treatment happens in a clinic. The final decision always belongs to the patient and, when appropriate, their loved ones. That's the way it should be.

I wasn't privy to the conversations my mother and father had after his diagnosis, but I can imagine how they might have navigated those early decisions. My dad was a risk taker, someone who believed deeply in the power of medicine. He feared death and would have wanted to pursue anything that offered even the possibility of slowing his disease. Clinical trials for amyloid or tau removal weren't available when he was alive, but I believe he would have enrolled without hesitation. He trusted the process, would have accepted the risks, and would have told his doctor, "If there's a chance to slow this disease, let's try it."

My mother, on the other hand, is cautious by nature. She worries about worst-case scenarios. I think she would have tried to protect my father from therapies she deemed too risky. She would have questioned the time spent traveling back and forth to an infusion center, arguing that those hours could be better spent together at home. She might have said, "Moe, even if the drug slows the disease, I don't think you'll appreciate the difference, and the side effects may not be worth it."

So, who would have been right—my mother or my father? The truth is, they both would have been. Each perspective carries weight and wisdom. There's no universal answer. The best decision is always personal, shaped by the patient's values, their family's input, and careful guidance from their medical team.

From a logistical standpoint, the role is demanding. Most studies are based in major cities at academic centers. Appointments often happen during business hours, requiring time off work or long drives. Many study partners are not compensated for their time, and trials can stretch across months or even years. It's a real sacrifice.

Study partners feel the investment is worthwhile, especially when the trial includes biomarker results or feedback that might improve their loved one's care. That makes sense. Anyone willing to take on such a commitment wants their time to matter. Without that sense of purpose, it can feel like they're giving up hours that might otherwise be spent on more productive or more enjoyable activities. No one wants to wait in hospital lobbies or sit through interviews that seem to drag on. Study partners want to know their efforts have meaning, not only for science but also for the person they love.

There's another, less obvious benefit as well. In contrast to hurried office visits, research environments are structured to allow more time for listening and connection. Staff members often have the time and training to offer thoughtful, compassionate support. Many study partners tell me they felt more heard and valued in a research setting than they ever had in a traditional clinic. That's not a criticism of clinical professionals but a reflection on the constraints they face. Research gives people room to breathe and to talk.

Being a study partner is hard work. It's hopeful work, too. Not only are you standing by your loved one, you're helping shape a future where earlier diagnoses, better treatment, and maybe even a cure are possible. The path is not easy, but you're helping to forge it.

Mrs. Chin Remembers—Being a Study Partner

Being in a drug trial helped Moe come to terms with his diagnosis. At the time, he didn't think he had Alzheimer's, but he knew his life was gradually changing. Participating reminded him he could still contribute to medicine—in a different way.

When researchers interviewed him to see if he was a good fit for the study, I don't recall asking any questions. I knew Moe was going to enroll. He was on a mission, and I admired him for that. The experience from beginning to end was for my husband, and it mattered deeply to him. I never wanted to say or do anything that might make it feel less important.

As a part of the study, we drove an hour to the hospital in Madison several times a month for his evaluations. We met with researchers separately, and we were together during the physical exam, procedures, and important conversations about the study. Moe always brought eggs from our chickens to give away. That gave him a lot of satisfaction, too. It was one more way he could continue to help and bring joy to others.

While Moe met privately with a researcher, I sat with a counselor. It wasn't always the same person, but they were consistently kind and attentive. They made audio recordings of our conversations, which I didn't love, but I understood they did this so they could concentrate on the conversation rather than taking notes. There's a balance between the scientific process and the humanity of caring.

No one told us whether Moe was receiving the placebo or study medicine. However, I began to suspect he was on the trial drug when he developed a rash that required a dermatologist's care. I surmised that the drug had no effect or one so small it could not be observed. I always told Moe that whatever the outcome, it made no difference to me. What mattered was that he was helping others, including our children and grandchildren. Being in the study lifted his spirits.

He would not have liked virtual visits, so traveling to Madison worked for us. The car rides gave us time to talk. Moe enjoyed chatting with nurses, the social worker, and other staff we met. He also liked being in the hospital. It reminded him of the career he loved so much. After each session, we ate in the café and talked about the choices on the menu. The disease never robbed us of our ability to enjoy the moment. We rediscovered the simple pleasures that are often ignored when life is rushed.

Moe knew his memory was fading. He anticipated doing poorly on the cognitive testing. On the way there, I would quiz him on everyday knowledge like the names of our family members, the date, who the president was. We were told not to do this, but it felt good to conspire with him. At each visit, the research coordinators separated us and asked us to recall events from the past week that the other person might mention. We also rehearsed those answers. On the way home, I would ask Moe what they asked him, and he would usually remember one or two of his answers. That always made him smile.

CAREGIVER RESEARCH: SUPPORTING THOSE WHO SUPPORT OTHERS

When people think about Alzheimer's research, drug trials come to mind. While developing medications is important, another vital area is caregiver research. When caregivers are better supported, their loved ones with dementia often stay at home longer and receive more consistent, higher-quality care. Reducing household stress can delay institutionalization, strengthen families, and preserve relationships.

When you're on the Alzheimer's caregiving journey, it can feel like you're barely keeping up, let alone contributing to the greater good. But participating in research is something you *can* do. It doesn't require you to be a perfect caregiver or to have it all figured out. It only requires a willingness to share your experience. Many who participate tell me it gave them a renewed sense of purpose. Helping out made them feel less alone, offered new tools, and gave them the confidence to become better caregivers. They began to see their role as a meaningful part of a larger effort to improve lives—not as a burden. They discovered that their story, no matter how painful or imperfect, had value.

The first challenge in caregiver research is that many people don't see themselves as caregivers. Volunteers for caregiver research could be the spouse who manages medications, the adult child who coordinates appointments, the neighbor who checks in regularly, or the friend who provides occasional meals. All these roles count as caregiving. The truth is that caregiving includes emotional support, reminder calls, transportation, decision-making, and advocacy. Only by recognizing the diverse functions caregivers perform will more people see themselves as eligible to volunteer for research.

You don't have to be a current caregiver either. You might be someone whose loved one has moved to a long-term care facility or who has passed away. These caregivers may now have time to participate in studies on mindfulness, wellness, or stress reduction. Every perspective brings something to the conversation.

As with other types of Alzheimer's research, you can choose from an incredible variety of studies. Some explore the health effects of caregiving by measuring stress levels, immune response, sleep quality, and heart health. Others examine carers' psychological and emotional journeys. Still others concentrate on support systems to understand why people reach out for help when they do and what assistance is most useful.

Researchers also want to know how families make difficult decisions about driving cessation, transitions to residential care, and advance care planning. Some studies design and test support systems such as mindfulness training, peer programs, and app-based tools to reduce caregiver burden.

Maybe you only have an hour a week to spare. Some studies respect that limitation. They may involve answering a few questions on the phone or filling out a short online survey. Others may have volunteers wear a smartwatch to measure how stress affects their heart rate.

One of the easiest ways to participate is by joining dementia caregiving registries. Their questionnaires can be answered online, by phone, or by mail. They cover caregiver burden, emotional health and depression, quality of life, social supports, health literacy, and responses to behavioral challenges. All responses are de-identified to protect privacy, and the data becomes part of a larger research effort to better understand real-world experiences.

In some peer-counseling studies, caregivers work one-on-one with researchers who were once care providers themselves. The caregiver receives guidance and support, and their story contributes to larger-scale research to improve caregiving. These studies do more than document experiences—they improve a caregiver's skills right then and there.

Every study should make clear what's involved, how much time it takes, what's expected emotionally, and what volunteers might receive in return. Some offer compensation. Others focus on the benefits of reflection, education, and connection. All these studies have one thing in common—they respect the reality that caregiving is already a full-time commitment.

THE LAST GIFT: HOW BRAIN DONATION POWERS ALZHEIMER'S RESEARCH

Brain donation is one of the most meaningful contributions a person can make. Despite exciting advances in the field of Alzheimer's biomarkers, brain tissue analysis after death remains the gold standard for diagnosis.

These microscopic examinations can confirm Alzheimer's with certainty and reveal much more than current tests do.

Donated brain tissue is also critical for developing future treatments and prevention strategies. It helps scientists understand how Alzheimer's progresses, how it interacts with other diseases, and what else may be happening inside the brain. Researchers also rely on brain donations from people who did not have dementia, which helps establish healthy baselines. That, too, is a valuable and needed contribution.

There's another urgent reason brain donations are needed. More than half of Alzheimer's cases involve other coexisting brain pathologies, such as Lewy body disease, TDP-43, and cerebrovascular disease. This mixed dementia is still poorly understood, particularly regarding how these diseases interact with Alzheimer's. Only an autopsy can conclusively reveal the presence of these diseases.

The insights gained from studying mixed pathology help pave the way for new diagnostic tools and treatment strategies for the conditions. Creating biomarkers for other brain disorders begins with the accurate identification of diseases during autopsies, and biomarkers that are validated against autopsy results represent the most reliable way to diagnose illness in living people. Eventually they open the door to less invasive tools, like blood tests. Treatments cannot be developed until the underlying biology is accurately identified. That process starts with donated brains.

While neuropathological assessment remains the gold standard, it is not perfect. Like all areas of medicine, it continues to evolve. Improvements in diagnostic precision, especially for complex or overlapping diseases, depend on continued brain donations. The more tissue available for study, the better scientists can refine the technology and methodology behind these evaluations.

Donating one's brain is, however, different from being an organ donor. When a person donates organs, they are immediately transplanted into recipients who need them. Donating your brain means it will be examined after death to identify amyloid plaques, tau tangles, and signs of other brain diseases. Brain donation does not interfere with most religious beliefs, but—as you would with organ donation—you may wish to discuss it with your spiritual leader.

A brain must be put on ice immediately after death. Without rapid cooling, the tissue begins to break down too quickly, making it unusable for research. That's the biological reality. Planning for brain donation ideally happens months or even years before death. When someone passes away, the emotional shock can be overwhelming. Thinking about research is far removed from what loved ones are experiencing in the moment. That's why it's critical to have these plans in place well in advance.

Some people worry about the logistics of brain donation. Will it disrupt funeral planning? Is an open casket no longer possible? The answer to both is no. The brain ideally is collected within hours of death, but the process is not rushed. The funeral home and research program work together. The body is transported to the hospital for the procedure before embalming. Skilled pathologists and morticians ensure there is no disfigurement, and families can move forward with the funeral they planned, including ones with open-casket services.

When my father died at home, my mother faced the unusual task of placing ice around his head—a surreal, almost unthinkable act just moments after losing her partner. But of course, this was not foremost on her mind when she called me before dawn to tell me he had died. The news, though expected, hit me like a hammer. I wasn't thinking clearly either. My wife was the capable one. She called my mother and gently reminded her what needed to happen. She was the one who contacted the university's brain retrieval team and the funeral home. Without her, I'm not sure the donation would have happened.

The funeral home knew exactly what to do. It transported my father to the hospital for the brain removal process. Later, his body was returned to the funeral home for preparation and cremation. If we had wanted an open-casket viewing, that would have been possible—there were no visible signs of the procedure thanks to the skilled medical and mortuary teams.

Conversations about brain donation require sensitivity. Trust must come first. When I talk with participants, I begin by answering questions and addressing common misunderstandings. Then I give people space. No one should feel pressured into making this decision. At the Wisconsin ADRC, we've learned that if a person hasn't agreed to donate in the first few years of participation, they're unlikely to do so later. That means the early relationship is essential—building trust, providing transparency, and helping participants understand the research center's mission.

Historical abuses in medicine have made this conversation even more delicate for some communities, particularly African American and Native American. Researchers today are committed to cultural humility and sensitivity. We often delay donation discussions with underrepresented participants until later in the study process, and we involve families and funeral homes in that conversation. Inclusion in research starts with connection, and that takes time.

Doctors often talk about brain donation like it's no big deal, but it is. Having lived through it, I can attest to how difficult it really was. When the time comes, families aren't thinking about science or future patients. They're thinking about their own loss and sorrow. In that moment, brain donation can feel distant, even irrelevant.

For many families, brain donation brings closure. After the procedure, they receive an autopsy report and can meet with a pathologist who can explain the findings. In Wisconsin, families may also attend a case conference at the medical school where the donation is presented as part of teaching. They see firsthand how the gift of brain tissue advances the work of future doctors and scientists. Knowing that their loved one's donation will contribute to a treatment, a cure, or a breakthrough gives families comfort. Brain donation is a final act of service. It transforms loss into progress.

I encourage you to consider this gift. It matters. It can help other families, fuel the fight against Alzheimer's, and move us closer to the answers we so desperately seek. To learn more about brain donation, talk to your doctor or visit the website of an Alzheimer's Disease Research Center (ADRC) near you. Another way to donate is through the Brain Donor Project at braindonorproject.org. Its motto is "Be the brain behind the breakthrough," and that's worth keeping in mind.

"A HURDLE WE FACE"

"When I was a medical student, hardly a page in my textbooks was dedicated to Alzheimer's because we knew nothing about it," recalls Dr. Sanjay Asthana, the founding director of Wisconsin's ADRC. The disease has been misunderstood, often conflated with the general idea of senility, and largely ignored in public health conversations. "In the last few decades, as a result of extensive research in Wisconsin, in the U.S., and around the world, we better understand what causes it, what genes are involved, and how it progresses—but we still don't have all the answers." Under Dr. Asthana's leadership, Wisconsin's research program has played a vital role in this progress, contributing to discoveries that are transforming how we detect, study, and ultimately understand the disease.

Despite the advancements that have been made, many unknowns continue to cloak Alzheimer's disease in mystery. No one knows why some people develop elevated amyloid or why others with amyloid develop symptoms while others remain cognitively unimpaired. We don't understand the protective factors that shield certain individuals. We have yet to find the mechanisms that drive the transition from amyloid accumulation to the elevated presence of the protein tau—which is always present in Alzheimer's brains—to eventual neurodegeneration. We need better biomarkers for other brain diseases, like frontotemporal dementia and Lewy body disease. We need prognostic tools that help clinicians better estimate risk—like the heart disease risk scores cardiologists use.

This next stage of discovery depends on one irreplaceable resource: people. "A hurdle we face is we are always looking for more people to participate in research," says Asthana. "Alzheimer's only affects human beings. The only way we can win against Alzheimer's is with people participating in research. We simply need more volunteers."

Participation is the backbone of Alzheimer's research. It's what allows scientists to test new drugs, evaluate new diagnostics, and track the natural course of the disease. Participation doesn't end with blood samples or brain scans. Researchers need brain donations. Only through autopsies can researchers definitively understand what happened in the minds of people who gave science the essence of themselves. Such gifts are the final and most profound gift to science and the future.

We cannot afford to slow down. In fact, despite the gains we've made, now is the time to accelerate. Without more volunteers, progress will stall—and with it, our hopes of relieving the strain on families, health systems, and future generations. The path ahead is promising, but only if people continue to walk it with us.

9

"Dying of Alzheimer's Is Just Dying"

LET'S TALK ABOUT THINGS NO ONE WANTS TO TALK ABOUT

What Happens in the Final Weeks, Days, and Hours • What Is "Paradoxical Lucidity"? • Hospice and Palliative Care • The Brain Donation Process • Difficult Decisions at the End

Dying with Alzheimer's is not a sudden catastrophe. It is a release. A letting go. A gradual, invisible surrender of systems that once sustained a vibrant life. The heart slows. The breath softens. The organs will yield. And then, in stillness, the sojourn ends.

But what has been remains: the stories told, the love shared, the hands held. The presence once offered by that person is not undone by this quiet end. In the grand scheme of biology, what is most profound is not that a loved one's body can forget how to carry on but that for so long it remembered how to live, and did so with vigor.

* * *

So far this book has been about the period of time immediately before, during, and after a diagnosis of Alzheimer's. So why include this chapter, especially when most people live for many years after they're diagnosed?

I want to talk about death and dying because questions about it are among the most common ones I hear. Even in the first or second visit, family members ask me, "How long is this person going to live?" Sometimes they ask sheepishly, when the patient has stepped out of the room. Other times, they are bolder. I have had spouses ask me, right in front of their recently diagnosed partners, "What is their death going to look like?"

Nonetheless, death in the twenty-first century is a taboo topic. A hundred years ago, when most people lived rural lives, they bore witness to farm animals being born, mating, and eventually being slaughtered. Most people began and ended their lives at home. They lived the seasonal rituals of planting, ripening, and harvesting. Children and adults experienced all of it. People lived this circle of life.

There was more of a connection to death, more of an acceptance of its inevitability—perhaps because death often came earlier in life. In the 1800s, 30 percent of children died before their first birthday, and 40 percent didn't survive past their fifth. Midwives tended births at home, and families prepared bodies for wakes right in their own houses. Death was part of life. It was visible, tangible, and communal.

Today, more people are dying in a facility of some sort and are quickly whisked away to the crematorium or funeral home. We've expedited the process and created a façade of hominess instead of actually being at home, where grief and community used to unfold together.

There is nothing inherently wrong with this modern way of dying. But it keeps us distant—from the presence of death and from its process.

This chapter will share my personal account of caregiving and grief. And it might give you an idea of what you and your loved one might experience in the final months, weeks, hours, and even minutes.

THE LONG GOODBYE

Alzheimer's has been called a long goodbye. It is the body forgetting itself. The disease begins as a quiet thief, stealing nouns and faces, tucking away memories into unreachable corners. At first, it seems like a disease of the mind—a cruel division between clarity and confusion. But over time, Alzheimer's reveals itself to be far more sweeping. It is not merely a loss of memory. The body forgets, too.

Misplaced keys and repeated questions get noticed first but the internal damage has been at work for years. The brain, our master conductor, ceases to conduct. And the music of the body—its rhythm and harmony, its synchronized pulse—fades into disarray.

We often think of the brain as the seat of thought and personality. It is also the silent overseer of heartbeat and breath, temperature and thirst, balance and digestion. Every organ, every cell, takes cues from the brain. When those signals dim, the systems that depend on them begin to drift unmoored.

The nervous system unravels. At the core of this slow collapse is the loss of innervation. In a healthy body, the autonomic nervous system acts as a messenger between the brain and the body, delivering instructions with elegant precision. Most notably, the vagus nerve serves as a highway of life, transmitting signals that regulate heart rate, digestion, immune responses, and other vital functions. As those nerve impulses become fainter, the body works with less cohesiveness and more disarray.

In Alzheimer's, the brain's communication with the body frays. The brainstem, the most primitive, deeply buried part of the brain, starts to disconnect. The hypothalamus, the tiny command center responsible for regulating the body's internal balance, also deteriorates. It's as if the body's thermostat is broken. Temperature regulation becomes unreliable. Thirst may disappear entirely. Signals that tell us to eat or rest or fight an infection grow faint or vanish.

As the disease spreads, voluntary muscle control erodes. People lose the ability to walk and then to stand and then to even sit upright. Finally, turning in bed becomes difficult. Muscles weaken not from injury but from disuse and disconnection. This atrophy extends throughout the entire muscular system. Smooth muscles that move food through the digestive tract slow down. Sphincters that control urination and defecation lose their tone. Incontinence becomes a part of daily life.

The esophageal sphincter fails. Stomach acid flows back into the throat, causing discomfort and increasing the risk of aspiration. Even the act of swallowing—something we do over five hundred times a day without thought—becomes dangerous. Dysphagia (difficulty swallowing) sets in. Food and fluids can slip into the lungs instead of the stomach, leading to aspiration pneumonia, a common cause of death in Alzheimer's. And yet, even as the body weakens, swallowing often lingers—a quiet instinct that endures, a last thread of agency before the body lets go. Many people will continue to eat and drink in small amounts until their last few days, when they slip into a state of deep rest and wakefulness becomes rare.

The greatest consequence of this progressive neural failure is the breakdown of homeostasis, the body's ability to maintain its internal stability, which encompasses a constant balance of temperature, hydration, pH, glucose, and oxygen. This ever-shifting harmony is what allows us to stay alive moment to moment through heat and cold, hunger and exertion.

In Alzheimer's, homeostasis is dismantled from within. The hypothalamus no longer commands the adrenal glands with precision. Interactions between and among the hypothalamus and the pituitary and adrenal glands falter. At first, stress hormones like cortisol may flood the body, contributing to damage. Later, cortisol production wanes. The adrenal glands, once vital for responding to stress, fatigue, and infection, fall silent.

This hormonal dysfunction continues across the body's systems. The thyroid may slow, bringing fatigue and cold intolerance. Sex hormones diminish, removing their neuroprotective support. Vasopressin, essential for water retention, declines, contributing to dehydration and unstable blood pressure. Signals to drink water or eat are muted or lost entirely.

Liver, kidneys, and the gut experience silent strain. The gut, slowed by poor neural input and muscle weakness, begins to stagnate. Peristalsis—the wavelike motion that pushes food through the intestines—diminishes. Waste sits longer in the bowels. Toxins reenter the bloodstream. Gut bacteria flourish in ways they shouldn't. The intestinal wall becomes more permeable, allowing inflammatory molecules to circulate.

The kidneys, deprived of steady blood pressure and hormonal regulation, filter less efficiently. Toxins like urea accumulate in the blood, a condition called uremia. Electrolyte balances shift unpredictably. The liver, already burdened by inflammation and low oxygen, slows its breakdown of metabolic waste and medications. Ammonia builds up, causing further mental fog. The body becomes more toxic.

The skin is the edge of life, and it is not spared either. Evaporation from the skin increases. Dehydration accelerates. The body's last reserves are spent trying to stay in balance. No longer nourished by robust blood flow, skin thins and dries. It loses its elasticity and protective oils. It cannot regulate heat or hold in moisture. Small pressure points become wounds. These sores, often called pressure ulcers or bedsores, can open paths for infection. And without a strong immune response, even minor infections can overwhelm the body's defenses.

Meanwhile, the heart's cadence grows wayward. Lacking appropriate hormonal and neural feedback, it beats irregularly. Mitochondria, the tiny engines producing energy within heart cells, become inefficient. The heart struggles to pump blood with the same force. Blood pressure drops. Organs receive less oxygen and nutrition. Fatigue deepens.

Breath by breath, the lungs lose their rhythm. Muscles involved in breathing weaken. The chest rises and falls more shallowly. Mucus accumulates and cannot be cleared. Alveoli—the tiny sacs in the lungs where gas exchange occurs—collapse. Oxygen levels fall while carbon dioxide builds up. This is called hypercapnia, and it causes confusion, drowsiness, and eventually unconsciousness. Breathing is one of the final acts of the body—a slow, shallow rhythm that persists long after awareness fades. For families, it offers reassurance that their loved one is still with them, and when the pattern changes, a quiet signal that death is drawing near.

The brain no longer responds to rising carbon dioxide. Outwardly, however, the person often appears calm. The struggle for air is silent. The systems are failing, but the person is not suffering.

Yet the body appears peaceful in the midst of this complex storm. To describe all this—the cellular collapse, the hormonal disarray, the organ failure—might suggest a brutal death. But that is not the truth.

Alzheimer's often removes the person from awareness of these processes. The cognitive decline that robs memory also protects against pain. The person is not distressed by weakened kidney function or toxic blood gases. She does not feel fear about wayward blood pressure or high cortisol levels. The person with Alzheimer's is often unaware of the body's slow fading, and in this way, she is spared.

Even in the final stages, joy is possible. A favorite song can bring a smile. A familiar touch can bring calm. A gentle breeze, the warmth of the sun, the presence of a loved one—small sensory gifts can still reach the person. Hearing and touch, remarkably, are often among the last senses to endure. Even when all else falls away, the soft brush of a hand or the sound of a voice may still be felt. This is a gift—it allows the family to maintain a meaningful bond with their loved one, knowing the person is cognizant of the moment, too. The body may be failing, but the moment still occurs and often that is enough. Paradoxical lucidity may occur. These are moments when a person's pre-Alzheimer's mind briefly returns—until life ebbs. (See page 354 for more on paradoxical lucidity.)

At last a mighty current pulls away the sand from where a person stood. The end has come, one that takes us all, as Shakespeare wrote, to "the undiscovered country from whose [boundaries] no traveler returns."

THE HONOR OF YOUR PRESENCE

It is an honor to help someone in their last days. You care for your loved one with your words, touch, presence, and humble service. This privilege can be difficult to live through, yet one ought not view it as a burden. You are sharing a sacred experience that humans have engaged in for time immemorial.

Everyone's departure from this world is a little different. Death is the natural passage shared by all living creatures. Of course, the process of dying is also a time of grief, yet even that is softened by the outpouring of the love we have for each other.

When I was growing up, my family stopped every year at a shop in Door County, Wisconsin—the Cape Cod of the Midwest—where thousands of vacationers flock. The store had a road sign that read: GRATITUDE IS ATTITUDE. I've thought about that maxim for years. Only now, having lived through loss, do I recognize its truth. It's hard in the moment to realize that there is always a reason to be grateful, but I encourage you to embrace this sentiment, even in times of sorrow.

Eventually, I learned to express thanks for all of life, the bad and the good. As I've written elsewhere in this book, life doesn't owe us anything. We owe life a duty to respond as best we can to its obstacles, hardships, and woes. I've seen this same recognition in my patients and their families.

Your experience as a caregiver may leave you feeling empty, bereft, desolate, or even angry. I will always remember when my mom asked me to help my dad call his older brother the month before he died. His sibling was not well enough to travel, and she wanted them to speak one last time. I dialed and put my dad on speaker phone. As my uncle told my father how much he loved him, all my dad could do was bellow his brother's name over and over. That raw emotion stays with me—it reminds me of the love my father and I shared, and the love he and his brother felt for each other.

Deep love takes many forms, and my practice of medicine is richer because of that experience and many others. Although it did not seem so at the time, my father's passing was a rite of passage, one that allowed me to fully appreciate my own blessings. It ignited in me a passion for life I had not known before. Tending to my dad over those years, as all caregivers understand, left little room for self-care and personal exploration. But through that experience, I found the inspiration to help others find the emotional space to embrace themselves, as well as their loved ones. That became my mission in my medical practice, my research, and in writing this book.

UNPLEASANT REALITIES

One of the earliest indications that death is looming is when patients with dementia begin losing significant weight. This can start months, even years, beforehand. In my clinical experience, this pattern is nearly universal and does not seem to depend on a person's prior level of fitness, body type, or other medical conditions. For loved ones, this can be very upsetting, but it is part of the process. The patient loses appetite and muscle mass. Some medications may abet this weight loss. What's happening is that people with Alzheimer's gradually lose their sense of smell and taste. They don't feel hungry, and often they no longer enjoy eating. Their stomachs contract, and in the final weeks of life, they often lose all desire to eat.

During my father's last two weeks, he stopped eating and mostly slept. His hospital bed was pushed up against my mom's twin mattress in what had been their bedroom. One of the tough decisions families face at the end of an Alzheimer's patient's life is whether to continue feeding. Doctors do not advise tube feeding someone with advanced dementia. The risk of aspiration remains high and can lead to pneumonia. By this point, the person is dying. Nothing more can be done, and there's no medical reason to insist on eating.

Of course, food should be offered. If the patient takes it, this is known as *comfort feeding*. My mother did this for my father. He loved eating. It was one of his passions—right alongside his love of work and travel. He continued eating until near the end, but in his last two weeks, he stopped. Although he wasn't receiving any hydration, his pain and antianxiety medications were given through a subcutaneous line, which carried a small amount of fluid along with them.

This is not a time to stress about nutrition. Feeding should be about comfort, enjoyment, and connection—not calories, carbs, or fat content. Let your loved one guide the experience. If they're interested in eating, offer food slowly. If they're not, don't push. Think about their favorite dishes, especially those tied to happy memories. And always consider consistency—soft foods are often safest to prevent choking. A spoonful of mashed potatoes, a sip of warm broth, a taste of ice cream may be more valuable than any supplement or meal replacement.

Your doctor and medical care team should do everything possible to make your loved one comfortable in their last days. It is a natural, normal part of dying for a patient to lose the ability to eat or have disinterest in eating.

The Weight of Care

One of the most visceral experiences I had helping care for my dad came during his final weeks. We could sense my dad was uncomfortable—he grimaced when we turned him, and he had stopped eating. My mom, always attentive, was carefully tracking his urination and bowel movements. He had been constipated for many days. We had tried stool softeners and prune juice, but nothing worked. Eventually, my mom made the difficult decision to manually remove the hardened stool.

When I arrived for one of my regular visits, she didn't tell me ahead of time what I was walking into. When she explained what we needed to do, I froze. I didn't know how to process it. I eventually obliged, holding my dad on his side while she did it.

He groaned loudly. His whole body trembled. I remember questioning, even in the moment, whether this was the right thing to do. It was horrible. But afterward, he felt better—he began talking and eating again. His relief was immediate and undeniable.

When I reflect on that moment, I am still in awe of my mother's strength—not just in making the decision but in having the courage to do it herself. It was moments like that when I fully realized I was the *secondary caregiver*. The *primary caregiver* carries a weight that is beyond measure.

CATHETERS, COMFORT, AND THE MOST COMMON CAUSES OF DEATH

In the final stage of Alzheimer's, urinary and fecal incontinence occur. This can begin years before, during the middle stage of the disease. In his final weeks, my bedridden father wore as few clothes as possible and was in Depends.

Do you put in a Foley catheter or not? (A Foley catheter allows urine to slowly drain out by means of a thin flexible tube inserted into the bladder that can remain in place for long periods.) By this point, the bladder musculature has withered away. Urinary sphincter control will diminish or disappear, and a person can no longer contract the muscles needed to urinate. There are several good reasons to use a catheter. It prevents the bladder from becoming distended and uncomfortable. It also reduces the risk of a patient's skin becoming irritated or infected from urine exposure. A catheter also allows caregivers to assess hydration based on the color of the urine. Downsides to catheterization include discomfort during insertion, increased risk of urinary tract infections, and restricted movement. If a catheter is not used, the need to change a patient's Depends will continue. This is a decision to discuss carefully with the medical team.

For patients who are not dying, long-term catheter use is not recommended because of infection risk. For dying patients, that rule no longer applies. By that point, the risk of infection is accepted because most people in advanced dementia will ultimately die from it. If it happens to be from a urinary tract infection, so be it. The cause of death is usually sepsis—a severe, whole-body infection of organs and tissues. This may sound callous, but when death is close at hand, the goal of medical care shifts. The focus is not on preventing death or extending life but rather on easing the natural dying process.

I watched this transition happen at home. A few days before my dad died, my mom asked the home nurse to catheterize his bladder. She had been gently massaging his abdomen and was concerned he might feel an uncomfortable fullness. At that point, it wasn't about eliminating infection risk but about relieving possible distress. Hospice was glad to oblige.

Pneumonia and urinary tract infections are common causes of death in Alzheimer's patients. Other causes include dehydration and malnutrition, falls, heart disease and strokes, blood clots, respiratory issues, and sepsis from pressure ulcers (bedsores) and dental issues. Whatever the precipitating cause, the disease itself is the underlying culprit. Brain atrophy and synaptic dysfunction have created cascading problems throughout the body. Autonomic nervous system dysfunction destabilizes breathing and heart rate. Loss of muscle tone creates respiratory issues. Hormonal regulation collapses. The immune system is ravaged and can no longer mount an effective defense. Death due to infection or some other cause is inevitable.

One of my University of Wisconsin–Madison colleagues, Dr. Shahriar Salamat, a neuropathologist, likens death in an Alzheimer's patient to a battery that is running down. "The brain is the driving system of the body," he says. "In Alzheimer's this central system has pruned its connections with its environment. In a sense, it has retracted into itself. The brain loses its connections with the critical functions of the body." Without the brain's leadership and guidance, the body fails.

The end is near when breathing becomes labored. This is known as Cheyne-Stokes breathing and involves long, irregular, guttural inhalations and exhalations. Though this is not distressing to the patient, you hear the struggle for breath. You eventually see the skin turn gray, a sign that the body is not getting enough oxygen. In addition, lips and nail beds turn bluish. This is when nurses know to call the doctor, because experience has taught them that death is at hand. The doctor's role will be to officially pronounce death.

PARADOXICAL LUCIDITY

Brief episodes of mental clarity are surprisingly common in Alzheimer's patients near death. Late in the disease—often at a point when you believe your loved one is incapable of meaningful communication—suddenly, it happens, moments of true clarity. The person is fully present, completely oriented, and astonishingly fluent. This episode may last just a few minutes, sometimes hours, and occasionally even longer.

In the hours and days before death, your loved one might suddenly want to play a long-forgotten musical instrument. She might ask to gather friends for lunch one last time and join them in casual conversation. He might remember your name and wish to talk, perhaps revisit old memories, or simply say goodbye.

This is not some internet rumor or pseudoscientific myth. Paradoxical lucidity has been reported countless times, and most doctors and hospice nurses will be well acquainted with this phenomenon. One study found that more than 90 percent of people who experience a lucid episode will die within a week. About 40 percent pass away within a day or two, and 15 percent will only live another few hours. Of course, paradoxical lucidity does not occur with every Alzheimer's patient.

This is yet another aspect of the disease that is actively being studied. Only a handful of researchers are investigating paradoxical lucidity, and we still don't fully understand why or how it happens.

The leading theory is that near the end of life a brief cognitive surge occurs. Neural networks begin to fire in a more synchronized way. After all, not all brain cells are dead. Many remain alive but have been disconnected. Somehow, in those final hours or days, a burst of neuroelectrical and neurochemical activity aligns—like green traffic lights suddenly syncing along a busy street. Everything lines up, and meaningful communication becomes possible.

When this happens, families often panic. They ask, "Were we wrong all this time? Maybe she didn't really have Alzheimer's after all!" The answer is no. The diagnosis was correct. Enjoy what's happening. It won't last. Speak what needs to be heard. Ask the questions you've been carrying. Don't question the moment. Don't feel guilty about a possible misdiagnosis. Simply be present and treasure the clarity while it lasts.

THE POWER OF TOUCH AND HEARING

Touching a dying person—massaging the hands or feet, gently stroking the temples and scalp, or simply holding hands—can be grounding, even reverent. This kind of care can soothe both the giver and the receiver. But the needs and preferences of the person you are ministering to should always lead the way. Every gesture is most meaningful when offered with sensitivity, presence, and deep respect.

When keeping vigil with someone who is dying, touch and presence often speak louder than words. In those moments, nonverbal communication becomes its own form of care. People who are unresponsive or comatose still retain some sense of bodily awareness. A 2021 study published in *Psychological Science* found that the brain can respond unconsciously to physical contact even when the sensory region is temporarily disrupted, suggesting that people may still perceive touch on some level. Similarly, findings from Mass General Brigham suggest that some unconscious patients retain hidden consciousness and can register external stimuli. This aligns with clinical observations from end-of-life care, where families and healthcare workers report subtle facial expressions or finger movements when a seemingly unconscious loved one's hand is held. If your loved one is sensitive to sound or becomes agitated by noise, you might try Reiki. Reiki is a Japanese healing practice based on the idea that gentle touch or hand movements can help balance the body's energy, promote relaxation, reduce stress, and facilitate natural healing.

Hearing is believed to be the last sense to remain active. A 2020 study from the University of British Columbia found that the brains of unresponsive, actively dying patients still registered auditory stimuli, suggesting that hearing persists near the end of life. I've seen dying patients, eyes closed and breath slowed, subtly respond to the voices of loved ones. I've been part of quiet prayer circles in patients' rooms where the stillness itself seemed to calm the mind. I've also watched relatives and friends chant around their loved ones' beds, with one person beating a drum, its steady rhythm mimicking a heartbeat.

In those last days, hours, and minutes, tell the person how much he means to you. Say his name. Let him hear your voice: "I love you" or "I'm here for you. I'm with you."

Will I Recognize My Loved Ones?

One of the greatest fears among Alzheimer's patients is that, as death nears, they won't recognize their loved ones. Many worry that they won't recognize their own children. When I counsel patients, I often say: *Even if you don't remember your children's names, I believe you will still know them. You will know they are special people who love you and have always been close to you.* I don't think my father remembered my name near the end, but I do believe he knew me and knew I was his son.

Patients tend to accept and be grateful for this counseling. I've found that sharing my personal story builds trust. It's hard to argue with a doctor who has walked this path. Of course, I always admit I can't know this for certain. No one can look inside the mind of someone with Alzheimer's and confirm what they know or recognize. But in this gray area of uncertainty, I choose to believe in the positive, and I ground that belief in my experience—with my father and with my patients. Maybe I am rationalizing. Still, I find comfort in what I believe, and my patients do, too.

THE DOCTOR'S ROLE IN THE FINAL WEEKS

The doctor's role in the final weeks varies depending on the patient's wishes. When a patient is dying unexpectedly, the doctor's job is to prevent death. This is the hospital setting depicted in countless movies and TV shows where Code Blues are run. If the person is dying but the situation is not an emergency, doctors are the ones giving medications, ordering tests, and still trying to prevent death. In both cases, it feels like a confrontation. The doctors are a force pushing back, until finally they or the patient says, "Enough." At that point, doctors pivot to providing comfort and reducing pain.

When people don't fight dying—when it is foreseen and planned for, as in a hospice—doctors provide education, lead the healthcare team, and focus on easing the patient's symptoms, addressing anxiety and sadness. They help with basic bodily functions, support the family with their grief, and assist with preparations for death and arrangements afterward. The doctors are only part of the team though. They tend to focus on medications and symptom management. The social worker, nurse, and chaplain are often the ones who step in to help with the emotional and spiritual needs, such as understanding and accepting grief, and the deeper aspects of the dying process. Once pain and symptoms are well controlled, the roles of the nurses, social workers, and chaplain often matter most.

Every physician reacts differently when a patient dies, but, even if they don't perceive it, death affects all doctors emotionally and psychologically. This impact changes as we age and mature, but losing a patient never becomes normal. Over time some grow more comfortable in death's presence; others resist getting used to the reality that it is natural and inevitable. It's hard for any doctor to lose patients they've become close to because they do become friends, and sometimes they feel like family.

Death is not foreign or unusual—it's part of our work. It occurs especially frequently for ICU and ER doctors, and geriatricians. We encounter it more often than most MDs, and we're well aware it's part of life. Still, you may be certain that doctors cry and grieve. Loss is loss, even when you see it every day.

HOW MUCH MEDICAL INTERVENTION?

Are Alzheimer's patients more likely to die with less medical intervention than people with other diseases, like cancer, where many battle aggressively until the end? It depends. Some patients and families decide early on that they don't want aggressive interventions. Instead of pursuing every option, they may choose to avoid emergency rooms, hospitalizations, or treatments—including common ones like antibiotics—that would prolong life. They shift their focus to comfort and letting nature take its course, with a clear priority on quality of life and symptom management.

Others, however, will demand all possible care and interventions. They might have their loved ones in a hospital on artificial life support, hoping and praying for a miracle. They focus on time and longevity. Such cases will have many medical interventions.

Many people find a compromise. Each individual circumstance is discussed carefully. Some medical interventions are chosen; some are declined. With cancer and other diseases, there tend to be more treatment options and therefore more interventions to attempt. In Alzheimer's and dementia, no medications reverse existing damage, and only a few directly target the Alzheimer's disease process itself. Instead, most medications target behaviors, mood changes, psychosis, and other factors like infections and nutrition. Because Alzheimer's leads to functional impairments, care shifts in the direction of support: turning the person in bed to prevent bedsores; assisting with standing and walking; reducing risk of falls; providing clean clothes; offering help with eating; managing medications; and supporting toileting. The focus is less on medication and more on simply living.

Hospice Versus Palliative Care—What's the Difference?

Palliative care and hospice care both focus on comfort, but they are not the same. Palliative care is about living well alongside illness. Hospice is about dying well when death is near. Both can provide tremendous support. Knowing when to use each—and how they differ—can make a profound difference for patients and their families.

Palliative Care:

- Can begin at any stage of a serious illness, even from the time of diagnosis.
- May be provided alongside curative and aggressive treatments.
- Focuses on relieving symptoms, reducing suffering, and improving quality of life.
- May be administered by someone other than the primary caregiver in a consulting role with the primary care doctor and other specialists.
- Can be available in hospitals, outpatient clinics, long-term care facilities, and sometimes at home.
- May be covered by insurance. Some private insurance plans may not fully cover it.

Hospice Care:

- Begins when a patient is expected to have six months or less to live, and the focus shifts entirely to comfort rather than cure.
- Happens when curative treatments are no longer pursued.
- Means that the hospice team often becomes the primary care team, coordinating nearly all aspects of care.
- Provides comprehensive support for the patient and family, including symptom management, emotional and spiritual care, and guidance through the dying process.
- Offers bereavement counseling after the person has passed.
- Takes place at home most often but can also be available in hospice centers, nursing homes, or hospitals.
- Is covered by Medicare, which means many people in the United States have full coverage for hospice services.

How They Connect:

- Hospice care falls under the umbrella of palliative care. All hospice is palliative care, but not all palliative care is hospice.
- In many settings, the same team may provide both palliative and hospice care, depending on the patient's stage and goals.

Doctors field many questions about pain and antianxiety medications at the end of life. Many loved ones worry about oversedating the person dying with Alzheimer's. Some even fear they might accidentally hasten death by giving too much morphine. A few worry about addiction. Rest easy—addiction is not a concern at the end of life, and study after study has shown that treating pain in dying patients will not accelerate the dying process. You won't accidentally kill someone with the prescribed doses of morphine. It would require a massive amount to be fatal.

More often, pain in Alzheimer's patients arises from being bedbound. Pressure ulcers—wounds from sitting or lying in the same position for too long—are unfortunately common, especially on the buttocks and at the coccyx, the last bone in the spine. The person's skin is weakened and wears down more easily, leading to the wound. Bones and joints can also ache from prolonged immobility. Sometimes the greatest pain comes from their back or an injury from decades ago.

Like many people, my dad was anxious toward the end. It was a quiet kind of unease, the sort that settles in when the body is working harder than the mind can explain. In the final days or hours, many people experience terminal delirium, a state of confusion and disorientation. This is not unusual. Physiologically, it makes sense a person would have nervousness or hesitation at the end because breathing can become more difficult. Antianxiety medications, like lorazepam,* can alleviate some of the agitation this causes.

If your loved one is dying at home, open yourself to the acceptance of death. It is an intimate experience that will leave its mark on you. Don't underestimate your own ability to bring comfort all the way to the end. Hospice can walk with you through questions and uncertainties. Your greatest gift in these final moments is simply to be present, to relieve pain and suffering when you can, and to maintain your vigil with love.

ENJOY THE TIME YOU HAVE

I visited my father every day after work during his last weeks, often bringing my mother ButterBurgers and frozen custard from Culver's, a family restaurant chain in Wisconsin. My mother and I spent those evenings chatting together in my parents' bedroom. My father had moments of lucidity, periods when he was clear, mostly focusing on my mom. We never left his room. I was overwhelmed every night, but I smiled through my tears so as not to distress him. I never knew if each goodbye would be the last, but I did know that in each of these moments, I was expressing a lifetime of gratitude for his love.

Even before his illness, my father never talked to me about dying, be it his own mortality or that of his patients. He would occasionally talk

* This is sold under the brand name Ativan.

about losing his father when he was young. His father owned a convenience store. A customer shot and killed him, and my father saw it happen. He also talked about his mother, who died of heart disease when he was in his early twenties.

My dad was fully aware of life's fragility. Perhaps that's why he was so focused on healing others, keeping them healthy and alive. I don't know if he didn't talk to me about death because he didn't like the subject, or because he didn't feel like talking *to me* about it. He knew my mother openly talked about it. Maybe he felt that was enough. Instead, my dad focused on the miracles of medicine and healthcare—how incredible it was that we could keep people healthy, heal them when they were sick, and bring them back from the brink of death. At his core, he believed in both Western and Eastern medicine, in harnessing the body's natural ability to heal and in helping that process with medications.

Even as a child, death was not foreign to me. My mom loves dogs and volunteered with the local humane society, serving on their board. Often, when she learned that a dog was about to be euthanized, she would rescue them. At one point, we had four dogs and a baby pig. (The pig eventually went to our local community-supported farm where I spent much of my childhood playing and helping.) The dogs were usually old and ailing. When they got sick, no extraordinary measures were taken. I had to say goodbye to many beloved dogs. I don't recall ever being there when they were "put down." My mom usually took them to the veterinary clinic while I was at school. I would come home, and they would be gone.

Modern society keeps death away from the home. Even our pets typically die at the vet's office. I wept for each one we lost. My mom would cry with me, and those are some of my clearest memories of her crying when I was a child. She was always honest with me about what had happened. She would explain, in simple terms, how my pets were given a medication, and that they would drift to sleep while she petted them and talked to them. She told me about heaven, the possibility of reincarnation, and of energy returning to Earth.

Losing these four-legged companions never got easier. In fact, it became harder as I grew older. Lorax, the first dog I owned as an adult, died of cancer at home a few months before my father passed away. It was unexpected and traumatic. We spent a great deal of money trying to prolong her life, even though we knew she was terminal. After her diagnosis, we fed her the most amazing food and took her with us on every trip throughout Wisconsin. For the last six months of her life, we never went anywhere without her.

On the day she died, I was at my clinic seeing patients. When my wife Erin called to tell me the bad news, I sobbed the entire ride home. I knew my dad would be next. In many ways, this felt like a dress rehearsal. I spent that night sleeping on the couch with Lorax on the den floor next to me, my hand resting on her side.

Before my grandmother died in her late eighties, she spoke of death every day. She was completely comfortable with it. She had been one of the first hospice nurses in Wisconsin, and I spent many hours with her talking about dying. Her peace with death always amazed me.

During one of our conversations, I told her I was afraid of dying. She smiled and said, "Oh, you have so much life to live. So many adventures and exciting things to accomplish. Don't fret about the end. Focus on now and the days ahead. When your time comes, you'll be ready, as I am, as long as you live to the fullest."

Years later, I would have a similar conversation with my mother. Oddly enough, she told me the same thing. "With every birth, there will be a corresponding death at a later date," she said. "We just don't know when, so you should take advantage of the time you have."

Both my grandmother and my mother had a remarkable comfort with death. Their openness imprinted on me as I grew up. Looking back, it wasn't just my father's career as a physician that prepared me for medicine—it was also this emotional familiarity with death that shaped me. I entered medicine with a more mature understanding of dying than many people my age. For me, death was never a topic to avoid. It was part of the conversation.

Then, finally, the day of my father's death came. Erin was with me that early morning when I got the call. Of course, I didn't go into work. As much as I had been expecting my father to die, the news was still a shock. When I arrived at my parents' home an hour after he died, I was able to sit with him, alone. My thoughts wandered. I felt an unexpected sense of relief. I held him gently in my arms and knew, in a profound way, that our time together as father and son was over.

Grieving Alzheimer's—Living with Ambiguous Loss

Grief from Alzheimer's is different from other kinds of loss. You don't grieve just once or twice. It comes in layers, over and over.

There is the sorrow that arrives after the diagnosis, when you realize your loved one is changing. You feel it again when they begin to forget important dates, familiar places, sometimes even you. You mourn the future you thought you would share, the memories you expected to make. Because Alzheimer's progresses slowly, the grieving stretches for months and years. And when death comes, you face yet another moment—the deep, familiar ache that settles in when someone you love is truly gone.

This layered experience is called ambiguous loss. Unlike a sudden death, where the loss is clear and final, ambiguous loss happens while the person is still physically present but slowly fading away in mind, memory, and ability. It is the heartbreak of holding on while letting go. This kind of grief is complicated because it doesn't follow a straightforward path. It rises, recedes, and resurfaces—often unexpectedly.

My grief became harder to manage when I moved home. Living far away, I could notice the changes in my dad's voice over the phone, but I didn't see it or feel it in the same way. Years later, when I sat with him, the losses became real and tangible. I bore witness to them. I carried them.

I now find myself grieving the most—not because I haven't accepted his death but because I miss him. I yearn to talk with him about my own children, my patients, and his life when he was my age. I want to hear his stories in a way I never could have appreciated when I was younger.

This is the grief that lingers. It doesn't disappear—it softens, it changes, it lives alongside you. Sometimes it fades into the background, sometimes it surges like a tsunami, but it becomes part of you. In time, you don't try to erase it. You simply feel it, accept it, and wipe it away like tears—until the next reminder brings it back.

CREATE FAMILY RITUALS

As the end approaches, each family finds its own way to show devotion to its loved one. Some bake a different pie each day of the week. Others might watch home movies or gather to sing favorite songs. These small acts can be a beautiful way to honor a family's story and life together. They also help children recognize and acknowledge what their parents are going through. Families should lean into these moments—they will only strengthen the bonds between siblings and loved ones.

The traditions we create, large and small, become sacred touchstones. These are not mere habits—they are acts of love and the bonds that weave us ever more tightly together. Rituals give us structure when the future feels uncertain. They help us stay present and create meaning amid the sadness. Some families may draw comfort from religious customs, others in cultural practices, and some from entirely new expressions of connection. There is no right or wrong way to honor this time.

You may find yourself doing things you never imagined you would do, if only to please a relative. My mom got into Reiki toward the middle and end stages of my father's disease. In this Japanese alternative healing practice, the practitioner places her hands on or just above another person with the goal of creating a state of calmness. My mother brought in a Reiki master, and we all sat around the living room, including my dad, who was still able to sit upright. The master talked about energy and Reiki to train us to be certified Reiki providers.

My sister is a family medicine doctor, and she and I exchanged glances. I know we both initially thought, *Oh, my God, we've hired a fortune teller. This is like something out of a movie about some goofy family.* We were humoring my mom, but I confess there was something to what was going on. Because we were all emotional about my dad, we all felt this sense of energy, love, and passion. Later, my mom had my sister and me perform Reiki on my dad, and we did so with full intention. We weren't faking it. It felt good. We were connecting as much with our mother as we were with our father.

My Sister Maggie's Reflections—One Year Later

My five-year-old son Jack is obsessed with getting older. It's with such pride that he announces to people that he is now five and one-quarter, then five and one-half as the months tick by. With kindergarten in full swing, he's already talking about birthday parties and the day he'll finally turn six.

It's hard for me not to share in his excitement. I'm continually in awe of this little person we created who grows, learns, and loves with such a big heart. And yet his birthday also marks one full year since my father passed away.

What is a year? I've lived over thirty-eight of them, spending more than sixteen of those with my husband Nat, and now almost six with my son. But for thirty-seven of those years, I had my dad. It seems like so much time, and yet it wasn't nearly enough.

Having a child makes you think much more about your own parents and childhood. I see now how adolescents pull away from their parents for reasons that have nothing to do with how "good" they were. The next decades are often spent looking outward—seeking new experiences, friendships, and careers. But when you have your own child, you start to look inward again and focus more on family and community. In my medical practice as a family physician, I see how patients gradually narrow their social circles to those they find most meaningful.

I'm not stuck on the unfairness of my dad's early death, but I grieve the loss. And perhaps I grieve it more because his death also changed my mom.

My mom is the strongest person I know. "Strong" sounds cliché, but for her, it's all encompassing. In our small family—where three out of the four of us are doctors—her strengths have probably outshined us. Her ability to understand others, her loyalty, her community building, her confidence and self-acceptance are the very qualities that allowed her to care for my dad for over seven years. I sometimes wonder, "Could I do that for my husband?" Then I feel it deep inside me—yes, I could—*because I am my mother's daughter.*

I haven't reflected on my dad's passing until now for many reasons. As the daughter who wasn't there day-to-day, I was distanced from the suffering my mom and brother carried. Instead, I carried guilt. It became such a constant companion that I stopped fighting it. So, when my dad died, I felt guiltily relieved that my mom and brother would finally have some release. I also felt my dad had a great life and, given the circumstances, an incredible end. While I would have loved to have had more time with him, I'm incredibly grateful for what he gave me, and I believe he knew that. I now struggle with how to support my mom.

In the months since my dad passed, my mom has sent me emails and videos about grieving. I've read them briefly but have left them bolded and unread in my inbox. I don't know how to respond to her grief, which is different from mine. I see those unread emails every day, and they remind me of her. I could unbold them, but this is how I punish myself.

I'm not sure I will ever fully understand what this experience has been for my mom. Maybe it would be like someday expecting Jack to understand the stress and sacrifice I now encounter trying to be both a great doctor and mother. Maybe the time for understanding just isn't now.

Some time after my father died, I took an intensive weeklong class in San Francisco where I learned how to relieve pain and stress with acupuncture. I did so as an homage to my father, who incorporated this form of Chinese medicine in his practice. I believe it stimulates the nervous system to release neurochemicals like endorphins while also modulating the responsiveness of the autonomic nervous system. It helps bridge the connection between body and mind. Like deep breathing, these practices can have both physiological and psychological effects.

Throughout this book, I've emphasized the value of habits and practices. When it comes to supporting someone at the end of life, you don't need to be an expert. Try different approaches and see what feels right. Take a class, whether in person or online. You may find someone or something that resonates with you and, more important, with the person for whom you're caring.

Faith-based rituals can offer deep solace. Praying, reading sacred texts, singing hymns, lighting candles, or simply sitting together in silence can become anchoring moments. Even for families who don't consider themselves religious, ritual can emerge through repetition and intention—gathering at the same time each day, sharing stories, listening to music, or holding hands before saying goodbye.

At the end, my mother spoke to my father about all the memorable times in their past. She traced their life story. She talked about his work, his childhood, and their marriage. My sister and I reminisced about our travels because, as much as my father loved his work, his memories of seeing the world remained vivid and clear to him. My mother repeated her stories again and again. It was beautiful for my sister and me to witness. For me, it was almost too much to take, but my mother made those visits down memory lane every day. All the while, my father sat there listening, mostly passively, with his eyes open. He was looking around, still verbalizing and making sounds of enjoyment. As if my mother's monologues weren't emotional enough, she almost always held my father's hand while she spoke.

Handholding, storytelling, touch—these small rituals are often more powerful than we realize. They create a sense of safety and presence for both the dying and the living.

Music is one of the most enduring rituals we can offer. It connects to deep memory, provides comfort, and can transcend words when language begins to fail. My family had another ritual—singing Christmas carols to my father. He loved Christmas songs. My mother began singing to him, sometimes gently and sometimes with gusto, in August five months before he died. Thanks to his embedded long-term memory, he sometimes sang along, too. Even four months before he passed away, he could remember his favorite stanzas and join in. "Silent Night" celebrates the birth of Christ, but when you are at your dying father's bedside murmuring, "Sleep in heavenly peace," the song takes on a different meaning.

I was raised in the Episcopal Church. I believe in an afterlife, though I don't know what it will look like, and my vision of it has evolved throughout my life. I don't believe the Earth and life on it happened by chance. There is something greater than us in the universe. My patients' stories—and now my own—have taught me not to look to the sky for proof but to find it in the people and the world around us.

If you think doctors might be less religious than other people because seeing so much suffering and death hardens them and makes them cynical, you would be wrong. A 2005 University of Chicago study of physicians' beliefs found that 76 percent of doctors believe in God, and 59 percent believe in some kind of life after death. Physicians witness so many births, deaths, and every possible human joy and grief in between that we as a profession are privileged to witness the holiness of life on a daily basis. As a result, perhaps we spend more time marveling at the mysteries of existence than other people. Can it be possible that we are here thanks to the operation of random chance over billions of years? Maybe so, but in my heart, I think there is more—something unseen, something we touch when we give a hug, share a meal, or say goodbye. I have come to believe that the sacred is not distant. It is right here, woven into the moments we share, the stories we tell, and the love we leave behind.

SIX HOSPICE MISCONCEPTIONS

How we die matters. We may not be able to control when we die, but we often have some say in how the process unfolds. More and more people are choosing to die at home, surrounded by the people and places they love. Hospice can play an important role in supporting that choice and providing comfort along the way. Here are six common misconceptions people have about this wonderful service:

1. **Hospice is a place people go to in their final months or weeks.** While some hospitals and nursing homes have dedicated hospice wards, hospice is more often a service that travels to wherever the patient is. For many families, the ideal choice is for their loved one to pass away in a peaceful, familiar setting while being cared for by family members.

   In larger cities, there are often several hospice agencies to choose from. While their offerings may vary slightly, all typically provide core services and will go to the patient's location.

   While under the care of hospice, members of an interdisciplinary team visit once or twice a week or more often if needed. They assess the patient, manage care, and deliver medications, medical supplies, and equipment. The hospice team is typically led by a physician, though it's the nurse you'll see most often. The team may also include a social worker, spiritual counselor, and volunteers. A member of the medical team is always on call twenty-four hours a day to answer questions and respond to emergencies.
2. **Hospice continues curative medical treatments.** That's not the case. Hospice care is a form of palliative care, which is designed to manage symptoms and improve quality of life. Palliative care can complement curative treatments, but when it reaches the hospice stage, the focus shifts solely to symptom management. (See the sidebar on page 359 for more on the differences between hospice care and palliative care.)
3. **Hospice hastens death.** Not so. Hospice focuses on providing comfort as life nears its end. It does not attempt to postpone death. Hospice simply accepts its inevitability and helps people live as fully and comfortably as possible during their remaining time.

   A patient can receive hospice care only if a doctor certifies that she is likely to live fewer than six months. Some patients—like former President Jimmy Carter and my father—live longer than expected. In those cases, the family and physician must seek hospice recertification every six months. (President Carter was in hospice nearly two years.)
4. **Hospice is costly.** That's not true. Hospice is fully covered for any-

one enrolled in Medicare. Medicaid covers hospice in many states, and private insurance plans also provide hospice benefits.

5. **Hospice nurses do all the work.** Hospice nurses and medical professionals visit regularly, but most of the hands-on daily care is provided by family or privately hired help. Hospice at home doesn't mean there's a live-in nurse or rotating nursing shifts.
6. **Hospice is just nursing care.** While families are the primary caregivers, hospice offers guidance and support, and staff will step in as needed. Many programs provide resources on meditation, music therapy, pet therapy, aromatherapy, and bereavement counseling. Hospice cares for the whole person and the entire family.

The greatest gift of hospice is the control it offers. In hospice, the patient and family guide the care—shaping it to reflect their values, priorities, and beliefs. Just as important is the atmosphere itself. Most hospice settings are intentionally designed to feel homey, soothing, and calm. There are no medical devices beeping, no intercoms blaring, and no middle-of-the-night checks of vital signs. Instead, the environment is quiet and reassuring, often filled with staff and volunteers who are clearly in the right jobs—people whose presence alone conveys steadiness and compassion. Being in a place where others are walking the same path, and where no one feels frantic about it, can create a quiet solidarity that eases the weight of the moment.

The sad reality is that most people are only in hospice care for an average of two weeks. Because of the stigma and misconceptions surrounding hospice, many wait too long to fully benefit from the support it can provide.

What the Doctor Needs to Know

When a patient is actively dying, the doctor's role changes. It's not about standing in the way of death with more tests, drugs, or procedures. Instead, the role shifts toward presence, steadiness, and support. Families look to the physician for guidance not only in managing symptoms but also in understanding what is happening and what to expect.

The first responsibility is to ensure that no one suffers. Pain, shortness of breath, and anxiety must be treated quickly and consistently. These interventions are not just medical; they communicate compassion and reassurance to families who may be frightened by what they see. When pain and agitation are under control, loved ones can redirect their energy toward being present, saying what needs to be said, and beginning the process of letting go.

Doctors also serve as a resource and a foundation for the rest of the care team. Nurses, social workers, chaplains, and aides all play essential roles in the final days, but the physician's steadiness can bring cohesion. By answering questions, clarifying the plan, and reaffirming the goals of care, the doctor anchors the team and the family.

Equally important is demeanor. If the physician shows fear, families will mirror it. If the physician demonstrates calm and confidence, it creates space for trust. This does not mean denying the gravity of the moment—it means holding it honestly and without panic.

What doctors need to know, above all, is that their presence matters. Even when the outcome is inevitable, how a doctor carries herself can shape the memory of a patient's final days. In the end, the work is not to treat death but to honor it with dignity, comfort, and the reassurance that no one is alone.

A GOOD DEATH

A good death is usually preceded by a thoughtful life. My mother believes this. She talks about it openly, perhaps too much, and always without fear. After losing my dad—her husband—she feels closer to the end, but not in despair about it. She misses him deeply, and it's obvious when I visit. In some ways, she feels more ready than I am. I want her to stay. I selfishly want more time—for me, and for my children.

She tells me to stop thinking so much, to feel more. Her advice is simple: Stop scripting memories and just live them. She says that death, when accepted, reminds us to appreciate the present moment. Awareness gives life its sharpness, its beauty. I'm still scared of death. I have little boys. I want more time. I want a long, meaningful life, one that is filled with moments I don't just capture but inhabit.

My mother wrote me the following message, and I've held onto it. At the time, I was overwhelmed—torn between the pull of a new career that gave me purpose and energy and that of being with my boys, whom I love more than anything. From my father's death, I had learned the true importance of being present with my family, and so I didn't know how to give fully to both, or even if it was possible. In those moments of tension, I tried to record everything I could.

> Don't always take snapshots with your cell phone. Those are just pictures stored externally. Truly capture what's in front of you, and blink—that operates the shutter of your mind. Keep your memories and their sensations close and tactile. These will serve you far better than any digital image. When your senses are fully alive in a visual experience, the memory becomes deeply ingrained. You will always have it in a way no photograph ever could.

My mom constantly researches information online. She's curious, relentless, and unafraid to dive deep into obscure corners of knowledge. She sends me Latin phrases she stumbles upon, such as *compos mentis*, which means "of sound mind." Then she'll tell me where the phrase comes from, reminding me that the Latin root of *mentis* is *mens*, which means "mind" or "intellect." She often says that even people with dementia have a form of *mentis*. Their inner vision shifts as the pathways in their brains change. But their being, perhaps even their essence, remains. The mind may be rewired, but the soul stays in subtle and profound ways. Dementia doesn't erase the mind. The external signs may fade, but what is essential remains.

In the end, her message is clear: Live thoughtfully. Love deeply. Feel fully. And when the time comes—may you have a good death, held in the arms of a life well lived.

So, while I wrestle with the idea of death, my mother embraces it. We continue to meet in the space between.

Afterword

THE NEW BEGINNING

When I moved home to help care for my dad, it marked the beginning of my transformation. It wasn't just a change in residence or medicine specialty—it was a reorientation in *how* I live. Gradually, I began to incorporate the brain health strategies outlined in chapter 5, starting with a daily run on a treadmill while listening to audiobooks and podcasts on dementia and brain science.

I fear Alzheimer's—as anyone with a family history does—but it has also been my teacher, reminding me to live fully and appreciate what's right in front of me. That awareness led me to ask: What does it really mean to live well? Not in theory, or ideally, but in our daily choices. We don't get to choose what takes us, but we do get to choose how we show up each day.

That question has been at the core of this book. It should be one you ask yourself every day, regardless of how old you are. I hope reflecting on it helps challenge the stigma surrounding cognitive aging and disease. It's vital that you understand which changes are normal and which ones are not. It's equally important to realize that there's much you can do to improve your brain and your life. Don't be afraid to ask questions. Talk to your family, your friends, your doctor. Seek an evaluation. Don't hide from fear—confront it head-on with curiosity and courage.

Too often, we settle for managing our health. We treat chronic conditions like obesity, high blood pressure, and depression with medications alone. But we need to move beyond that mindset. Optimizing our health—sometimes even reversing disease—begins with whole foods. Eat nourishing meals and recognize that what you eat is more than sustenance—it's an investment in your future. Move your body every day. You don't have to train like an Olympian to feel the benefits—regular physical activity is one of the most powerful tools we have for lifelong brain and body health.

Exercise, in turn, often improves sleep and reduces stress—two of the most underrated yet foundational habits for brain resilience. Prioritize rest. Try to live with a sense of calm. Connect with others, nurture relationships, and cultivate a supportive community.

Even during the writing of this book, the field of Alzheimer's took monumental steps forward. The FDA approved the first-ever blood test to help confirm Alzheimer's disease, removing the uncertainty in a diagnosis. PET scans became more widely used in clinics due to the rollout of two novel disease-modifying therapies that slow progression. Research is accelerating, with prevention trials that advance the goal of delaying or even preventing symptoms before they appear. Remarkable work is underway.

Despite these breakthroughs, trust in science has eroded—in part due to pandemic misinformation and a polarized political climate. Two Pew polls, in 2023 and 2024, showed that fewer Americans express confidence in scientists than they did before Covid-19. Meanwhile, healthcare has grown more expensive, more complex, and harder to access. No wonder—it's burdened by administrative hurdles, insurance restrictions, and pressures on care providers that limit how much time they can spend with patients. Many clinicians want to focus on prevention, lifestyle, and social-environmental influences of health, but the system remains centered on disease after it appears and driven by financial margins.

We cannot depend on healthcare alone to meet all our needs. We must advocate for ourselves and our loved ones by investing in our health, seeking out knowledge, and being committed to take action. That doesn't mean chasing trends—it means asking thoughtful questions, seeking real evidence, and taking responsibility for the decisions that shape our lives.

This book began with a different question: What do we do when memory begins to fade? As you've read each page, I hope you've found more than facts and advice. I hope this book has given you a new perspective on what to expect at every stage—from early signs to full support for Alzheimer's and dementia. A diagnosis isn't the end. The path ahead may not be what you anticipated or wanted, but it can be beautiful and fulfilling. Life doesn't stop having purpose unless you let it. So, live with intention and gratitude—and never, ever give up hope.

Hope is not just a feeling—it's a practice. A commitment we make to ourselves again and again.

Acknowledgments

This book would not be possible without the steadfast love and support of my family. From the first sentence to the final draft, they made space for this work in every sense of the word.

My wife Erin carried the weight of this project just as much as I did—though in different, and arguably more difficult, ways. She took on more responsibilities at home, gave me the time and room to write, and held our family together through the moments when I wasn't fully present. She endured the emotional turbulence this process sometimes brought out in me, offering patience, compassion, and grace even when I probably didn't deserve it. I'm grateful I married a woman with such strength and tenacity—I needed every bit of it during this writing process while she cared for everything else in our lives. I love her more than I can express.

Our sons Auggie and Bennett brought a kind of support all their own. They never voiced resentment about the time I gave to this project. Instead, they found ways to become part of it. I will never forget walking into my office to find one of them sitting in my chair, tapping away at the keyboard and announcing they were writing "just like Daddy." Their laughter, curiosity, and love reminded me why this work mattered in the first place. They kept me grounded and gave me lightness when I needed it most.

My mother Karen is an inspiration to me. She is the living definition of resilience and dedication. While she wasn't always gentle—and at times, quite blunt—when reviewing my drafts, her honesty made the book stronger and brought depth and humanity to its pages. She didn't want to be mentioned here at all, so as a compromise, I'll simply say, *thank you.*

My sister Maggie got lovingly roped into this process—as only a sibling can be. I leaned on her for advice, and she offered feedback on chapters, both as a primary care physician and as a fellow family member affected by the disease. She helped me think through ideas and remember family stories. We still debate as passionately with each other as we do with our mom, and I wouldn't want it any other way, or with any other person.

I am also grateful to my aunt Kathryn Weaver, attorney and my mom's twin sister, who generously read several chapters—especially those dealing with legal issues. Her clear-eyed guidance strengthened this book and kept me out of trouble.

I was also fortunate to have the support of my mother-in-law Cathy Ruegg and our nanny Amelia Stoeberl, who helped care for our boys with such warmth, devotion, and deep affection. Their love for our children gave me the peace of mind and focus to write.

Outside my family, I was supported by a number of people who believed in the book. My agent Linda Konner and my editor Elizabeth Beier saw potential in my writing and in me. Their belief and encouragement were instrumental in bringing this project to life. Elizabeth, in particular, brought an invaluable editorial perspective during the review process—her instincts and revisions elevated the book to another level.

I am thankful to my friends Jeni Synnes, Tammy Heinrichs, and Dave Cieslewicz, who provided thoughtful feedback on chapters and helped sharpen my voice and refine the message. Their care, time, and insight left a lasting mark on the final version.

I also deeply appreciate the editing expertise of Ann Shaffer and Dustin Beilke. They helped me fine-tune my message and keep the writing clear, accessible, and light on medical jargon.

I've been lucky to work under the guidance of leaders who have profoundly shaped my career. Dr. Sanjay Asthana, the founding director of the Wisconsin Alzheimer's Disease Research Center, has long been a mentor like no other. His trust in me and the space he created for my growth gave me the foundation to rise into roles I once only dreamed about. He never doubted the path I was on—or the impact I could make. That kind of certainty is a rare and precious gift. Dr. Sterling Johnson has been one of the best colleagues I could hope for. His confidence in me, his generosity, and his steady support have made all the difference. He's a visionary in the field and a man I continue to learn from, and his unflinching belief that research is a public service—meant to be shared widely—is inspiring. I wouldn't want to face the next ten years of research working alongside anyone else.

I also want to thank collaborators and colleagues who helped improve the content of this book. Tori Williams, Adrienne Johnson, Cindy Carlsson, Andrea Gilmore-Bykovskyi, and Bonnie Nuttkinson all offered insights that helped me shape the narrative into something more grounded, inclusive, and honest.

This book also owes a quiet debt to the many conversations I've had as host of the *Dementia Matters* podcast. The guests—researchers, clinicians, advocates—continue to enrich my perspective. Every interview makes me more thoughtful, more reflective, and more hopeful. To our listeners, thank you for your encouragement, and for letting me know that this work matters to you. Your support strengthens my resolve.

The work I do is only possible because of the people I do it in partnership with. The physicians, social workers, nurses, medical assistants, schedulers, nurse practitioners, and clinic managers I collaborate with each day have shown me—through unspoken acts and consistent presence—what it truly means to care for another human being. They remind me that compassion isn't simply a virtue—it's a practice, refined daily through dedication, patience, and empathy.

Equally essential are those we care for. Our patients, research participants, and their families and friends have entrusted us with their stories and their vulnerability. Their courage gives me light and direction, especially when the path forward feels uncertain. I carry their voices with me in everything I do, and this book is, in many ways, an extension of that shared experience.

This book wouldn't exist without the steady partnership of my cowriter George Spencer. We met when the University of Wisconsin's alumni magazine asked him to profile me. He encouraged me to write this book, and what began as a spark turned into more than a year of collaboration—at times messy, sometimes challenging, but always rewarding. We've created something lasting, and I'm grateful for his talent, insight, and friendship.

At the heart of all this stands my father, Moe Chin. He gave his life to his family, his patients, and his calling. He is the reason I have a meaningful career. I can never fully thank him for helping me find my own purpose and voice. His life continues to guide mine—quietly, steadily, and always forward.

Resources

These organizations, websites, podcasts, and books are recommended by my Alzheimer's Disease Research Center and UW Health memory clinic, and they reflect sources I've turned to in caring for patients, conducting research, or writing this book.

NATIONAL AGENCIES AND GOVERNMENT-SPONSORED INITIATIVES

National Institute on Aging (NIA)
https://www.nia.nih.gov
Comprehensive federal resource on brain aging, dementia research, clinical trials, and caregiving.

Alzheimers.gov (Managed by NIA)
https://www.alzheimers.gov
Centralized access to Alzheimer's and dementia information, support for patients and families, and research updates.

Alzheimer's Disease Education and Referral (ADEAR) Center
https://www.nia.nih.gov/health/alzheimers-and-dementia
Extensive resources for health professionals, families, and the public.

Administration for Community Living (ACL)
https://acl.gov
Support for older adults and people with disabilities, including dementia-related services.

National Library of Medicine—MedlinePlus

https://medlineplus.gov

Plain-language summaries of medical conditions, medications, and diagnostic procedures.

Alzheimer's Disease Research Centers (ADRCs)

I work at the Wisconsin ADRC—https://adrc.wisc.edu

Thirty-six academic hubs offering opportunities for research participation and access to expert care.

LEADING ALZHEIMER'S ORGANIZATIONS

Alzheimer's Foundation of America (AFA)

https://www.alzfdn.org | (866) 232-8484

Caregiver education, memory screening tools, and daily virtual support programs. Offers a national helpline staffed by licensed social workers and resources to promote brain health and dementia awareness.

Alzheimer's Association

https://www.alz.org | 24/7 Helpline: (800) 272-3900

National leader in education, research, community programs, and advocacy. Offers support groups, care consultations, and a chapter locator.

Community Resource Finder

https://www.communityresourcefinder.org

Searchable database sponsored by the Alzheimer's Association and AARP for care services, housing, and support in your area.

ALZConnected

https://www.alzconnected.org | (800) 272-3900

Online community for people living with dementia and caregivers to share support.

UsAgainstAlzheimer's

https://www.usagainstalzheimers.org | (202) 410-5199

Focus on advocacy, public policy, and health equity. Connects families, caregivers, and communities to resources and opportunities to advance progress against Alzheimer's.

CONDITION-SPECIFIC ORGANIZATIONS

Lewy Body Dementia Association (LBDA)

https://www.lbda.org

Education, support, and clinical updates specific to Lewy body dementia.

Association for Frontotemporal Degeneration (AFTD)

https://www.theaftd.org

Focused on early-onset and atypical dementias, including behavioral and language variants of FTD.

Parkinson's Foundation

https://www.parkinson.org

Dedicated to improving care and advancing research for people living with Parkinson's disease. Offers expert resources on symptoms, diagnosis, treatment, and dementia-related progression.

CAREGIVER SUPPORT AND TOOLS

Family Caregiver Alliance (FCA)

https://www.caregiver.org

Legal, financial, emotional, and practical guidance for caregivers of older adults with cognitive impairments.

Caregiver Action Network

https://www.caregiveraction.org | (855) 227-3640

Caregiver tips, depression screening tools, respite care resources, and post-loss support.

AARP—Caregiving and Brain Health

https://www.aarp.org/caregiving

https://stayingsharp.aarp.org/about/brain-health/the-science/

Legal, financial, and wellness tools for caregivers and aging individuals.

Dementia-Friendly Toolkit (UW-Madison CARE Center)

https://wai.wisc.edu/for-caregivers

Training videos and communication strategies for engaging with people living with dementia.

Assisting Cognitively Impaired Individuals with Voting
https://www.americanbar.org/groups/law_aging/resources/voting_cognitive_impairments/
Prepared by the American Bar Association Commission on Law and Aging and the Penn Memory Center. Gives guidance for supporting voting rights of cognitively impaired individuals.

EDUCATIONAL AND MEDIA RESOURCES

***Dementia Matters* Podcast (Hosted by the Wisconsin ADRC and Dr. Nathaniel Chin)**
https://www.adrc.wisc.edu/dementia-matters
Interviews with researchers, clinicians, and caregivers.

***GeriPal* Podcast**
https://geripal.org/geripal-podcast/
Geriatric and palliative care perspectives with humor and compassion.

***Spotlight on Care* Podcast (Hosted by UCI MIND and the California Caregiver Resource Center)**
https://mind.uci.edu/mindcast/#spotlight
Candid conversations about the realities of caregiving, featuring experts and care partners.

BrainStorm
https://www.usagainstalzheimers.org/brainstorm
Podcast by UsAgainstAlzheimer's exploring the lived experience of brain health.

ISTAART Voices
https://istaart.alz.org/podcasts
Expert conversations on the science and impact of Alzheimer's disease.

World Alzheimer's Report
https://www.alzint.org/what-we-do/research/world-alzheimer-report/
Annual research summaries and global dementia trends from Alzheimer's Disease International.

Alzheimer's Association Annual Report
https://www.alz.org/about/annual-report
Tracks progress in advocacy, care, and research funding.

Teepa Snow—Positive Approach to Care
https://teepasnow.com
Dementia education, caregiving techniques, and communication strategies.

Being Patient
https://www.beingpatient.com
Digital newsroom dedicated to Alzheimer's news, personal stories, and expert commentary.

National Sleep Foundation
https://www.thensf.org
Information on the intersection of sleep health and cognitive disorders.

Lorenzo's House
https://lorenzoshouse.org
Connects individuals living with younger-onset dementia and their families through care partner education, youth programs, community, and innovative support models.

Voices of Alzheimer's
https://www.voicesofad.com
A platform dedicated to amplifying the voices of people living with Alzheimer's disease.

Brain Donor Project
https://braindonorproject.org
Advice on brain donation for research into neurological diseases.

MindCare Collective
https://www.mindcare.org.au
Multilingual comics and videos about dementia tailored to culturally and linguistically diverse communities.

GENERAL AGING AND ELDERCARE RESOURCES

AgingCare
https://www.agingcare.com
Online resource for family caregiving, eldercare, and support networks.

Eldercare Locator
https://eldercare.acl.gov
Connects caregivers with local services and community agencies.

RECOMMENDED BOOKS

High-Octane Brain by Dr. Michelle Braun
Remember by Lisa Genova
The Power of Habit by Charles Duhigg
Atomic Habits by James Clear
Why We Sleep by Matthew Walker
Wherever You Go, There You Are: Mindfulness Meditation in Everyday Life by Jon Kabat-Zinn
The Blue Zones by Dan Buettner
Mayo Clinic on Alzheimer's Disease and Other Dementias, Revised and Updated by Dr. Jonathan Graff-Radford and Angela Lunde
Super Brain by Deepak Chopra and Rudolph Tanzi
Keep Sharp: Build a Better Brain at Any Age by Dr. Sanjay Gupta
Memory Rescue by Dr. Daniel Amen
My Two Elaines by Martin J. Schreiber
Until My Memory Fails Me by Sharon Lukert
Creative Care by Dr. Anne Basting
The Problem of Alzheimer's: How Science, Culture, and Politics Turned a Rare Disease into a Crisis and What We Can Do About It by Dr. Jason Karlawish

Glossary

CHAPTER 1

Alzheimer's disease—A progressive brain disorder and the most common cause of dementia, affecting memory, thinking, and behavior.

amyloid—A sticky protein that can build up in the brain and is part of the biological definition of Alzheimer's disease.

apathy—A lack of motivation or interest, common in many types of dementia.

atrophy—Shrinking or wasting away of body tissue, such as the brain in dementia.

autopsy—An examination of the body after death to determine cause of death or disease.

axon—The long part of a nerve cell that sends signals to other cells.

biomarker—A measurable sign, like a protein or brain image, that indicates disease is present.

cerebrovascular disease—A group of conditions—including stroke and small vessel disease—that affect blood flow to the brain and can lead to dementia.

cognition—The mental processes of learning, memory, attention, and problem-solving.

cognitive change/cognitive decline—A noticeable difference in how someone thinks, remembers, or processes information.

cognitive disorder—A medical condition that affects a person's ability to think, remember, or make decisions.

cognitive domain—A specific area of mental function in the brain, such as memory, attention, or language.

cognitive screening tests—Short assessments used to check for problems with memory, language, or thinking.

dementia—A general term for decline in memory and thinking that is severe enough to affect daily life.

delirium—A sudden, temporary state of confusion, often caused by illness or medication.

dendrite—A branch-like part of a nerve cell that receives signals from other cells.

executive function—Mental skills that help with planning, decision-making, and reasoning.

hippocampus—A small, curved structure deep in the brain that plays a major role in forming new memories and helping with learning and navigation; it is one of the first areas affected in Alzheimer's disease.

hospice—Care that focuses on comfort and quality of life for people nearing the end of life.

Lewy body disease—A type of progressive dementia caused by abnormal protein deposits in the brain, often involving hallucinations, movement issues, and fluctuating cognition.

mixed dementia—A type of dementia involving more than one cause, such as the combination of Alzheimer's and vascular disease.

mild cognitive impairment (MCI)—A condition of noticeable cognitive decline that doesn't yet interfere significantly with daily functioning.

neurogenesis—The brain's ability to create new nerve cells.

neurotransmitters—Chemical messengers that carry signals between nerve cells in the brain.

pathologist—A doctor who studies body tissues and organs to understand disease.

posterior cortical atrophy (PCA)—A rare dementia that affects visual processing first, making it hard to read or judge distances.

primary progressive aphasia (PPA)—A type of dementia where language abilities gradually decline, often before memory is affected.

short-term memory—The ability to remember information from moments ago.

social determinants of health—Life factors like education, income, and housing that influence a person's health.

synapse—The small gap between nerve cells where messages are passed between axons and dendrites.

tau—A protein in the brain that can form tangles and is part of the biological definition of Alzheimer's disease. Different forms also contribute to other dementias.

visual-spatial skill—The ability to understand where objects are in space.

CHAPTER 2

ADRC—Alzheimer's Disease Research Center, where scientists study dementia and its treatment.

autosomal dominant Alzheimer's—A rare, inherited form of Alzheimer's passed through families.

donanemab—A monoclonal antibody drug that targets amyloid buildup in the brain.

lecanemab—A monoclonal antibody drug that targets amyloid buildup in the brain.

monoclonal antibody treatments—Lab-made proteins designed to target harmful substances such as amyloid in the brain.

WRAP study—Wisconsin Registry for Alzheimer's Prevention, a long-term research study focused on identifying early signs of Alzheimer's disease.

young-onset dementia—Dementia that begins before the age of sixty-five.

CHAPTER 3

ADLs—Activities of daily living, like bathing, dressing, eating, and using the bathroom.

advance care planning—Making decisions in advance about the kind of medical care you want later in life.

anticholinergic—A property of some medications that can interfere with memory and thinking by blocking a key brain chemical (acetylcholine).

brain disease—Any illness or disorder that affects brain structure or function.

chronic health condition—A long-lasting medical problem like diabetes or heart disease.

cognitive evaluation—A detailed assessment to determine if memory and thinking symptoms are related to age or represent an underlying abnormal process.

collateral historian—Someone who provides reliable information about a patient.

comorbid—Medical conditions that often coexist and affect a person's health, like having high blood pressure and high cholesterol.

functional history—A description of how a person manages daily activities and routines.

function—The ability to perform tasks and live independently.

general practitioner—A primary care doctor who treats a broad range of health issues.

geriatrician—A doctor who specializes in the care of older adults.

IADLs—Instrumental activities of daily living, such as cooking, shopping, and managing money.

memory clinic—A center that evaluates and treats people with memory problems.

memory specialist—A clinician who focuses on diagnosing and treating memory problems.

neurodegenerative disease—A disease that causes brain cells to break down or die.

neurologist—A doctor who treats conditions of the brain and nervous system.

neuron—A brain cell that sends and receives information through electrical and chemical signals.

neuropsychological evaluation—A set of tests that measure various aspects of thinking and memory.

neuropsychologist—A specialist who tests brain function through standardized assessments.

reversible or modifiable causes—Factors that can be treated to improve memory or thinking.

sleep apnea—A condition where breathing stops briefly during sleep.

social worker—A professional who helps with emotional support, resources, and care coordination.

CHAPTER 4

advance directive—A document stating a person's medical wishes in case they can't speak for themselves.

autonomy—The ability to make personal decisions independently.

caregiver burnout—Physical, emotional, and mental exhaustion from long-term caregiving.

cognitive impairment—Trouble with thinking or memory that is greater than normal aging.

entrainment—The brain's ability to form patterns and rhythms through repetition.

healthcare power of attorney (HCPOA)—A type of power of attorney that lets someone make medical decisions when a person can't.

intestate—Dying without a legal will in place.

neuroplasticity—The brain's ability to change and adapt through learning or after injury.

power of attorney (POA)—A legal document that lets someone make decisions on another's behalf.

respite—Temporary relief for caregivers, giving them time to rest or take a break.

social isolation—A lack of regular, meaningful interaction with others.

staging (of Alzheimer's)—A way to describe the progression of the disease in defined steps.

trust—A legal arrangement allowing a third party to manage assets for someone else.

CHAPTER 5

habit stacking—Building a new habit by linking it to an existing one.

keystone habit—A habit that triggers positive changes in other areas of life.

lifestyle intervention—A program aimed at improving health behaviors like diet and exercise.

neural pathways—Connections between brain cells formed through repeated actions or thoughts.

sedentary behavior—Spending a lot of time sitting or refraining from activity.

synaptogenesis—The process by which new synapses (connections between nerve cells) are formed in the brain, allowing neurons to communicate and supporting learning, memory, and brain development.

CHAPTER 6

amyloid cascade hypothesis—A theory that amyloid buildup starts a harmful chain of events in the brain.

APOE—A gene that can affect a person's risk of developing Alzheimer's disease.

ARIA (amyloid-related imaging abnormalities)—A side effect from some Alzheimer's treatments that includes brain swelling or bleeding.

deprescribe—To safely reduce or stop medications that may no longer be needed.

Memory Café—A social event for people with memory loss and their care partners.

respite care—Short-term care for someone with dementia to give the caregiver a break.

selection bias—A problem in studies where the participants don't represent the general population.

CHAPTER 7

behavioral symptom—A change in mood, behavior, or personality caused by dementia.

caregiver—A person who helps someone with a chronic illness or disability.

executive function—Mental skills that help with planning, decision-making, and self-control.

mild-stage dementia—The early phase of dementia when symptoms begin to affect more complicated aspects of daily life, such as instrumental activities of daily living, but not basic activities of daily living.

moderate-stage dementia—The middle phase of dementia when symptoms are more noticeable, disability develops in some basic activities of daily living, and support is often needed.

processing speed—How quickly the brain can understand and respond to information.

triage—The process of deciding who needs medical attention first.

CHAPTER 8

clinical trial—A study that tests how well a treatment or procedure works.

informed consent—Agreeing to take part in research after learning about the risks and benefits.

lumbar puncture—A test where spinal fluid is collected from the lower back to look for signs of disease.

observational study—Research that observes people without giving them an intervention or treatment.

open-label extension—A study phase where everyone, including those on the placebo, gets the real drug.

PET scan—An imaging test that detects small amounts of radioactive tracer to highlight brain activity or specific proteins, such as amyloid or tau.

placebo-controlled—A type of study where some participants get the real treatment and others get a harmless one that has no curative ability.

study partner—A friend or relative who helps someone participating in a research study.

CHAPTER 9

alveoli—Tiny air sacs in the lungs where oxygen and carbon dioxide are exchanged.

aspiration—When food, fluid, or saliva enters the lungs instead of the stomach.

aspiration pneumonia—A lung infection caused by inhaling food, drink, or stomach contents.

autonomic nervous system—The part of the nervous system that controls automatic functions like breathing and heart rate.

bedsores (pressure ulcers)—Skin wounds caused by staying in one position for too long.

dysphagia—Difficulty swallowing, often due to weak muscles or nerve damage.

esophageal sphincter—A muscle at the top of the stomach that keeps food and stomach acid from flowing back up the throat.

homeostasis—The body's way of keeping its internal systems balanced and stable.

hormonal dysregulation—A disruption in the balance of hormones that affects many body functions.

hypercapnia—A buildup of carbon dioxide in the blood, which can cause drowsiness and confusion.

hypoxia—A condition where there's not enough oxygen in the body's tissues.

innervation—The supply of nerves to a body part that allow it to move or feel.

paradoxical lucidity—A brief period of clarity in someone with advanced dementia near the end of life.

peristalsis—Muscle movements that push food and waste through the digestive system.

pituitary gland—A small gland in the brain that controls many of the body's hormones.

swallow reflex—An automatic movement that helps food pass from the mouth to the stomach.

terminal restlessness—Agitation or distress some people experience near the end of life.

uremia—A condition where waste builds up in the blood because the kidneys are not working well.

vagus nerve—A nerve that helps control vital functions like heartbeat and digestion.

Bibliography

CHAPTER 1

Barrett C. When the air hits your brain. BMJ. 2008 Jun 21;336(7658):1441. doi: 10.1136/bmj.39611.510127.4E. PMCID: PMC2432179.

Boyle PA et al. Much of late life cognitive decline is not due to common neurodegenerative pathologies. Ann Neurol. 2013 Sep;74(3):478–489. doi: 10.1002/ana.23964. Epub 2013 Jul 10. PMID: 23798485; PMCID: PMC3845973.

Centers for Medicare & Medicaid Services (CMS). Nursing home data compendium 2015 edition. 2015. https://www.cms.gov/medicare/provider-enrollment-and-certification/certificationandcomplianc/downloads/nursinghomedatacompendium_508-2015.pdf

Cleveland Clinic survey: men will do almost anything to avoid going to the doctor. Cleveland Clinic. 2019 Sep 4. https://newsroom.clevelandclinic.org/2019/09/04/cleveland-clinic-survey-men-will-do-almost-anything-to-avoid-going-to-the-doctor

Handcock, M. "It'll get better on its own": men and their resistance to seeing a doctor. Health Policy Partnership. 2022 Jun 14. https://www.healthpolicypartnership.com/itll-get-better-on-its-own-men-and-their-resistance-to-seeing-a-doctor/

Mayeda ER, Glymour MM, Quesenberry CP, Whitmer RA. Inequalities in dementia incidence between six racial and ethnic groups over 14 years. Alzheimers Dement. 2016 Mar;12(3):216–24. doi: 10.1016/j.jalz.2015.12.007. Epub 2016 Feb 11. PMID: 26874595; PMCID: PMC4969071.

Mormino EC, Papp KV. Amyloid accumulation and cognitive decline in clinically normal older individuals: implications for aging and early Alzheimer's disease.

J Alzheimers Dis. 2018;64(s1):S633–S646. doi: 10.3233/JAD-179928. PMID: 29782318; PMCID: PMC6387885.

Mukherjee S. Emperor of all maladies: a biography of cancer. Scribner; 2010.

Native Americans and Alzheimer's. Alzheimer's Association; [accessed 2025 Sep 27]. https://www.alz.org/help-support/resources/native-americans

Neprash HT et al. Measuring primary care exam length using electronic health record data. Med Care. 2021 Jan;59(1):62–66. doi: 10.1097/MLR.0000000000001450. PMID: 33301282.

Sarcopenia. Cleveland Clinic; [last reviewed 2022 Jun 3]. https://my.clevelandclinic.org/health/diseases/23167-sarcopenia

Schwartz, TH. Gray matters: a biography of brain surgery. Dutton; 2024.

Tang W et al. Concern about developing Alzheimer's disease or dementia and intention to be screened: an analysis of national survey data. Arch Gerontol Geriatr. 2017 Jul;71:43–49. doi: 10.1016/j.archger.2017.02.013. Epub 2017 Mar 1. PMID: 28279898; PMCID: PMC5995109.

Trojanczyk C et al. P4-623: Lessons from a research collaboration with the Oneida nation of Wisconsin. Alzheimer's & Dementia. 2019;15:P1565–P1566. https://doi.org/10.1016/j.jalz.2019.08.172

Vertosick, F, Jr., MD. When the air hits your brain: tales from neurosurgery. W. W. Norton; 1996.

CHAPTER 2

Chin N, host. Dementia Matters, podcast. Let's talk: navigating family conversations about dementia through shared decision-making. Campbell T, guest. 2024 May 14. https://www.adrc.wisc.edu/dementia-matters/lets-talk-navigating-family-conversations-about-dementia

Kaplan M. SPIKES: a framework for breaking bad news to patients with cancer. Clin J Oncol Nurs. 2010 Aug;14(4):514–516. doi: 10.1188/10.CJON.514–516. PMID: 20682509.

Radziewicz R, Baile WF. Communication skills: breaking bad news in the clinical setting. Oncol Nurs Forum. 2001 Jul;28(6):951–953. PMID: 11475881.

CHAPTER 3

Aging and alcohol. National Institute on Alcohol Abuse and Alcoholism; [updated 2024 Dec]. https://www.niaaa.nih.gov/alcohols-effects-health/alcohol-topics/older-adults

Gray SL et al. Cumulative use of strong anticholinergics and incident dementia: a prospective cohort study. JAMA Intern Med. 2015 Mar;175(3):401–407. doi: 10.1001/jamainternmed.2014.7663. PMID: 25621434; PMCID: PMC4358759.

Han BH, Moore AA, Ferris R, Palamar JJ. Binge drinking among older adults in the United States, 2015 to 2017. J Am Geriatr Soc. 2019 Oct;67(10):2139–2144. doi: 10.1111/jgs.16071. Epub 2019 Jul 31. PMID: 31364159; PMCID: PMC6800799.

Kumar RR, Singh L, Thakur A, Singh S, Kumar B. Role of vitamins in neurodegenerative diseases: a review. CNS Neurol Disord Drug Targets. 2022;21(9): 766–773. doi: 10.2174/1871527320666211119122150. PMID: 34802410.

Langa KM et al. A comparison of the prevalence of dementia in the United States in 2000 and 2012. JAMA Intern Med. 2017 Jan 1;177(1):51–58. doi: 10.1001/jamainternmed.2016.6807. PMID: 27893041; PMCID: PMC5195883.

Leopold VJ et al. Is elective total hip arthroplasty safe in nonagenarians? an arthroplasty registry analysis. J Bone Joint Surg Am. 2023 Oct 18;105(20):1583–1593. doi: 10.2106/JBJS.23.00092. Epub 2023 Aug 25. PMID: 37624906.

Sommer I et al. Vitamin D deficiency as a risk factor for dementia: a systematic review and meta-analysis. BMC Geriatr. 2017 Jan 13;17(1):16. doi: 10.1186/s12877-016-0405-0. PMID: 28086755; PMCID: PMC5237198.

Understanding binge drinking. National Institute on Alcohol Abuse and Alcoholism; [updated 2025 Feb]. https://www.niaaa.nih.gov/publications/brochures-and-fact-sheets/binge-drinking

Vyas CM et al. Effect of multivitamin-mineral supplementation versus placebo on cognitive function: results from the clinic subcohort of the COcoa Supplement and Multivitamin Outcomes Study (COSMOS) randomized clinical trial and meta-analysis of 3 cognitive studies within COSMOS. Am J Clin Nutr. 2024 Mar;119(3):692–701. doi: 10.1016/j.ajcnut.2023.12.011. Epub 2024 Jan 18. PMID: 38244989; PMCID: PMC11103094.

Wang Z, Zhu W, Xing Y, Jia J, Tang Y. B vitamins and prevention of cognitive decline and incident dementia: a systematic review and meta-analysis. Nutr Rev. 2022 Mar 10;80(4):931–949. doi: 10.1093/nutrit/nuab057. PMID: 34432056.

CHAPTER 4

CDC releases updated maps of America's high levels of inactivity. Centers for Disease Control and Prevention; 2022 Jan 20 [accessed 27 Sep 2025]. https://archive.cdc.gov/#/details?url=https://www.cdc.gov/media/releases/2022/p0120-inactivity-map.html

Ma T et al. Social support and cognitive activity and their associations with incident cognitive impairment in cognitively normal older adults. BMC Geriatr 2024 Jan 9;24(38). https://doi.org/10.1186/s12877-024-04655-5

Munson R. Ingenious: a biography of Benjamin Franklin, scientist. W. W. Norton; 2025.

CHAPTER 5

Alcohol and cancer risk 2025. The U.S. Surgeon General's Advisory. Office of the U.S. Surgeon General; [last reviewed 2025 Jan 17]. https://www.hhs.gov/sites/default/files/oash-alcohol-cancer-risk.pdf

Agarwal P et al. Association of Mediterranean-DASH Intervention for Neurodegenerative Delay and Mediterranean diets with Alzheimer disease pathology. Neurology. 2023 May 30;100(22):e2259–e2268. doi: 10.1212/WNL.0000000000207176. Epub 2023 Mar 8. PMID: 36889921; PMCID: PMC10259273.

Barnes LL et al. Trial of the MIND diet for prevention of cognitive decline in older persons. N Engl J Med. 2023 Aug 17;389(7):602–611. doi: 10.1056/NEJMoa2302368. Epub 2023 Jul 18. PMID: 37466280; PMCID: PMC10513737.

Biddinger et al. Association of habitual alcohol intake with risk of cardiovascular disease. JAMA Netw Open. 2022;5(3):e223849. doi:10.1001/jamanetworkopen.2022.3849

Boyle PA et al. Effect of purpose in life on the relation between Alzheimer disease pathologic changes on cognitive function in advanced age. Arch Gen Psychiatry. 2012 May;69(5):499–505. doi: 10.1001/archgenpsychiatry.2011.1487. PMID: 22566582; PMCID: PMC3389510.

Bracci EL, Davis CR, Murphy KJ. Developing a Mediterranean healthy food basket and an updated Australian healthy food basket modelled on the Australian Guide to Healthy Eating. Nutrients. 2023 Mar 30;15(7):1692. doi: 10.3390/nu15071692. PMID: 37049532; PMCID: PMC10096976.

Cené CW et al. Effects of objective and perceived social isolation on cardiovascular and brain health: a scientific statement from the American Heart Association. J Am Heart Assoc. 2022 Aug 16;11(16):e026493. doi: 10.1161/JAHA.122.026493. Epub 2022 Aug 4. PMID: 35924775; PMCID: PMC9496293.

Chen H et al. Association of the Mediterranean Dietary Approaches to Stop Hypertension Intervention for Neurodegenerative Delay (MIND) diet with the risk of dementia. JAMA Psychiatry. 2023 Jun 1;80(6):630–638. doi: 10.1001/jamapsychiatry.2023.0800. PMID: 37133875; PMCID: PMC10157510.

Chin N, host. Dementia Matters, podcast. MIND diet for healthy brain aging. Morris MC, guest. 2017 Oct 24. https://www.adrc.wisc.edu/dementia-matters/mind-diet-healthy-brain-aging

Chin N, host. Dementia Matters, podcast. Mindfulness: what is it, what are the benefits, where to begin. Minichiello V, guest. 2020 May 27. https://www.adrc.wisc.edu/dementia-matters/mindfulness-what-it-what-are-benefits-where-begin

Chin N, host. Dementia Matters, podcast. Gut feelings: the links between gut health and Alzheimer's disease. Bendlin B, Ulland T, guests. 2024 Aug 28. https://www.adrc.wisc.edu/dementia-matters/gut-feelings-links-between-gut-health-and-alzheimers-disease

Devanand DP et al. Computerized games versus crosswords training in mild cognitive impairment. NEJM Evid. 2022 Dec;1. doi: 10.1056/evidoa2200121. Epub 2022 Oct 27. PMID: 37635843; PMCID: PMC10457124.

Du L et al. Associations between self-reported sleep patterns and health, cognition and amyloid measures: results from the Wisconsin Registry for Alzheimer's Prevention. Brain Communications. 2023;5(2);fcad039. https://doi.org/10.1093/braincomms/fcad039

Echouffo-Tcheugui JB et al. Circulating cortisol and cognitive and structural brain measures: the Framingham Heart Study. Neurology. 2018 Nov 20;91(21):e1961–e1970. doi: 10.1212/WNL.0000000000006549. Epub 2018 Oct 24. PMID: 30355700; PMCID: PMC6260201.

Fioroni S, Foy D. Americans sleeping less, more stressed. Gallup; 2024 Apr 15. https://news.gallup.com/poll/642704/americans-sleeping-less-stressed.aspx?utm_source=alert&utm_medium=email&utm_content=morelink&utm_campaign=syndication

Gaitán JM et al. Brain glucose metabolism, cognition, and cardiorespiratory fitness following exercise training in adults at risk for Alzheimer's disease. Brain Plast. 2019 Dec 26;5(1):83–95. doi: 10.3233/BPL-190093. PMID: 31970062; PMCID: PMC6971821.

Gerardin E et al. Partially overlapping neural networks for real and imagined hand movements. Cereb Cortex. 2000 Nov;10(11):1093–1104. doi: 10.1093/cercor/10.11.1093. PMID: 11053230.

Goyal L, Gupta S, Perambudhuru Y. Association between periodontitis and cognitive impairment in adults. Evid Based Dent. 2023 Sep;24(3):123–124. doi: 10.1038/s41432-023-00915-2. Epub 2023 Jul 11. PMID: 37433922.

Griep Y et al. Can volunteering in later life reduce the risk of dementia? A 5-year longitudinal study among volunteering and non-volunteering retired seniors. PLoS One. 2017 Mar 16;12(3):e0173885. doi: 10.1371/journal.pone.0173885. PMID: 28301554; PMCID: PMC5354395.

Han SH, Roberts JS, Mutchler JE, Burr JA. Volunteering, polygenic risk for Alzheimer's disease, and cognitive functioning among older adults. Soc Sci Med. 2020 May;253:112970. doi: 10.1016/j.socscimed.2020.112970. Epub 2020 Apr 2. PMID: 32278238; PMCID: PMC7527033.

Healthy living with MCI: clear the air about cigarettes and the aging brain. Wisconsin Alzheimer's Disease Research Center. YouTube; uploaded 2022 Feb 28. https://www.youtube.com/watch?v=0-hSmDfV23g

Howard L. Volunteering in late life may protect the brain against cognitive decline and dementia. UC Davis Health; 2023 July 20. https://health.ucdavis.edu/news/headlines/volunteering-in-late-life-may-protect-the-brain-against-cognitive-decline-and-dementia/2023/07

Is a spider's web a part of its mind? Deep Look, season 7, episode 16. PBS; 2020 Sep 22. https://www.pbs.org/video/is-a-spiders-web-a-part-of-its-mind-rj9awk/

Jonaitis E et al. Cognitive activities and cognitive performance in middle-aged adults at risk for Alzheimer's disease. Psychol Aging. 2013 Dec;28(4):1004–1014. doi: 10.1037/a0034838. PMID: 24364404; PMCID: PMC4029346.

Kapogiannis D et al. Brain responses to intermittent fasting and the healthy living diet in older adults. Cell Metab. 2024 Aug 6;36(8):1668–1678.e5. doi: 10.1016/j.cmet.2024.05.017. Epub 2024 Jun 19. Erratum in: Cell Metab. 2024 Aug 6;36(8):1900–1904. doi: 10.1016/j.cmet.2024.07.012. PMID: 38901423; PMCID: PMC11305918.

Kylkilahti TM et al. Achieving brain clearance and preventing neurodegenerative diseases—a glymphatic perspective. J Cereb Blood Flow Metab. 2021 Sep;41(9):2137–2149. doi: 10.1177/0271678X20982388. Epub 2021 Jan 18. PMID: 33461408; PMCID: PMC8392766.

Lazar SW et al. Meditation experience is associated with increased cortical thickness. Neuroreport. 2005 Nov 28;16(17):1893–1897. doi: 10.1097/01.wnr.0000186598.66243.19. PMID: 16272874; PMCID: PMC1361002.

Lee CS et al. Association between cataract extraction and development of dementia. JAMA Intern Med. 2022;182(2):134–141. doi:10.1001/jamainternmed.2021.6990

Lin FR et al. Hearing intervention versus health education control to reduce cognitive decline in older adults with hearing loss in the USA (ACHIEVE): a multicentre, randomised controlled trial. Lancet. 2023 Sep 2;402(10404): 786–797. doi: 10.1016/S0140–6736(23)01406-X. Epub 2023 Jul 18. PMID: 37478886; PMCID: PMC10529382.

Livingston G et al. Dementia prevention, intervention, and care: 2024 report of the Lancet standing commission. Lancet. 2024 Aug 10;404(10452):572–628. doi: 10.1016/S0140–6736(24)01296–0. Epub 2024 Jul 31. PMID: 39096926.

Lotze M et al. Activation of cortical and cerebellar motor areas during executed and imagined hand movements: an fMRI study. J Cogn Neurosci. 1999 Sep;11(5):491–501. doi: 10.1162/089892999563553. PMID: 10511638.

Luong TV et al. A 3-week ketogenic diet increases global cerebral blood flow and brain-derived neurotrophic factor. Journal of Clinical Endocrinology & Metabolism, 2025 Apr 2;dgaf207. https://doi.org/10.1210/clinem/dgaf207

Miller K. Habit stacking is the expert-approved method to making your new year's resolutions stick. Times Weekly; 2024 Dec 31. https://thetimesweekly.com/2024/12/habit-stacking-is-the-expert-approved-method-to-making-your-new-years-resolutions-stick/

Moore AA, Whiteman EJ, Ward KT. Risks of combined alcohol/medication use in older adults. Am J Geriatr Pharmacother. 2007 Mar;5(1):64–74. doi: 10.1016/j.amjopharm.2007.03.006. PMID: 17608249; PMCID: PMC4063202.

Morris MC et al. MIND diet slows cognitive decline with aging. Alzheimers Dement. 2015 Sep;11(9):1015–22. doi: 10.1016/j.jalz.2015.04.011. Epub 2015 Jun 15. PMID: 26086182; PMCID: PMC4581900.

Office of the Surgeon General (OSG). Our epidemic of loneliness and isolation: the U.S. Surgeon General's advisory on the healing effects of social connection and community. Washington (DC): US Department of Health and Human Services; 2023. PMID: 37792968. https://www.hhs.gov/sites/default/files/surgeon-general-social-connection-advisory.pdf

Okonkwo OC et al. Physical activity attenuates age-related biomarker alterations in preclinical AD. Neurology, 2014;83(19): 1753–1760.

Pascoe MC, Thompson DR, Jenkins ZM, Ski CF. Mindfulness mediates the physiological markers of stress: systematic review and meta-analysis. J Psychiatr Res. 2017 Dec;95:156–178. doi: 10.1016/j.jpsychires.2017.08.004. Epub 2017 Aug 23. PMID: 28863392.

Phillips MCL et al. Randomized crossover trial of a modified ketogenic diet in Alzheimer's disease. Alzheimers Res Ther. 2021 Feb 23;13(1):51. doi: 10.1186/s13195-021-00783-x. PMID: 33622392; PMCID: PMC7901512.

Renjun L et al. Intermittent fasting and neurodegenerative diseases: molecular mechanisms and therapeutic potential. Metabolism. 2025 Mar;164:156104. ISSN 0026-0495. https://doi.org/10.1016/j.metabol.2024.156104

Sagal P. Here's looking at you, grid: a history of crosswords and their fans. New York Times. 2020 Mar 17. https://www.nytimes.com/2020/03/17/books/review/thinking-inside-the-box-crosswords-adrienne-raphel.html

Said-Sadier N et al. Association between periodontal disease and cognitive impairment in adults. Int J Environ Res Public Health. 2023 Mar 7;20(6):4707. doi: 10.3390/ijerph20064707. PMID: 36981618; PMCID: PMC10049038.

The science. AARP Staying Sharp; [accessed 2025 Sep 27]. https://stayingsharp.aarp.org/about/brain-health/the-science/

Seidler K, Barrow M. Intermittent fasting and cognitive performance—targeting BDNF as potential strategy to optimise brain health. Front Neuroendocrinol. 2022 Apr;65:100971. doi: 10.1016/j.yfrne.2021.100971. Epub 2021 Dec 18. PMID: 34929259.

Sutin AR, Aschwanden D, Luchetti M, Stephan Y, Terracciano A. Sense of purpose in life is associated with lower risk of incident dementia: a meta-analysis. J Alzheimers Dis. 2021;83(1):249–258. doi: 10.3233/JAD-210364. PMID: 34275900; PMCID: PMC8887819.

Vogt NM et al. Gut microbiome alterations in Alzheimer's disease. Sci Rep. 2017 Oct 19;7(1):13537. doi: 10.1038/s41598-017-13601-y. PMID: 29051531; PMCID: PMC5648830.

Wagner M et al. The association of MIND diet with cognitive resilience to neuropathologies. Alzheimers Dement. 2023 Aug;19(8):3644–3653. doi: 10.1002/alz.12982. Epub 2023 Feb 28. PMID: 36855023; PMCID: PMC10460833.

Zhang T et al. Associations between different coffee types, neurodegenerative diseases, and related mortality: findings from a large prospective cohort study. Am J Clin Nutr. 2024 Oct;120(4):918–926. doi: 10.1016/j.ajcnut.2024.08.012. Epub 2024 Aug 19. PMID: 39168304.

CHAPTER 6

Atri A, Rountree SD, Lopez OL, Doody RS. Validity, significance, strengths, limitations, and evidentiary value of real-world clinical data for combination therapy in Alzheimer's disease: comparison of efficacy and effectiveness studies. Neurodegener Dis. 2012;10(1–4):170–174. doi: 10.1159/000335156. Epub 2012 Feb 10. PMID: 22327239; PMCID: PMC3702018.

Beaney A. FDA AdCom to question efficacy and safety concerns with Eli Lilly's Alzheimer's drug. Clinical Trials Arena; 2024 Jun 7. https://www.clinicaltrialsarena.com/news/fda-releases-report-adcom-donanemab-trial/?cf-view

Betthauser TJ et al. Multi-method investigation of factors influencing amyloid onset and impairment in three cohorts. Brain. 2022 Nov 21;145(11):4065–4079. doi: 10.1093/brain/awac213. Erratum in: Brain. 2023 Feb 13;146(2):e11. doi: 10.1093/brain/awac390. PMID: 35856240; PMCID: PMC9679170.

Bocher L. 1906: The dawn of Alzheimer's disease. Nature. 2024 Sep 26. https://www.nature.com/articles/d41586-024-02881-w

Brouillette J et al. Neurotoxicity and memory deficits induced by soluble low-molecular-weight amyloid-β_{1-42} oligomers are revealed *in vivo* by using a novel animal model. J Neurosci. 2012 Jun 6;32(23):7852–7861. doi: 10.1523/JNEUROSCI.5901-11.2012. PMID: 22674261; PMCID: PMC6620963.

Cannon-Albright LA et al. Relative risk for Alzheimer disease based on complete family history. Neurology. 2019 Apr 9;92(15):e1745–e1753. doi: 10.1212/WNL.0000000000007231. Epub 2019 Mar 13. PMID: 30867271; PMCID: PMC6511086.

Chin NA, Widera E, Brangman SA, Karlawish J. Monoclonal anti-amyloid antibodies for the treatment of Alzheimer's disease and the hesitant geriatrician. J Am Geriatr Soc. 2024 Feb;72(2):643–645. doi: 10.1111/jgs.18652. Epub 2023 Nov 1. PMID: 37909226.

Chin N, host. Dementia Matters, podcast. Changing the narrative: one man's journey to Alzheimer's diagnosis and treatment. Zuendel M, guest. 2025 Mar 26. https://www.adrc.wisc.edu/dementia-matters/changing-narrative-one-mans-journey-alzheimers-diagnosis-and-treatment

Churchill W. Never give in, never, never, never, 1941. America's National Churchill Museum; [accessed 2025 Sep 28]. https://www.nationalchurchillmuseum.org/never-give-in-never-never-never.html

Cody KA et al. Characterizing brain tau and cognitive decline along the amyloid timeline in Alzheimer's disease. Brain. 2024 Jun;147(6):2144–2157. https://doi.org/10.1093/brain/awae116

Crook H, Edison P. Incretin mimetics as potential disease modifying treatment for Alzheimer's disease. Journal of Alzheimer's Disease. 2024;101(s1):S357–S370. doi:10.3233/JAD-240730

Deckers K et al. Target risk factors for dementia prevention: a systematic review and Delphi consensus study on the evidence from observational studies. Int J Geriatr Psychiatry. 2015 Mar;30(3):234–246. doi: 10.1002/gps.4245. Epub 2014 Dec 12. PMID: 25504093.

Edison P. GLP-1 drug liraglutide may protect against dementia. Alzheimer's Association; 2024 Jul 30. https://aaic.alz.org/downloads2024/AAIC-2024-GLP-1-Ph2-trial.pdf

Edison TA. The beginnings of the incandescent lamp. Scientific American Supplements 57, no. 1480supp (May 1904): 23711. https://doi.org/10.1038/scientificamerican05141904-23711bsupp

Eisai presents full results of lecanemab phase 3 confirmatory clarity ad study for early Alzheimer's disease at Clinical Trials on Alzheimer's Disease (CTAD) conference. Eisai Global; 2022 Nov 30. https://www.eisai.com/news/2022/news202285.html

Farrer LA et al. Effects of age, sex, and ethnicity on the association between apolipoprotein E genotype and Alzheimer disease: a meta-analysis. JAMA. 1997;278(16):1349–1356. doi:10.1001/jama.1997.03550160069041

Franceschi C, Campisi J. Chronic inflammation (inflammaging) and its potential contribution to age-associated diseases. J Gerontol A Biol Sci Med Sci. 2014 Jun;69 Suppl 1:S4–S9. doi: 10.1093/gerona/glu057. PMID: 24833586.

Gamba P et al. Oxidized cholesterol as the driving force behind the development of Alzheimer's disease. Front Aging Neurosci. 2015 Jun 19;7:119. doi: 10.3389/fnagi.2015.00119. PMID: 26150787; PMCID: PMC4473000.

Greger M. Oxidized cholesterol as a cause of Alzheimer's disease. NutritionFacts.org. 2018 May 30;42. https://nutritionfacts.org/video/oxidized-cholesterol-as-a-cause-of-alzheimers-disease/

Grill JD, Rabinovici GD. The bad medicine of *Doctored*. JAMA. 2025 May 27;333(20):1771-1772. doi: 10.1001/jama.2025.3372. PMID: 40095593.

Haass C, Selkoe DJ. Soluble protein oligomers in neurodegeneration: lessons from the Alzheimer's amyloid beta-peptide. Nat Rev Mol Cell Biol. 2007 Feb;8(2):101–112. doi: 10.1038/nrm2101. PMID: 17245412.

Hartz SM et al. Assessing the clinical meaningfulness of slowing CDR-SB progression with disease-modifying therapies for Alzheimer's disease. Alzheimer's Dement. 2025; 11:e70033. https://doi.org/10.1002/trc2.70033

Hendriks S et al. Global prevalence of young-onset dementia: a systematic review and meta-analysis. JAMA Neurol. 2021;78(9):1080–1090. doi:10.1001/jamaneurol.2021.2161

Honig LS et al. Updated safety results from phase 3 lecanemab study in early Alzheimer's disease. Alzheimers Res Ther. 2024 May 10;16(1):105. doi: 10.1186/s13195-024-01441-8. Erratum in: Alzheimers Res Ther. 2024 Jul 10;16(1):159. doi: 10.1186/s13195-024-01507-7. PMID: 38730496; PMCID: PMC11084061.

Hwang JH, Laiteerapong N, Huang ES, Kim DD. Lifetime health effects and cost-effectiveness of tirzepatide and semaglutide in US adults. JAMA Health Forum. 2025;6(3):e245586. doi:10.1001/jamahealthforum.2024.5586

Kinney JW et al. Inflammation as a central mechanism in Alzheimer's disease. Alzheimers Dement (N Y). 2018 Sep 6;4:575–590. doi: 10.1016/j.trci.2018.06.014. PMID: 30406177; PMCID: PMC6214864.

Kohler J, Turbitt E, Biesecker B. Personal utility in genomic testing: a systematic literature review. Eur J Hum Genet 2017;25: 662–668. https://doi.org/10.1038/ejhg.2017.10

Koscik RL et al. Amyloid duration is associated with preclinical cognitive decline and tau PET. Alzheimers Dement (Amst). 2020 Feb 13;12(1):e12007. doi: 10.1002/dad2.12007. PMID: 32211502; PMCID: PMC7085284.

Kramarow EA. Diagnosed dementia in adults age 65 and older: United States, 2022. National Health Statistics Reports. 2024 Jun 13;203. https://www.cdc.gov/nchs/data/nhsr/nhsr203.pdf

Mucke L, Selkoe DJ. Neurotoxicity of amyloid β-protein: synaptic and network dysfunction. Cold Spring Harb Perspect Med. 2012 Jul;2(7):a006338. doi: 10.1101/cshperspect.a006338. PMID: 22762015; PMCID: PMC3385944.

Perry G. CONy 2021 | Amyloid-β in Alzheimer's disease: pathogenic or protective? VJ Neurology; 2021 Sep 28. https://www.vjneurology.com/video/_lp5nzp2fs8-amyloid-%ce%b2-in-alzheimers-disease-pathogenic-or-protective/

Reagan R. Reagan's letter announcing his Alzheimer's diagnosis. Ronald Reagan Presidential Library and Museum; 1994 Nov 5 [accessed 2025 Sep 28]. https://www.reaganlibrary.gov/reagans/ronald-reagan/reagans-letter-announcing-his-alzheimers-diagnosis

Rogers SL, Doody RS, Pratt RD, Ieni JR. Long-term efficacy and safety of donepezil in the treatment of Alzheimer's disease: final analysis of a US multicentre open-label study. Eur Neuropsychopharmacol. 2000 May;10(3):195–203. doi: 10.1016/s0924-977x(00)00067-5. PMID: 10793322.

Rogers SL, Friedhoff LT. Long-term efficacy and safety of donepezil in the treatment of Alzheimer's disease: an interim analysis of the results of a US multicentre open label extension study. Eur Neuropsychopharmacol. 1998 Feb;8(1):67–75. doi: 10.1016/s0924-977x(97)00079-5. PMID: 9452942.

Rountree SD, Atri A, Lopez OL, Doody RS. Effectiveness of antidementia drugs in delaying Alzheimer's disease progression. Alzheimers Dement. 2013 May;9(3):338–345. doi: 10.1016/j.jalz.2012.01.002. Epub 2012 Oct 24. PMID: 23102979.

Selkoe DJ. Soluble oligomers of the amyloid beta-protein impair synaptic plasticity and behavior. Behav Brain Res. 2008 Sep 1;192(1):106–113. doi: 10.1016/j.bbr.2008.02.016. Epub 2008 Feb 17. PMID: 18359102; PMCID: PMC2601528.

Sims JR et al. Donanemab in early symptomatic Alzheimer disease: The TRAILBLAZER-ALZ 2 randomized clinical trial. JAMA. 2023 Aug 8;330(6):512–527. doi: 10.1001/jama.2023.13239. PMID: 37459141; PMCID: PMC10352931.

Smith A, Widera E, hosts. GeriPal, podcast. Amyloid antibodies and the role of the geriatrician: Nate Chin, Sharon Brangman, and Jason Karlawish. Chin N, Brangman S, Karlawish J, guests. 2023 Aug 17.

Study defines major genetic form of Alzheimer's disease. National Institutes of Health; 2024 May 14. https://www.nih.gov/news-events/nih-research-matters/study-defines-major-genetic-form-alzheimer-s-disease#:~:text=One%20of%20the%20strongest%20genetic,AD%20dementia%20by%20age%2085

A study of donanemab (LY3002813) in participants with early Alzheimer's disease (TRAILBLAZER-ALZ 2). ClinicalTrials.gov. National Library of Medicine; [last updated 2025 Aug 29]. https://www.clinicaltrials.gov/study/NCT04437511

Tang H et al. GLP-1RA and SGLT2i medications for type 2 diabetes and Alzheimer disease and related dementias. JAMA Neurol. 2025;82(5):439–449. doi:10.1001/jamaneurol.2025.0353

Wang W et al. Associations of semaglutide with first-time diagnosis of Alzheimer's disease in patients with type 2 diabetes: target trial emulation using nationwide real-world data in the US. Alzheimers Dement. 2024 Dec;20(12):8661–8672. doi: 10.1002/alz.14313. Epub 2024 Oct 24. PMID: 39445596; PMCID: PMC11667504.

Widera EW, Brangman SA, Chin NA. Ushering in a new era of Alzheimer disease therapy. JAMA. 2023 Aug 8;330(6):503–504. doi: 10.1001/jama.2023.11701. PMID: 37459123.

Xie Y, Choi T, Al-Aly Z. Mapping the effectiveness and risks of GLP-1 receptor agonists. Nat Med. 2025;31:951–962. https://doi.org/10.1038/s41591-024-03412-w

Yadollahikhales G, Rojas JC. Anti-amyloid immunotherapies for Alzheimer's disease: a 2023 clinical update. Neurotherapeutics. 2023 Jul;20(4):914–931. doi: 10.1007/s13311-023-01405-0. Epub 2023 Jul 25. PMID: 37490245; PMCID: PMC10457266.

CHAPTER 7

Allen, K. Alzheimer's disease: the magic of pets. Alzheimer's Disease Research; 2024 Feb 9. https://www.brightfocus.org/resource/alzheimers-disease-magic-pets/

Ho JY. Life course patterns of prescription drug use in the United States. Demography. 2023 Oct 1;60(5):1549–1579. doi: 10.1215/00703370-10965990. PMID: 37728437; PMCID: PMC10656114.

Hough K, Kotwal AA, Boyd C, Tha SH, Perissinotto C. What are "social prescriptions" and how should they be integrated into care plans? AMA J Ethics. 2023 Nov 1;25(11):E795–E801. doi: 10.1001/amajethics.2023.795. PMID: 38085581.

Klimova B, Toman J, Kuca K. Effectiveness of the dog therapy for patients with dementia—a systematic review. BMC Psychiatry 2019;19(276). https://doi.org/10.1186/s12888-019-2245-x

CHAPTER 8

Blumen HM et al. Randomized controlled trial of social ballroom dancing and treadmill walking: preliminary findings on executive function and neuroplasticity from dementia-at-risk older adults. J Aging Phys Act. 2022 Dec 14;31(4):589–599. doi: 10.1123/japa.2022–0176. PMID: 36516851; PMCID: PMC10264554.

Cummings JL et al. Alzheimer's disease drug development pipeline: 2025. Alzheimers Dement (N Y). 2025 Jun 3;11(2):e70098. doi: 10.1002/trc2.70098. PMID: 40463637; PMCID: PMC12131090.

Learn about studies. National Library of Medicine; [last updated 2024 Jun 10]. https://clinicaltrials.gov/study-basics/learn-about-studies

NIH clinical research trials and you: the basics. National Institutes of Health; [last reviewed on 2025 Apr 24]. https://www.nih.gov/health-information/nih-clinical-research-trials-you/basics

CHAPTER 9

Batthyány A, Greyson B. Spontaneous remission of dementia before death: results from a study on paradoxical lucidity. Psychology of Consciousness: Theory, Research, and Practice. 2021;8(1):1–8. https://doi.org/10.1037/cns0000259

Blundon EG, Gallagher RE, Ward LM. Electrophysiological evidence of preserved hearing at the end of life. Sci Rep. 2020;10:10336. https://doi.org/10.1038/s41598-020-67234-9

Bodien YG et al. Cognitive motor dissociation in disorders of consciousness. N Engl J Med. 2024 Aug 15;391(7):598–608. doi: 10.1056/NEJMoa2400645. PMID: 39141852; PMCID: PMC7617195.

Curlin FA, Lantos JD, Roach CJ, Sellergren SA, Chin MH. Religious characteristics of U.S. physicians: a national survey. J Gen Intern Med. 2005 Jul;20(7):629–634. doi: 10.1111/j.1525-1497.2005.0119.x. PMID: 16050858; PMCID: PMC1490160.

Ro T, Koenig L. Unconscious touch perception after disruption of the primary somatosensory cortex. Psychol Sci. 2021 Apr;32(4):549–557. doi: 10.1177/0956797620970551. Epub 2021 Feb 26. PMID: 33635728.

AFTERWORD

Pew Research Center. Americans' trust in scientists, positive views of science continue to decline. Nov 2023. https://www.pewresearch.org/science/2023/11/14/americans-trust-in-scientists-positive-views-of-science-continue-to-decline/

Pew Research Center. Public trust in scientists and views on their role in policymaking. Nov 2024. https://www.pewresearch.org/science/2024/11/14/public-trust-in-scientists-and-views-on-their-role-in-policymaking/

Index

About the Author

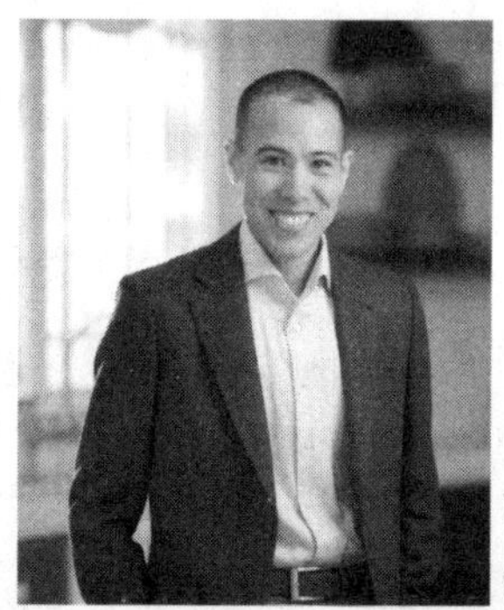

Clint Thayer

NATHANIEL A. CHIN, MD, is an associate professor of medicine at the University of Wisconsin School of Medicine and Public Health and a geriatrician specializing in memory care. He serves as the medical director of the Wisconsin Alzheimer's Disease Research Center (ADRC), the Wisconsin Registry for Alzheimer's Prevention (WRAP), and the ADRC Consortium for Clarity in ADRD Research Through Imaging (CLARiTI). In addition to his leadership roles, he sees patients each week and serves as associate program director of the UW Health Geriatric Memory Clinical Program.

Dr. Chin's clinical and research efforts focus on early detection of cognitive impairment, the use of biomarkers in diagnosis, and improving quality of life after diagnosis through comprehensive, person-centered care. He is also interested in understanding how modifiable factors—such as lifestyle, environment, and health behaviors—affect biomarkers and the underlying mechanisms of Alzheimer's disease. A passionate communicator, he is the creator and host of *Dementia Matters*, a nationally recognized podcast exploring Alzheimer's research, caregiving, and brain health. His work has been featured in *The New England Journal of Medicine*, *JAMA*, and *Scientific American*, as well as in national outlets such as NPR, *The New York Times*, and *Forbes*.

Nathaniel lives in Madison, Wisconsin, with his wife and childhood friend, Erin, their sons, Augustine and Bennett, and their dog, Wendell. His mother, Karen, lives just across the isthmus.

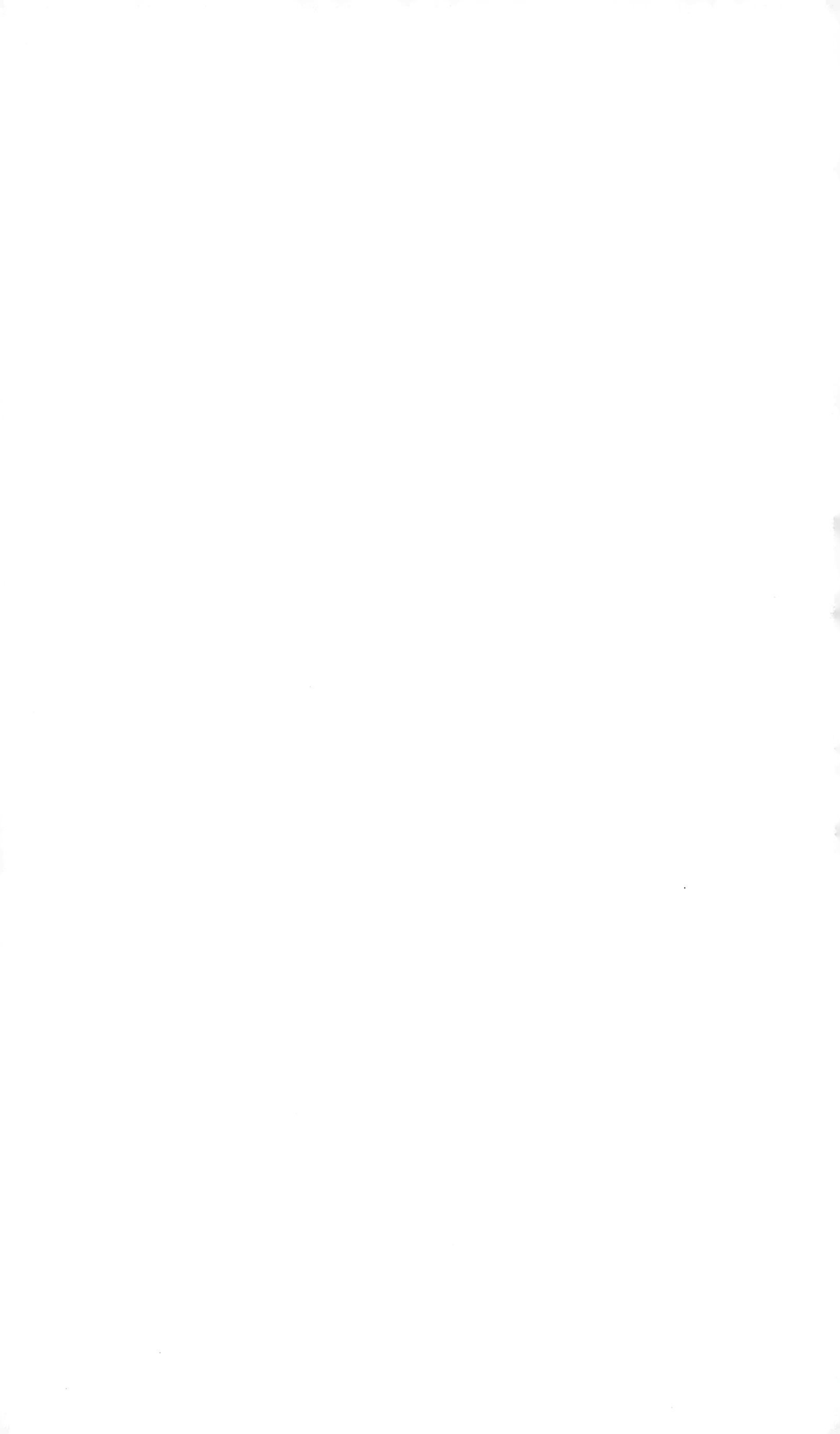